The Herbalist's Bible

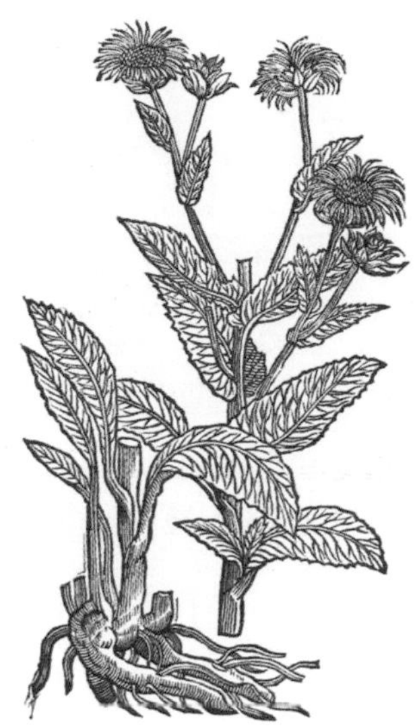

Above: woodcut of Elecampane (*Inula helenium*) from *Theatrum Botanicum* (1640), p654; overleaf: hand-coloured frontispiece from *Theatrum Botanicum*, by permission of the Bodleian Libraries, The University of Oxford, B.1.17 Med. Seld., title page

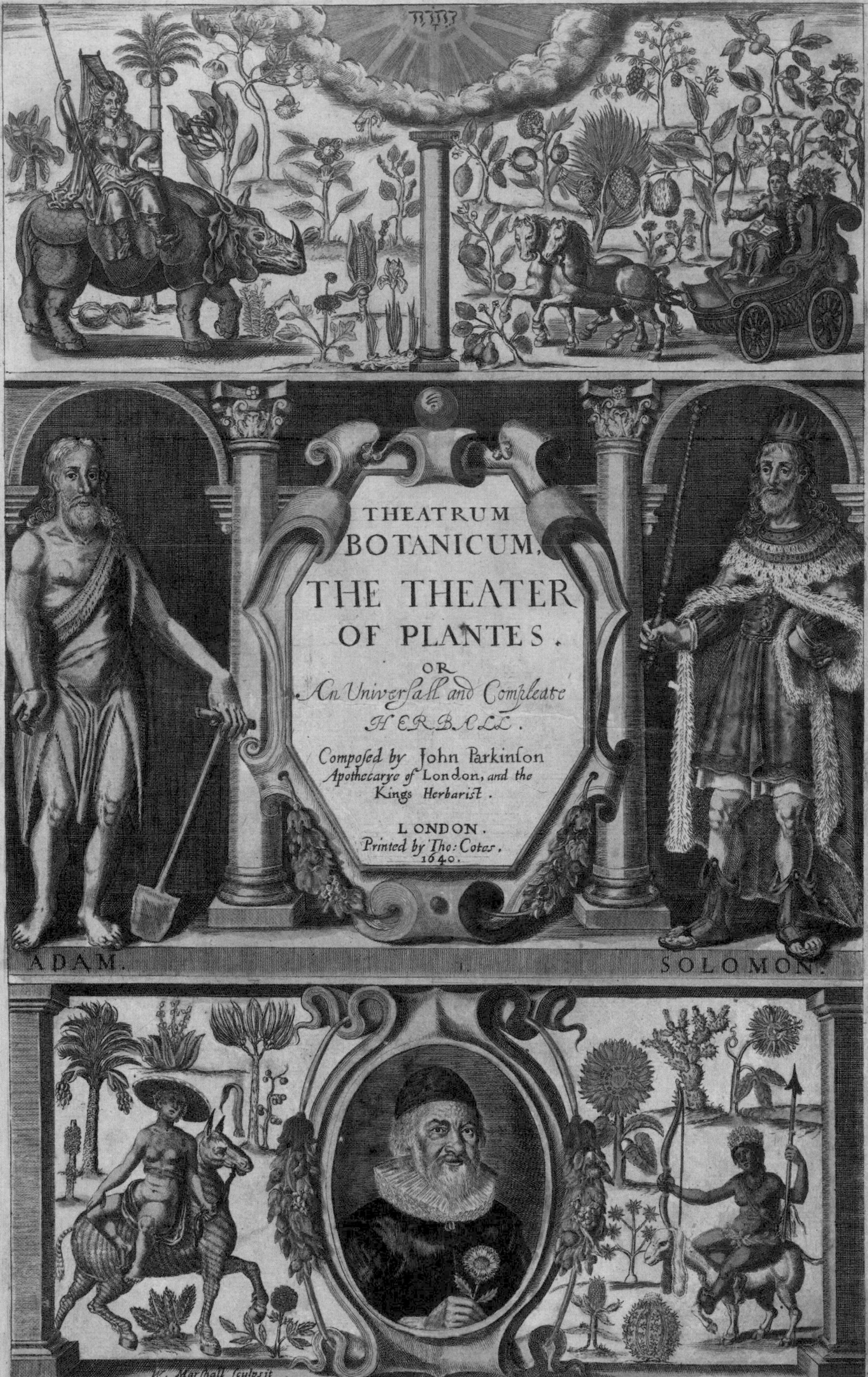

יהוה
THEATRUM
BOTANICUM,
THE THEATER
OF PLANTES.
OR
An Universall and Compleate
HERBALL.
Composed by John Parkinson
Apothecarye of London, and the
Kings Herbarist.
LONDON.
Printed by Tho: Cotes,
1640.
ADAM.
SOLOMON.
W. Marshall sculpsit

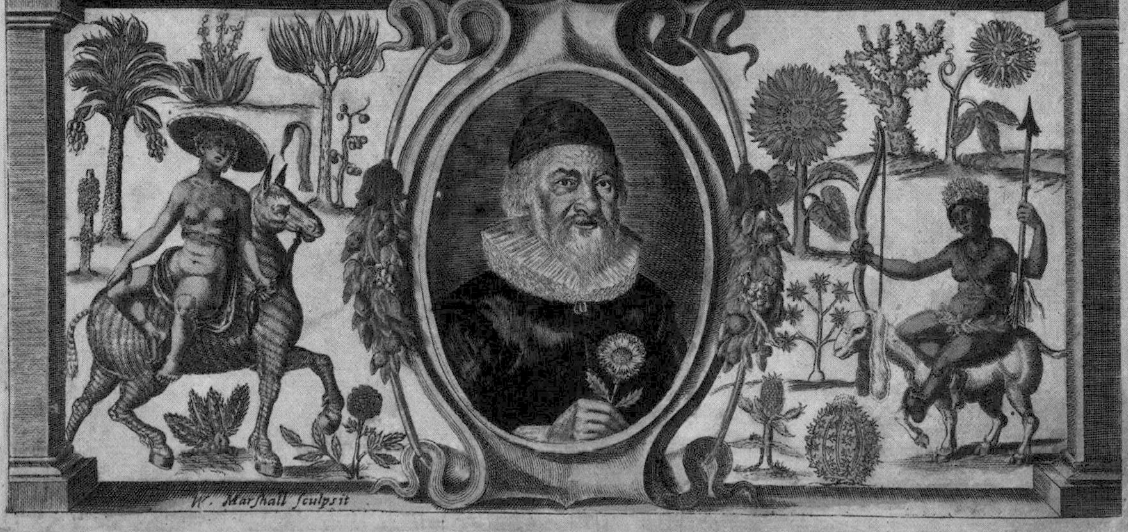

THE HERBALIST'S BIBLE

John Parkinson's Lost Classic— 82 Herbs and Their Medicinal Uses

Theatrum Botanicum (1640)
A selection and commentary
by

Julie Bruton-Seal & Matthew Seal

SP

Skyhorse Publishing

Skyhorse paperback edition published 2019

First published in the United Kingdom by Merlin Unwin Books Limited. This USA Edition of *The Herbalist's Bible* is published by arrangement with Merlin Unwin Books Limited.

Skyhorse Publishing books may be purchased in bulk at special discounts for sales promotion, corporate gifts, fund-raising, or educational purposes. Special editions can also be created to specifications. For details, contact the Special Sales Department, Skyhorse Publishing, 307 West 36th Street, 11th Floor, New York, NY 10018 or info@skyhorsepublishing.com.

Skyhorse® and Skyhorse Publishing® are registered trademarks of Skyhorse Publishing, Inc®, a

Delaware corporation.

Visit our website at www.skyhorsepublishing.com.

10 9 8 7

Library of Congress Cataloging-in-Publication Data is available on file.

Designed and typeset in Adobe Caslon Pro Regular (Parkinson's text) and Helvetica Neue Light (commentary) by Julie Bruton-Seal and Matthew Seal

Photographs by Julie Bruton-Seal, unless otherwise stated

Cover design and endpapers by Merlin Unwin

ISBN: 978-1-5107-4039-6
Ebook ISBN: 978-1-62914-983-7

Printed in China

Please note:

The information in *The Herbalist's Bible* is compiled from a blend of historical and modern scientific sources and from personal experience. It is not intended to replace the professional advice and care of a qualified herbal or medical practitioner. Do not attempt to self-diagnose or self-prescribe for serious long-term problems without first consulting a qualified professional. Heed the cautions given, and if already taking prescribed medicines or if you are pregnant, seek professional advice before using herbal remedies.

CONTENTS

Dedicated to

JOHN PARKINSON

(1567–1650)

Writer, gardener, herbalist, botanist, apothecary

❦

Phoebus hath fifty times lash't through the *signes*,
Since thou intend'st this *Iubilee* of lines.
And *now* 'tis extant; and shall swiftly scou're
Through darke oblivion to the world's last houre. ...
Keepe thy *Hesperides*; may thy herbes with thee
Still bloome; by *Prester* never blasted bee.
And seeing by thy hands the *day* is wonne,
No *night* of Age shall cloude bright *Parke-in-sunne.*

John Harmer, Oxford

(writing in the preliminary pages of *Theatrum Botanicum*, 1640)

❦

Worthy sir,

You have built us a Botanicke Theater; with such excellent skill and advantage to the Spectator; that at one view he commands the prospect of both Hemisphers; and all their vegetables in the pride of beauty: ranged in their proper orders, decking the Hils, Plaines, Valleyes, Medowes, Woods, and Bankes, with such a world of shapes and colours, so delightfull to the eye, so winning upon the rationall Soule which feeds on rarities! that we cannot hope for a more compleate Paradise upon earth, till Nature have found out a new stocke for more variety; what can be added to this I see not; nor is it (I beleeve) yet knowne to the best of Artists that have made search.

John Speed, Med.D., Oxon

(writing in the preliminary pages of *Theatrum Botanicum*, 1640)

right: John Parkinson's dedication to King Charles I of his 'Manlike Worke of Herbes and Plants', in *Theatrum Botanicum*, 1640. He had become the royal herbalist a few months before publication

TO THE KINGS MOST EXCELLENT MAIESTIE.

HAving by long paines and endeavours, composed this Manlike Worke of Herbes and Plants, Most gracious Soveraigne (as I formerly did a Feminine of Flowers, and presented it to the Queenes most excellent Majesty) I could doe no lesse then submissively lay it at your Majesties feet, to be approved or condemned, and if thought fit and worthy a publique passage, to offer it on the Altar of your Majestyes many favours to me, to be commanded as well as commended unto all for their owne good. For as your Majesty is *Summus Pater patriæ*, the chiefe of your people under God, that not onely provideth for their soules health, that they may have the pure Word of God, whereby to live ever, wherein we justly claime the prerogative above any Nation under Heaven, and most devoutly praise God for the same, and desire religiously to live thereunder: but many wayes also for their bodily estates, by good and wholesome Lawes, that every one may live obediently and peaceably under their owne Vine and Figtree, and by protection, &c. And I doubt not of your Majesties further care of their bodies health, that such Workes as deliver approved remedyes may be divulged, whereby they may both cure and prevent their diseases. Most properly therefore doth this Worke belong to your Majesties Patronage both to further and defend, that malevolent spirits should not dare to cast forth their venome or aspertions, to the prejudice of any well deserving, but that therby under God and good direction, all may live in health, as well as wealth, peace, and godlines, which God grant, and that this boldnesse may be pardoned to

Your Majestyes
Loyall Subject,
Servant, and Herbarist,
John Parkinson.

PREFACE

Our connection with John Parkinson began in late 2005 when we first saw a copy of his *Theatrum Botanicum* (1640) in the Collection of Rare Botanical Books at the John Innes Foundation in Norwich. It was our good luck to have found a collection of old botanical and herbal books within four miles of where we were living, and we made full use of it.

The book itself was a huge folio of 1,788 pages of illustrated text, with a sturdy leather cover, and weighing in at 11 lb (5 kg). It is not a book to be treated lightly, in any sense of the word. We did hear that some twenty or thirty years previously the book could then be borrowed from the open shelves of the John Innes Library, and that one person cycled home with a copy in an open rucksack on his back, later returning it complete with rain spatters.

Such old volumes were being treated with rather more care by the time we visited, with climate control and close supervision. Indeed, *Theatrum* now had the status and charisma of a rare book, the original edition of 1640 never having been reprinted.

Open its first few pages and you find the descriptive title page, in the 17th century manner, with some 180 words describing this 'herball of a large extent'. It is actually the biggest herbal ever to be published in English, so Parkinson didn't over-sell himself here.

Opposite the title is a frontispiece (which we reproduce in a hand-coloured version) by the engraver William Marshall, with central panels showing Adam as the original gardener, with a spade, and Solomon, the wise authority, with a crown and sceptre. At the four corners are four naked ladies from different continents who are riding on appropriate steeds and surrounded by native plants.

But what hits the eye among this careful mythology is the inset likeness at the foot of the page of John Parkinson himself, aged 73. He has short hair under an apothecary's skullcap and is dressed dourly in black, with a plain ruff, and holding a thistle. He is slender in build, unsmiling, somewhat tired and lightly bearded – and looks uncannily like Julie's father!

Three excellent indexes (of Latin names, English names and 'vertues', or medicinal uses) help you navigate his vast tome. But open it at any page, or look at random at the e-book. You can hardly fail to be impressed by the depth of knowledge on display, expressed calmly and with quiet dignity in supple but practical prose (while Parkinson preferred Latin titles for his books he always wrote in English). This is no mere book of spells, a grimoire, or quaint folklore, you realize; in its descriptions of some 3,800 plants and their names but especially in the 'vertues', this is a book of living herbalism from a time when herbs *were* orthodox medicine.

All but forgotten from the 18th to the 20th centuries, with a few passionate defenders and accusers to keep its memory alive, the book has taken on a new life in the twenty-first. *Theatrum* now has an online presence (though we still prefer to navigate the physical book), and since 2007 John Parkinson now has a biography, for the first time, written by the journalist, BBC producer and probable descendant, Anna Parkinson. Anna has made her own journey with Parkinson, and at this point we would like to express our appreciation of her thorough and fruitful research, which we draw on here with her permission.

We have been trying out Parkinson's recipes for some years, taking things further by purchasing a brass alembic in 2012 (see p206) to replicate some of the many distillations and aromatic waters he describes.

Our Parkinson relationship took a new turn in early 2006 when we looked online speculatively to see if there were any copies of *Theatrum* to be had. Most were for sale in the United States and seemed prohibitively expensive, but Bow Windows Bookshop in Lewes, East Sussex had a slightly damaged but cheaper copy. We made a phone call, dropped everything and drove through the February snow from Norfolk. We cashed in a savings plan – better a special book now rather than money in the bank for unspecified future use! We duly made the purchase and gingerly carried the precious volume to the car, promising each other we would drive carefully and not tell anyone how we had blown our savings.

It has proved to be our precious companion ever since, and now we are thrilled to have the chance to write about it and share its profound herbal knowledge with a wider readership. It is Julie's 'go-to' book for herbal inspiration, and we hope you too will benefit from this selection from Parkinson's life's work.

Julie Bruton-Seal & Matthew Seal
Ashwellthorpe, Norfolk, UK March 2014

INTRODUCTION

In his lifetime John Parkinson (1567–1650) was a royal herbalist, a practising London apothecary and early luminary of the new Society of Apothecaries, a renowned experimental gardener and plantsman. His lasting achievement, though, we believe, was as an author, in each of his main areas of activity – as one of the team that revised the first *Pharmacopoeia* for apothecaries; as sole author of the delightful *Paradisi in Sole* (1629), the first book in English devoted to gardening for pleasure; and his life's work, the *Theatrum Botanicum* (1640), the largest and last great English herbal.

IOANNIS PARKINSONI PHARMACOPŒI LONDINENSIS
EFFIGIES·LXII ÆTATIS ANNVM AGENTIS·A NATO CHRISTO

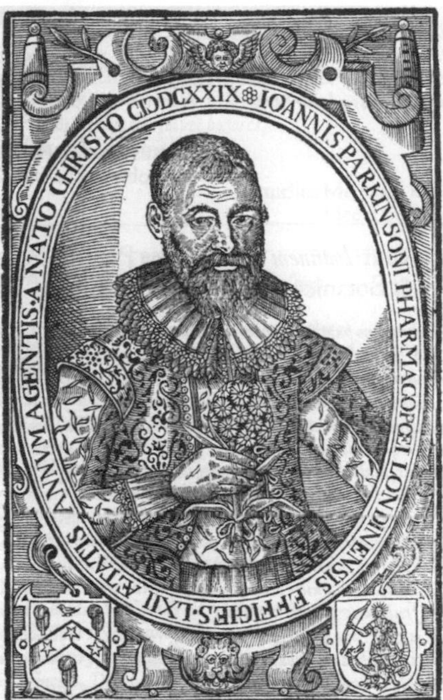

John Parkinson in 1629, aged 62, wearing court clothes. He is holding a 'sweet John' flower, and is described as 'apothecary of London'; his family coat of arms is bottom left, with those of the Society of Apothecaries opposite. He was a founder member of the Society, a plant breeder and garden innovator, and author of the biggest herbal to be published in English and the most loved gardening book (illustration from *Paradisi in Sole*)

Yet before his long life ended Parkinson had lost his king, his garden and his son, and nearly had *Theatrum* snatched away from him by an erstwhile friend who rushed to publish a competing work; within five years of his death he had been vehemently accused of being a plagiarist of the work of his mentor Matthias de l'Obel.

But the *Theatrum* was used as a medical textbook for nearly a century after its publication,[1]* and its author had notable defenders. A generation after Parkinson's death, John Ray, perhaps the greatest of English botanists, rated him among the international pioneers of scientific plant studies;[2] in 1790 a survey of English botanists by Richard Pulteney considered Parkinson to stand above John Gerard and alongside William Turner.[3]

Parkinson largely disappeared from view in the Victorian period but there was a revival of interest, with a short-lived Parkinson Society, towards the end of the 19th century (see p240). In 1922 the Oxford scholar Robert Gunther discovered Parkinson's papers and included him in his ground-breaking book, *Early English Botanists*;[4] in 1947 Canon C.E. Raven's magisterial study of English botanical history declared Parkinson's the last of the true herbals.[5]

But Parkinson was then forgotten once more, and only came to attention again in the 21st century. The *Theatrum* is now available as an e-book and, after more than 350 years, the first biography of Parkinson has appeared, Anna Parkinson's *Nature's Alchemist* (2007);[6] and, in a survey of the Western herbal tradition, published in 2011, Parkinson was one of four chosen to represent the 17th century.[7]

Parkinson's *Paradisi* has been reprinted as a facsimile more than once, but the first edition of 1629 and the second of 1656 remain valuable rare books; the *Theatrum* has never been reprinted after its first edition in 1640, even in a reduced version.

Its fate contrasts sharply with that of Parkinson's younger contemporary Nicholas Culpeper, whose much shorter *English Physitian* of 1652 has gone through dozens of editions and versions, and has never yet been out of print.[8] Culpeper is enduringly popular, yet Parkinson's book is the better herbal, and was indeed heavily copied by Culpeper. Perhaps, though, Parkinson is back in favour once more.

Studying the *Theatrum*, trying out its ideas and making some of its recipes has convinced us that it is a wise and unduly neglected book, which has valuable insights to offer the herbalist of today and indeed anybody interested in English and European botanical or medical history. It was a medical reference book of its day, and now, some 375 years later, it could have a new life as a herbal reference 'bible'.

The five sections of the Introduction set the scene, followed by a Note to the Reader.

* Notes to the Introduction are on pp234–6 below.

1 A brief life of John Parkinson

John Parkinson has been a mysterious figure. He was famous in his time as an apothecary, gardener and author, with a tangential role at court, but he preferred his garden to public life. His library, his working papers, even his will (presuming he had made one) were all lost in the maelstrom of the civil war.

But Anna Parkinson's research and book have fleshed out the bare bones. It is now established that he was born in Whalley, Lancashire in January 1567, the second son of James and Joan Parkinson.[9]

The Parkinsons were a large clan of tenant farmers in south Lancashire and across the Pennines, and they were mostly Catholic. John had three brothers and five sisters, with two of the children dying in infancy. His father probably ran a sheep farm on the moors and traded in wool. His mother Joan was well versed in herbs and midwifery, and was John's first plant teacher.[10] John himself learned Latin in a local school.

The nurturing markers were set: he had an early love of plants and their medicinal values, and was fluent in the international language of science. It is to his credit that he made so much of his early skills.

At 14, John he set off to London to become an apprentice apothecary. Anna Parkinson sees a family hand here: the Parkinsons were related to the Houghtons in London; Peter Houghton was a well-to-do grocer apothecary, and Roger Houghton was a steward for William Cecil, the secretary of state.[11]

From 1584 to 1592 Parkinson was apprenticed to Francis Slater, a grocer apothecary with a shop near St Mary Colechurch. John was trained in pharmacy, learning to make and administer medicines. He would assist in and clean his master's shop, accompany him to see patients and physicians, and along with preparing herbs might assist with blood-letting, enemas, embalming or a post-mortem.

Apothecary apprentices were expected to know their plants, and part of their training was to visit the great London gardens. At one such garden Parkinson met the renowned Flemish botanist Matthias de l'Obel (1538–1616). De l'Obel took to the young apprentice, in 1605 calling him 'the most excellent and honest of London apothecaries, and the most excellent scholar of the medicinal properties of plants'.[12]

Another lifelong influence was the royal physician, Sir Theodore de Mayerne (1573–1655). Once physician to Henri IV in France, he now lived in London as physician to his daughter, Queen Henrietta Maria, the

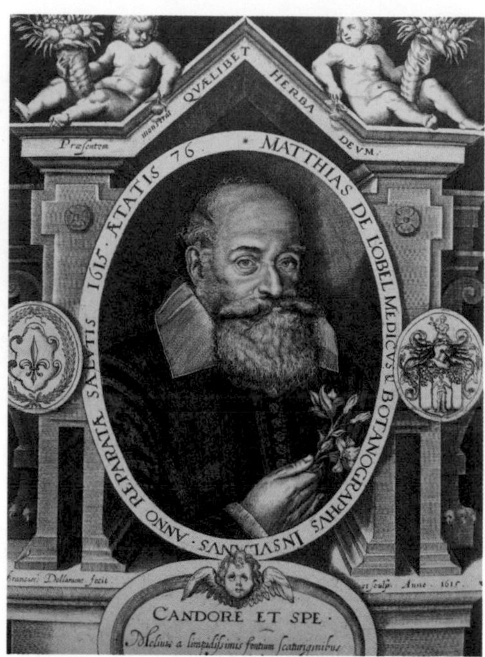

Matthias de l'Obel, aged 76, from a portrait by Francis Dellarme, 1615

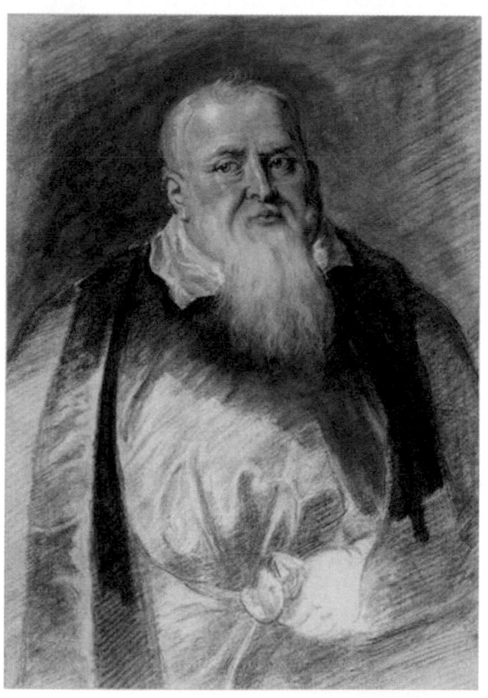

Sir Theodore de Mayerne in his late 50s, from a coloured sketch by Peter Paul Rubens, c. 1631

young bride of Charles I. Sir Theodore also became Parkinson's neighbour in Long Acre, and, like de l'Obel, he warmed to the young apothecary. In 1629 de Mayerne wrote that he was 'the most skilful [botanist], the most well practised, and ... with the most discerning nose'.[13] In 1640 de Mayerne secured for Parkinson the title he most wanted: herbalist to the king, and helped him get the huge *Theatrum Botanicum* into print.

In 1587 John's parents both died suddenly, within eight days of each other. The same year he met Mary Hutchens, the young widow of a coppersmith. Mary owned a house, shop and land at Cripplegate,[14] and their match provided security and prospects for both of them. They ran a successful apothecary's shop in Ludgate Hill as partners while John built his reputation as apothecary and gardener. Their first child, Richard, was born in 1601, followed by Katherine in 1603.

John began making notes while still an apprentice for what was to become his life's work, an encyclopaedia of all known medicinal herbs, written in English, based on writings of ancient and modern authors but filtered through his own experience.[15]

In January 1592 he was examined in Galenic medicine at the Grocers' Hall, found proficient, and so became a licensed apothecary and freeman of the City of London.[16] There was not yet an independent Society of Apothecaries so he was affiliated to the Grocers' Company, which then supervised the apothecaries, as did the College of Physicians.

The shop was doing well enough for Parkinson to take on apprentices, in 1594 and 1597.[17] The apprentice fees enabled him to afford a larger garden, which he now sought. Parkinson's kinsman Roger Houghton was steward to the Cecil family's London household – perhaps Roger's good offices secured two acres on the north of Long Acre for Parkinson, not only as a distant relative but for his reputation as a society gardener. The Long Acre garden, which he worked until 1640, made Parkinson famous.[18]

The year 1617 was eventful for him. First Matthias de l'Obel, aged 78, died in March. Then, some two months later, Mary Parkinson also died. Buried on 29 April 1617, Mary had been his partner and the driving force of the Ludgate Hill shop, both commercially and domestically, while John was spending increasing amounts of time at the Long Acre garden.

The children were teenagers (Richard 15 and Katherine 13), and John was heavily involved in the fledgling Society of Apothecaries. He chose not to remarry, while planning for Richard to take over the shop in due course. The disappointment of his life was that Richard estranged himself. He left home, professed himself an open Catholic, and in early 1640 possibly moved to Ireland. John mourned the loss.[19]

The years 1614 to 1622 for Parkinson were dominated by apothecary matters. Then, after the mid-1620s, he interrupted his flourishing shop and garden businesses to write a gardening book for Queen Henrietta Maria. The delightful *Paradisi in Sole* appeared in 1629. The 1630s, Parkinson's sixties, were spent trying to complete the *Theatrum*. Then in 1640, thanks to Sir Theodore, Parkinson at last became the king's herbalist, and his book appeared.

Parkinson did not follow his king and the court when they decamped to Oxford, and himself moved out of Long Acre. Perhaps he was being protected by gardener friends. John Morris, isolated in Isleworth, wrote to the merchant Johannes de Laet in Leiden, in 1646, that 'the crop of true Botanists nowadays is thin', with the death of Thomas Johnson, killed in the war, and (he thought) of Parkinson.[20] John Parkinson, however, lived longer than his king. Charles I was executed in January 1649, while Parkinson held on until August 1650, when he died of old age.

We do not know why, but a small packet of papers were Parkinson's only surviving possession. An old friend, the gardener John Goodyer, collected them from St Martin in the Fields; later these meagre memorials would join Goodyer's papers, safe in an Oxford college, and lie unseen until the 20th century. But there was a touching footnote – on the burial records of St Martin's by Parkinson's name is added, in a later hand, in pencil: 'A famous Botanist'.[21]

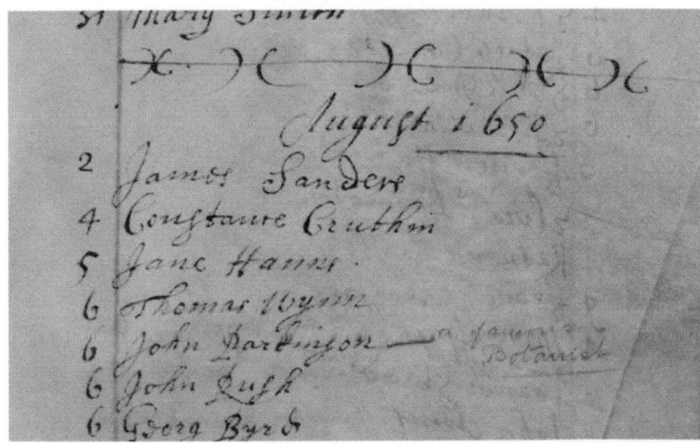

John Parkinson's burial notice in the parish register of St Martin in the Fields, 6 August 1650, to which is added a comment in a later hand, 'A famous Botanist'

2 The Society of Apothecaries: Parkinson as an apothecary

When John Parkinson became an apothecary and freeman in 1592 he had perforce joined the Worshipful Company of Grocers. An ancient City of London guild, it began as the Guild of Pepperers in 1180. In 1316 the Pepperers were linked to the Spicers, but eventually (as would happen with the apothecaries), their interests diverged. The Pepperers moved into wholesale importing ('grocer' comes from 'en gros'), winning incorporation as a City guild of Grocers in 1428. The spicers focused on selling spiced wines, perfumes and confectionery, while also mixing and selling drugs and herbs to the public in their shops.[22]

The spicers, in effect, were becoming apothecaries. But they were subject to two forms of irksome control: by the Grocers (who wanted to regulate more products and also to dispense drugs) and to the discipline of the College of Physicians, who since 1518 had been the senior medical establishment. It was an increasingly uneasy three-way relationship.

In absolute numbers the apothecaries were few, but expanding: from about 15 in England at the beginning of Elizabeth's reign in 1558 to a hundred or so at her death in 1603; the new independent Society of Apothecaries had over 130 members in the 1630s.[23]

London's trade was accelerating at an unprecedented rate, particularly once the Spanish Armada was defeated in 1588; Amsterdam and London now became the world's leading ports. Botanical wealth was among the forms of capital London swallowed up, both for gardens and for medicine.[24] The trade of apothecary was in demand and was, for some, well rewarded, but the restrictions on it were compromising the availability of qualified medical care to Londoners (there were also numerous unlicensed 'chemical' practitioners – quacksalvers – as well as midwives, wise women and so on).

A small group of apothecaries had petitioned the Grocers in 1588 to allow them some independence in order to control standards of drugs. This failed, but the efforts would be repeated. The next year, the Physicians tried to catch up with Continental European practice by compiling a pharmacopoeia, or list of sanctioned medical treatments, for apothecaries to dispense. This also foundered, not least on issues of secrecy: nobody wanted to divulge their best formulations, when some were big moneyspinners. For example, 'de Laune pills' for scurvy, dropsy, worms, etc, enabled leading royal apothecary Gideon de Laune to leave some £90,000 at his death, in 1659 (current values are easily a hundred times more).[25]

Independence of the apothecaries from the Grocers was won by incoporation of the Society of Apothecaries in 1617, but legal challenges by the Grocers persisted even beyond the City's recognition of the Society in 1630 by the award of its livery.

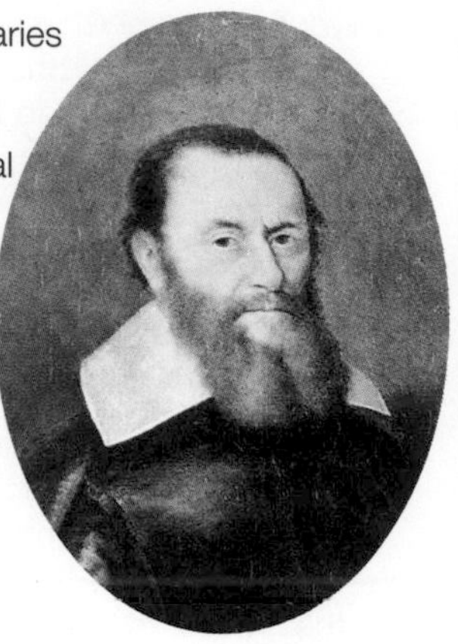

Gideon de Laune, founder member, Master and benefactor of the Society

The equally bitter contestation with the Physicians lasted until 1704, when the House of Lords in the *Rose* case gave apothecaries the right to practise and prescribe medicine. Thereafter some apothecaries would become general practitioners, others pharmacists.

Parkinson played no part in these processes until 1614. His previous most public encounter was in July 1596, when he was summoned to a censorial hearing of the College of Physicians.[26] He was accused of illegal practising, of extorting money from a lady and causing the death of her husband. She had come to Parkinson's shop, paid him to mix medicines to the doctor's prescription, but her husband had subsequently died. The distraught widow demanded her money back from Parkinson; he refused, and she complained to the College.

The solemn hearings were in Latin. Parkinson defended himself ably, all charges were dropped and the case was dismissed. He did not face a court of discipline again; actually most apothecaries would be charged from time to time with 'practising' without the Physicians' approval.

The politics of the breakaway were complex and fluid, but in brief the decade of the 1610s brought together more powerful forces for reform than for the status quo. The cause of the apothecaries was a pet one for James I, both for improving the health of his people and for defying parliament.[27] Leading royal Physicians, like Sir Henry Atkins and Sir Theodore de Mayerne, wanted apothecaries independent of the Grocers but more dependent on themselves. The apothecaries, led by de Laune, wanted freedom from the Grocers, ability to regulate themselves and a more equal relationship with the Physicians (who were their main clients, of course). The final factor was the machinations of Lord Keeper Francis Bacon, lobbying for reform.[28]

These were the protagonists for change, but the Grocers and the City of London were powerful opponents, along with more conservative Physicians and apothecaries.

In 1614 Parkinson joined a group of 75 reform-minded apothecaries who resigned from the Grocers and petitioned the king for independence. When this was finally granted in December 1617, Parkinson took his place as one of 20 Assistants (committee members); he was also an active member of a group of five to be invited by the Physicians to revise the defective draft *Pharmacopoeia* that other Physicians had compiled.

Parkinson, Daniel Darnelly and Gabriel Sheriff actively worked with the Physicians to make the *Pharmacopoeia Londinensis* usable. Parkinson also joined another group, consisting of Darnelly, De Laune and Edward Cooke, to prepare a schedule of medicines for the apothecaries' own use (both were in Latin). In 1649 Nicholas Culpeper, a non-qualified apothecary, would publish an English version of the *Pharmacopoeia.*[29]

Parkinson was further involved as a treasurer and for one year as a warden, visiting apothecary premises and supervising discipline. But by 1622 he felt he had fulfilled his obligations to the Society and secured his family's own future, and simply resigned. He still wanted to write, but not as part of a committee. He would play little part in the Society thereafter, except to give evidence in the *Quo Warranto* case brought by the Grocers in the 1630s,[30] but he always thought of himself as an apothecary.[31]

The Society grew steadily, and could pay for a hall in the 1630s (Parkinson did not subscribe); survived the civil war, largely thanks to de Laune's bottomless pockets; rebuilt its hall after the Great Fire of 1666; and started the Chelsea Physic Garden in 1673. It ranked 58th of Livery companies of the City; it was and is still a survivor.

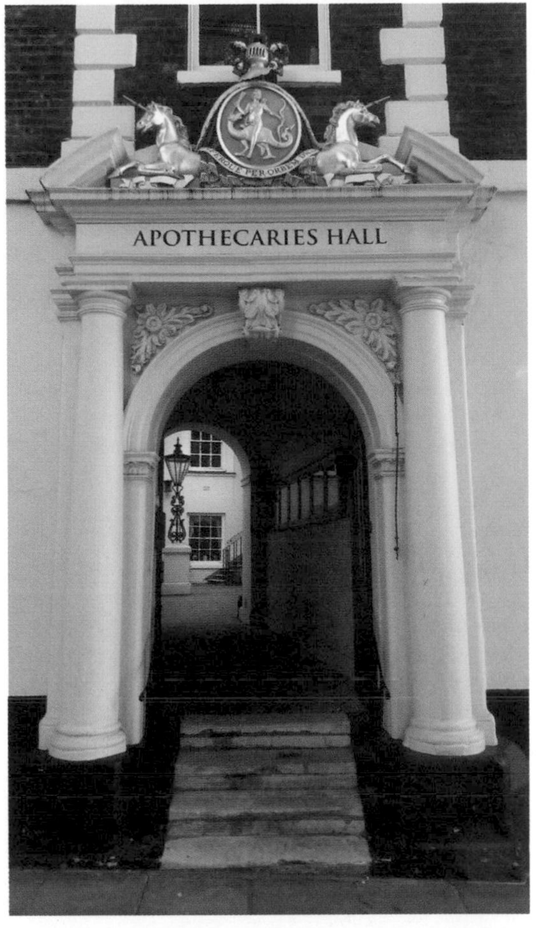

Apothecaries Hall, in Blackfriars, London, dates from 1672; the original hall of 1633 burnt down in the Great Fire of 1666; below: some of the 76 reformers of 1614; de Mayerne and Atkins head the list, and Parkinson's name is in the central column

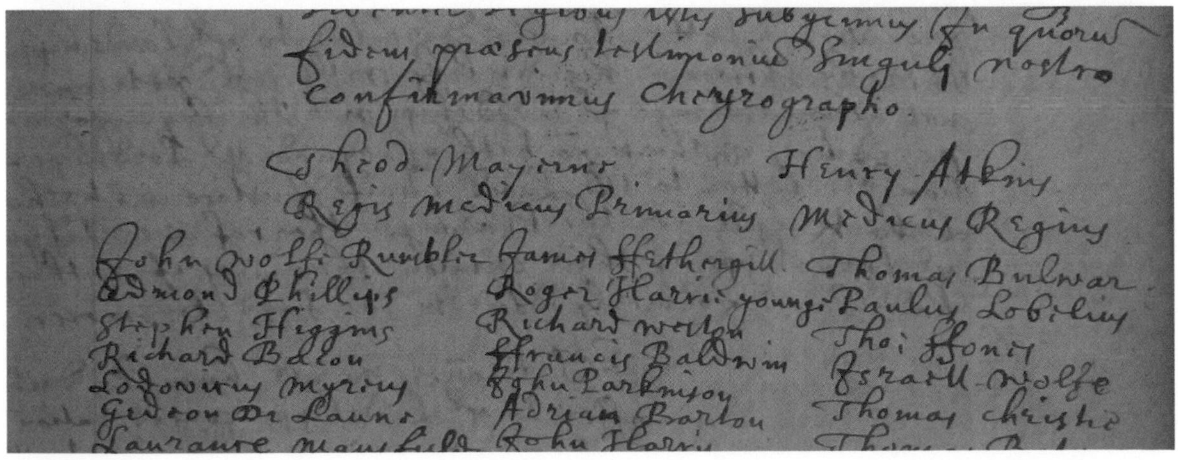
fidem praesens testimonium singuli nostro
confirmavimus chirographo.

Theod. Mayerne Henry Atkins
Regis medicus Primarius Medicus Regius

Thomas Bulwar
Stephen Higgins Richard Weston
Francis Baldwin
John Parkinson
Adrian Barton Thomas
John Harris

3 **Paradisi in Sole**: Parkinson as a gardener

Parkinson would probably be surprised, if not upset, to discover that his lasting fame has been, at least until now, for his quickly written gardening book, *Paradisi in Sole*, rather than his fifty-year herbal magnum opus, *Theatrum Botanicum*. But the earlier, shorter book has a charm, completeness, easy authority and lightness of touch he found harder to duplicate as the page count of the *Theatrum* rose, while he grew older and could not draw it to a close.

We are not sure how *Paradisi* came to be written, but by the mid-1620s Parkinson had become well known in royal circles. King James (who died in 1625) had already granted him a coat of arms and a lease of land on St Martin's Lane.[32] James's son and successor, Charles I, knew of Parkinson and his garden from Parkinson's Long Acre neighbour, Sir Theodore de Mayerne, the king's favourite physician. Perhaps a royal hint was dropped that the new queen, Henrietta Maria (they married in 1625, she being a bride of 16), might like a gift of a book on paradise gardens. Sir Theodore was adept at persuasion, and might well have suggested to Parkinson that such a book be of *English* gardens and written in English.

The idea of the book took fire in Parkinson's mind, and he heeded de l'Obel's advice to publish when he could.[33] The book would be dedicated to the Queen, though its real audience was 'gentlemen and gentlewomen', people who wanted their gardens to be beautiful as well as productive.[34] Progress was rapid, and by 1629 the book was ready for the press, with what became over 630 pages of text, three indexes, and 612 woodcut illustrations. His German engraver Albert Switzer had copied older illustrations where available, but many were new and drawn from life, these often being Parkinson's own garden 'rarities'. Switzer also drew Parkinson's courtly portrait and his own imaginative Garden of Eden as the frontispiece – his skill deserves more appreciation.

Parkinson writes here with ease and is relaxed, explaining what he knows from experience, always his great test. He seeks initially to charm his young queen, who knew great gardens in the Paris of her father, Henri IV, but found precious few in London. Parkinson would therefore make his paradise in words and offer her a 'speaking garden'.[35] He writes without fear, confident in his own ability to do the job well.

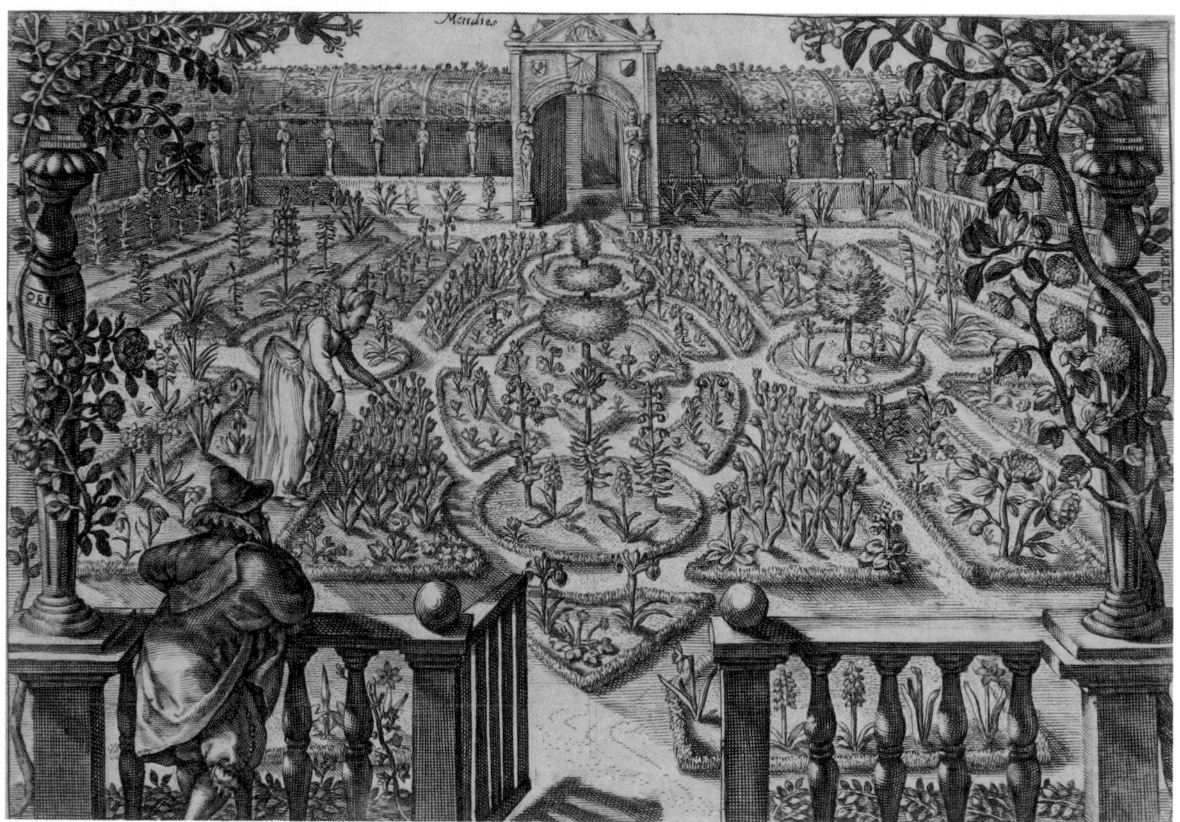

He begins his charm offensive with the title, with perhaps the best-known pun in British gardening history. His Latin title translates as Paradise in the Sun, or, with a near synonym, Park-in-son. He takes the irony further: in his portrait he holds a 'sweet John'; more tangential, if still with irony, is its other name, 'pride of London'. Whether the queen enjoyed the puns is not known.

The book itself is far more than a courtier's offering. In his 'Epistle to the Reader', Parkinson spells out why it is new. He says most Latin writers (he excepts Charles de l'Ecluse, Clusius) have not described the diversity of flowers. Previous English herbals by Turner, Lyte (translator of Dodoens) and Gerard tried, but all were now out of date. None featured beautiful flowers, 'fit to store a garden of delight and pleasure'. Also they lacked descriptions of the flowers, 'the greatest hinderance of all mens delight'.[36]

Parkinson promised he would give full plant names, noting some of the errors of previous authors, while 'reserving what else might be said to another time & worke' (i.e. the *Theatrum*). He had provided new illustrations, and briefly described plant 'vertues' and their cooking potential.

But he was too close to the book to see what is really new – his own passion for his plants. Sheer delight had not been the expressed motive for a flower book before.

For example, he introduces gilliflowers, 'the pride of our English gardens', nearly 100 sorts of daffodils, 50 of iacinthes (hyacinths), 20 crocus or saffron flowers, 20 lilies, including crown imperials, an 'almost infinite' number of tulips, and so on. His introductory pages of flowers – and likewise herbs and roots, kitchen garden vegetables, and an orchard of fruits and trees in later sections of the *Paradisi* – are prolifically impressive. He also promised a fourth part, 'a garden of Simples', which would become the monster *Theatrum*.[37]

Perhaps he was lucky that his era had more genetic diversity coming into the garden than at any time before. But he also made his luck. Let us pause for a moment and

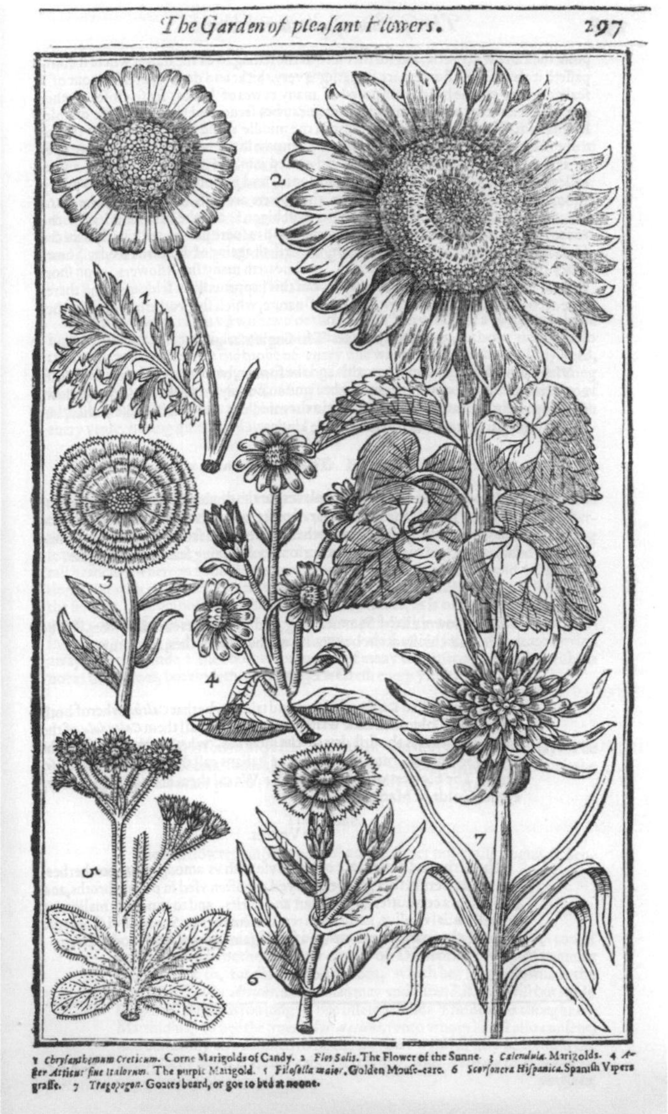

The Garden of pleasant Flowers. 297

1 *Chrysanthemum Creticum*. Corne Marigolds of Candy. 2 *Flos Solis*. The Flower of the Sunne. 3 *Calendula*. Marigolds. 4 *Aster Atticus sive Italorum*. The purple Marigold. 5 *Filosella maior*. Golden Mouse-eare. 6 *Scorsonera Hispanica*. Spanish Vipers grasse. 7 *Tragopogon*. Goates beard, or goe to bed at noone.

Above: **Parkinson's woodcuts of marigolds and relatives are dominated by his 'golden flower of Peru', a sunflower – a 'goodly and stately plant, wherewith every one is now a dayes familiar'. He had grown it 'ten foote high', with the flower 'breaking forth from a great head ... like unto a single great Marigold'. He finds 'there is no use in Physicke with us', i.e. no medicinal use. Some people, he adds, eat them 'as Hartichokes are' and call them 'good meate, but they are too strong for my taste'. Left: the Spring garden from *Hortus Floridus*, 1615, by Dutch artist Crispin I de Passe (1564–1637). The garden is in French parterre style, with raised beds, statuary and a colonnade; the well-dressed lady is picking tulips, with crown imperials, hyacinths and roses nearby, along with a male onlooker (is this perhaps us, the watchers?). These superb copperplates were hugely popular and remain so today**

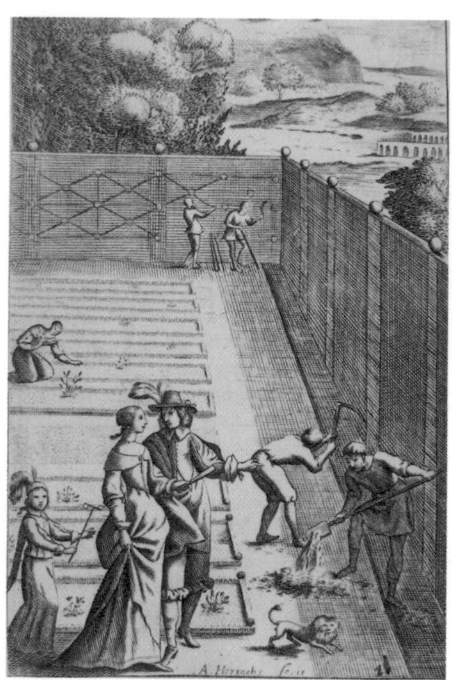

Illustrations from John Evelyn's *The French Gardiner*, 1658. Top: the owner, his wife, daughter and dog visit their walled garden, while a trellis is erected at the back; below: the kitchen garden, with enclosed raised beds for melons, a parterre and fruit trees

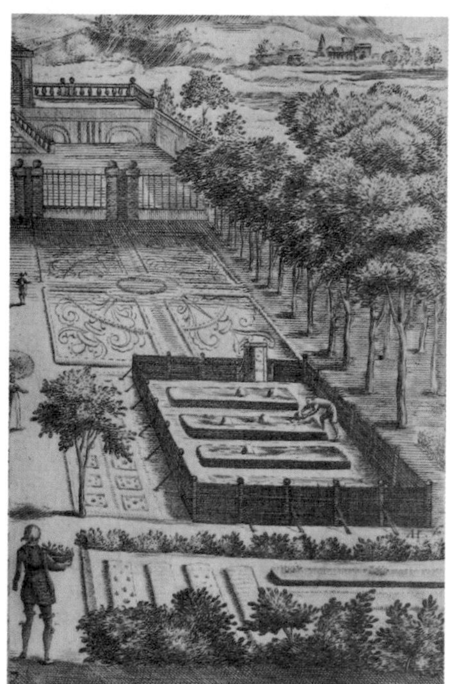

read his actual words. The rhythms of Parkinson's prose take a while to become familiar, but his love for his flowers is evident at once. You may well want to dash to the garden centre or go online and buy everything he describes! So, at random:

The ***Anemones*** *likewise or Windeflowers are so full of variety and so dainty, so pleasant and so delightsome flowers, that the sight of them doth enforce an earnest longing desire in the mind of any one to be a possessour of some of them at the least:*

For without all doubt, this one kinde of flower, so variable in colours, so differing in forme (being almost as many sorts of them double as single), so plentifull in bearing flowers, and so durable in lasting, and also so easie both to preserve and to encrease, is of it selfe alone almost sufficient to furnish a garden with their flowers for almost halfe the yeare, as I shall shew you in a fit and convenient place (p9).

All the time he was writing, Parkinson was gardening Long Acre vigorously, and had been since at least 1607.[38] It had become a tourist attraction, and was visited by many apothecaries and apprentices. Botanist John Goodyer records gathering seeds of *Astragalus lusitanicus* there in 1616,[39] while William Broad, a young botanist apothecary, marvelled at Parkinson's productivity in the late 1620s. In a short Latin poem for the prefatory pages of the *Paradisi*, Broad (writing as Guilielmus Brodus) finds himself unable to know whether to admire book or garden more, for 'the whole world that is in the garden is in this book of yours'.[40]

It was common knowledge that Parkinson did not travel far. He was always in his shop or garden, probably never returned to Lancashire, indeed seldom left London. How, then, did he build up such an impressive garden? It was known he had been given access to de l'Obel's papers after de l'Obel's death in 1617, so perhaps he had 'done a Gerard' and published someone else's work as his own? The *Paradisi*, remarkably, contains the confession of one such sceptic, the grocer William Atkins, who states in the opening pages that he had doubted, but now sees for himself that Parkinson is genuine, and apologises profoundly.[41]

Parkinson in fact paid plant-hunters, such as William Boel, to go to Spain and other places to find new plants for him. Parkinson was miffed that Boel took his money but also sold some of his Iberian plants to rival gardener William Coys, of Stubbers, Essex.[42] Francis le Veau was a 'root gatherer' Parkinson relied on.

Other travelling gardener friends, like John Tradescant the Elder, brought back new species from Russia and Virginia. Royal Physician Dr Matthew Lister sent seeds of 'true or English rhubarb' from Venice, and Dr Fludd, the alchemical Physician, the Great White Sea Daffodil from Pisa. There was a constant trade in plants and information between gardener friends and rivals. One of his more unusual plant suppliers was Thomasin Tunstall, from Lancashire, who found him the lady's slipper orchid. She was exactly the sort of 'gentlewoman' he was writing for (see p244).

4 THEATRUM BOTANICUM: PARKINSON AS A HERBALIST

The *Paradisi* had been a successful and enjoyable diversion for Parkinson, but the main task of his life remained to be completed. He summarized this half-century journey in introducing hyssop, the first plant in the *Theatrum* [p1]: *From a Paradise of pleasant Flowers, I am fallen* (Adam *like) to a world of profitable* [i.e. medicinal] *Herbes and Plantes, ... namely those Plants that are frequently used to helpe the diseases of our bodies*.

The *Theatrum* was the final part of his publication project, trailed in the *Paradisi* as a Book of Simples. Parkinson's ambition had now become more encyclopaedic, and the book bore a new name, the *Theater of Plants* (he used what we now think of as American spelling).[43] It would take the form of a traditional herbal, with sections on the names, distribution, growing times and 'vertues' of each plant.[44] Most would be illustrated with woodcuts. It would be as definitive a global plant reference work as Parkinson could make it, for readers who included apothecaries, physicians and gardeners, male and female – though it would have few formulas or recipes, which his readers could find elsewhere.[45]

In Parkinson's Epistle to the Reader in the *Theatrum*, you can feel his pride and relief at finally getting into print, but also pain and anguish.[46] He laments the separation from his son Richard, and says the book is his 'artificiall' legacy, since he has no 'Naturall' son. He blames the 'disastrous times' for the delay in publication, but also 'much more wretched and perverse men ... [whose] extreame covetousnesse had well nigh deprived my country of the fruition'.[47]

What made the normally gracious and equable Parkinson so angry was the outright commercialism of a rapidly produced, new and enlarged edition of Gerard's *Herball* (1597). It was universally known that Parkinson was working methodically on his great book, the first serious herbal in English since Gerard. The market was ready, and the publishers of the original Gerard, the Nortons (Mistress Joyce Norton and Bonham Norton), along with Adam Islip and Richard Whitaker, rushed into the gap in 1633.

The rising apothecary Thomas Johnson (1600–44) was their chosen author, and he did a remarkable job of completing a thorough revision and expansion in one year.[48] Johnson had visited the Long Acre garden with John Goodyer in 1616, and later, and had written a commendatory verse for the *Paradisi*. Parkinson saw him as a colleague and friend, so the sense of personal betrayal was acute.

What made it worse was that Johnson had published previously with the brothers Thomas and Richard Cotes, Parkinson's printers.[49] Goodyer, another friend, meanwhile, unknown to Parkinson, had provided Johnson with 25 pages of revisions – Parkinson felt it to be another stab in the back.

Parkinson's printer Richard Cotes had registered the intended *Theatrum* with the Company of Stationers on 3 March 1634, but it was too late.[50] Johnson's Gerard, as it became known, was already in print. The knife was to turn further when the book needed to be reprinted in 1636. Parkinson now had to wait until the market could bear another large, expensive herbal.[51]

Meanwhile exciting new plants and new books were still appearing, and Parkinson needed to insert them into his endless text. His Tribe 15, the 'Unordered Tribe', he admitted, was a *gathering Camp to take up all those straglers that have lost their rankes* (TB, p1325). The last Tribe, no. 17, the 'Strange and Outlandish Plants', was an alphabetical rather than systematic list of drugs and perfumes, foreign herbs and spices, from ambergris to unicorn's horn.[52]

There are few records of Parkinson meeting his king. But sometime in the 1630s Parkinson, Sir Theodore and Dr William Harvey, the king's 'physician in ordinary', were called to assess the king's 'unicorn horn'. All three men knew the unicorn was a myth, and that the king's horn, weighing 40 lb (18 kg), was probably from a 'sea unicorn', or narwhal, an Arctic whale. But it was valuable, and how do you tell a king he has been duped? Parkinson carefully describes the meeting (TB, p1611) – they told the king the truth.

It is not clear how Parkinson paid for such a large printing job as the *Theatrum* must have been. We know he gave the manuscript in completed sections to the Cotes to print: John Morris writes to Johannes de Laet in excitement on 12 January 1638 that he has seen the pages up to 1142 and expects as many again in the final version.[53] Perhaps Sir Theodore, Morris or another of Parkinson's wealthy friends came to his help, but there is no evidence of a subscription process or an appeal for funds. Parkinson may have sold the Ludgate Hill shop before 1640, and the proceeds put towards paying Cotes. Perhaps by this time he had become independently wealthy through his garden and nursery business. He probably spent more on his plants than he did on himself.

The book was finally sold at a pricy 36s, with 3s for binding (these figures are from the fly leaf of Goodyer's own copy, dated August 1640, in the Magdalen College library).[54] It was far later appearing than Parkinson had intended, but 1640 turned out to be the very final date he could have published.

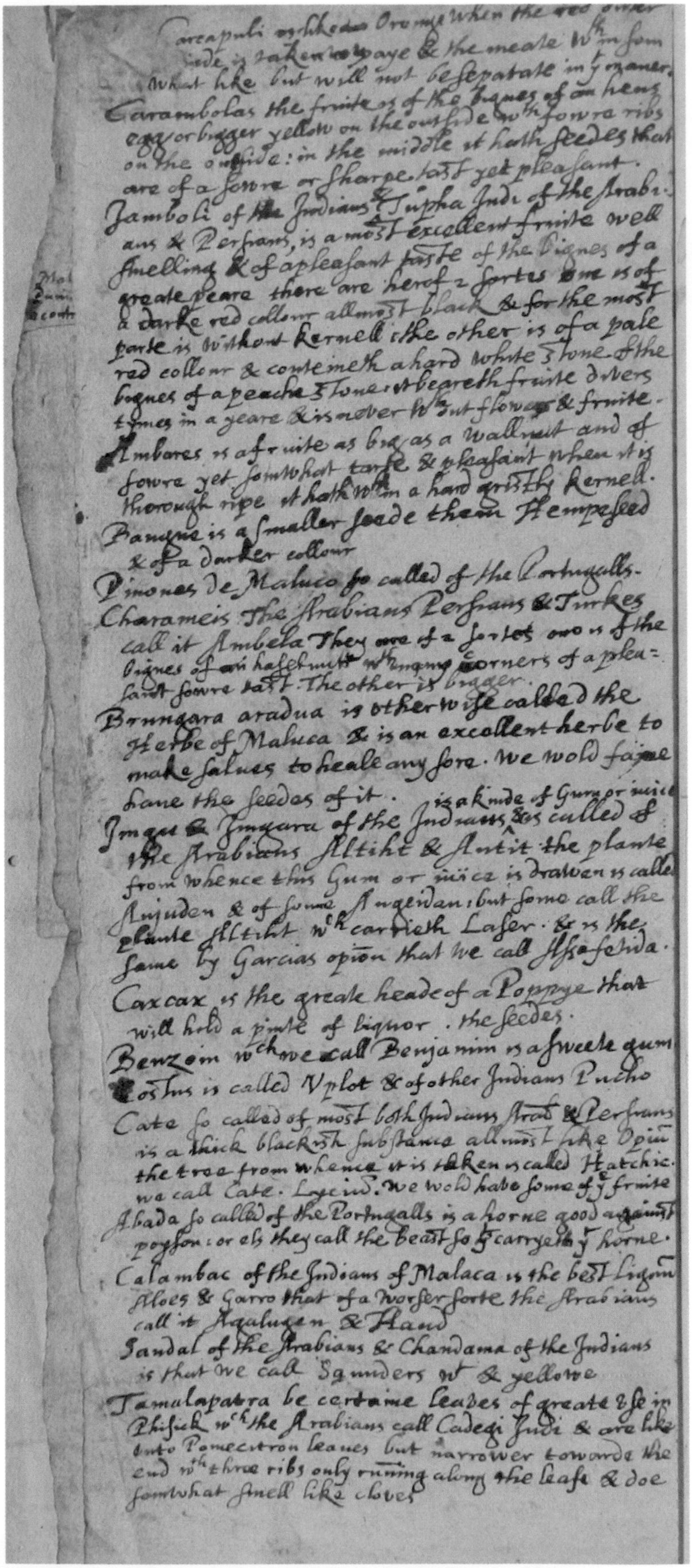

Sir Theodore had prevailed upon the King, at a rare good moment in 1639, to give Parkinson the official recognition that his unofficial fame merited. Parkinson now achieved what de l'Obel and Gerard before him had claimed, but not been formally granted, the title of 'King's Herbarist'. With this gift (there was no salary to go with it) Parkinson could now dedicate the book formally to Charles[55] and proceed into print. Any more delays would have made publication impossible: for one thing, in civil war conditions from 1642 onwards printers were no longer free to print commercial titles.

The *Theatrum* was to be the last in a century-long series of English-language herbals. The so-called *Grete Herbal* of 1526 described 207 species; Turner's three volumes (1551–68) had roughly 1,000; Gerard in 1597 had under 2,000; Johnson's revision grew to 2,850; Parkinson had 3,800. It was the biggest: was it the best?[56]

Its reputation has suffered by its publication falling between two perennial favourites of English herbalism, Gerard's *Herball*, in both 1597 and 1633 versions, and Culpeper's *English Physitian* of 1652 (later and still sold as *Culpeper's Herbal*).[57] They have enduring charm and charisma, but as practical herbals are inferior to Parkinson in accuracy, comprehensiveness and above all in detail of plants' names and medicinal values. Only by examining Parkinson's plant 'vertues' in detail, as we do in this book, are his forgotten scholarship and lasting relevance as a herbal reference book revealed.

Left: 'We wold faine have the seedes of it' [the 'Herbe of Maluca']: part of a list of his plant 'wants', probably for an agent visiting the East Indies, in Parkinson's best hand. Goodyer Papers, MS 324, fo. 165v, unpublished

William How's extraordinary personal attack on Parkinson, now among the Goodyer papers in Oxford, MS 324, unpublished

A good case can also be made that Parkinson is more original than either. It was known in 1597 that Gerard had taken over an almost completed English translation by Dr Priest of Rembert Dodoens' *Pemptades Sex* (1583), added to it and passed it off as his own work.[58] Culpeper meanwhile lifted chunks of Parkinson's *Theatrum*, often word for word, for his own herbal, with no credit given, though adding his own astrology. It seems entirely unfair that Culpeper is renowned and Parkinson forgotten.[59]

One young botanist, after Parkinson's death, saw in the *Theatrum* only the theft of de l'Obel's work. William How (1619–56) had come to own de l'Obel's papers, and published a selection in 1655, listing Parkinson's 'errors'. Yet Parkinson mentions in the *Theatrum* (in his account of peas, p1060) that he had bought the papers and made use of them; he acknowledges this debt to de l'Obel in the extended title of the *Theatrum* itself; and de l'Obel plainly saw him as his literary heir.

How's version (see above) is that Parkinson had bought a finished book by de l'Obel – How writes: *The Title! Epistle! and Diploma affix'd!* – then suppressed and copied it as his own. How claims that Parkinson *murdered his genuine scrutiny in treacherous oblivion, erecting upon this despoyled Fabrick that Theater, on wch is personated ye great Rhapsodist*. These words are scribbled in anger on the back of a page from de l'Obel, which is affixed by a rusty pin, upside down, in the Goodyer papers. But How was excessive and mistaken, and Parkinson emerges with reputation intact, Canon Raven judging that Parkinson 'has taken very little [of de l'Obel] for the simple reason that very little was worth taking'.[60]

Parkinson was the last man who could have produced a herbal such as the *Theatrum*. Rex Jones in 1984 put it well: Parkinson had made 'an admirable and final attempt to keep an exploding body of knowledge within a single volume'.[61] But the next fifty years in England see botany becoming a new discipline, with new classificatory precision; medicine itself turns more chemical; apothecaries win their freedom from the physicians; science is formalized, with a new national institution, the Royal Society. The old world has changed; herbals are old-fashioned, and woodcuts are replaced by the newer technology of copper engravings.[62]

But Parkinson could and did hold it together. He had written what John Ray in 1678 called 'the most full and comprehensive book of that subject [a herbal] extant'.[63] Parkinson's secret, concludes Canon Raven, is his 'authentic passion for a garden and the quiet wisdom of a gardener, than which there are few things more precious'.[64] The image below is suitably Parkinsonian: a grizzled gardener in his 'paradise'.

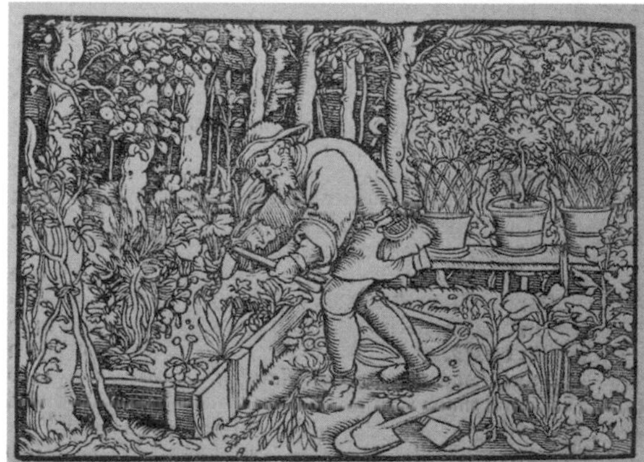

An elderly German gardener, absorbed in creating a garden of pleasure. The garden tools, raised beds, pots on a stand, vine on a trellis and pear tree would all be familiar to Parkinson a century later (by Christian Egenolph, *Lustgarten und Pflantzungen*, 1530)

5 Parkinson's medicine

Parkinson's herbalism often seems so current, despite the archaic language, that it is easy to forget how different medicine was in his day. His herbal was a mainstream medical text when it was written. The new 'chymical' medicine inspired by Paracelsus (1493–1541) was starting to come into fashion, but had not yet replaced Galenic medicine, and botany and medicine were still essentially one discipline.

How medicine was divided up

In London during Parkinson's lifetime, professional medicine was split between three main groups of practitioners. There were the university-trained physicians, and the more practically trained, apprenticed apothecaries and barber-surgeons.

There were also a range of other people, including midwives, who provided unofficial health care.

Medical theory

The prevailing medical model was still based on the writings of Hippocrates and Galen, and the theory of the four humours, which dominated Western medical theory for more than 2,000 years.[65] Illness was seen as arising when the humours got out of balance, and the aim of medical treatment was to restore the body to its natural equilibrium.

The four humours of Hippocratic medicine are black bile (*melan chole*) – which gives the word 'melancholy' – blood (*haima*), phlegm (*phlegma*) and yellow bile (*chole*). It has been suggested that the idea of four humours came from watching blood separate in a glass container. After about an hour it forms into four layers, corresponding to the colours of the humours.[66]

The humours came to be associated with four temperaments, depending on the predominant humour in an individual – respectively, melancholic, sanguine, phlegmatic and choleric.

Methods of restoring balance by reducing the excess humour included purging and blood-letting, which remained accepted medical practices into the 20th century. Medicines were also used to increase excretion through urination, sweat and saliva.

Herbs were classified as hot or cold, moist or dry, and prescribed accordingly. The degree of heat or cold was generally given as a range from one to four, with the hottest herbs (such as chilis) being hot in the fourth degree, and the coldest herbs (such as opium) being cold in the fourth degree. Heat or cold in the first degree would be very mild. Usually, the mildest herbs that would achieve the desired effect were the ones chosen. Heating herbs increase metabolic activity, cooling herbs decrease activity.

Herbs were also given other actions, such as vulnerary (wound healing), astringent (binding), diuretic (increasing urinary flow), diaphoretic (increasing sweating) and aphrodisiac ('provoking unto venery').

Complicated recipes with lots of expensive ingredients were favoured by physicians, and made more money for apothecaries. These included the theriacs and other antidotes to poisons, which often assembled dozens of ingredients. The use of pearls, gemstones, gold and expensive exotic spices was usually preferred by the wealthy rather than the simple local herbal remedies that most country people relied upon. One can't help but think that the poorer people who had access to these plants and a knowledge of 'simples' were better off than their wealthier counterparts, being expensively bled and purged.

Chemistry and alchemy were becoming more popular, with the use of metals such as mercury and antimony in various forms. Theodore de Mayerne had trained in Montpellier, where the new chemical medicine was taught, and he prescribed chemicals as well as herbs.

Diseases of the times

Many of the health problems that faced people in the 1500s and 1600s were the same as those that face us today, but there were notable exceptions.

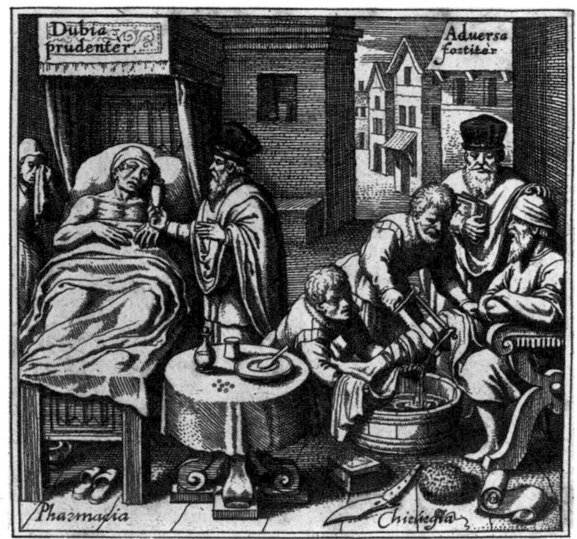

An apothecary administers medicine to a patient in bed, while surgeons, watched by a physician, perform an amputation (a 1646 engraving by Matthaeus Merian)

Plague was still a real problem, with several serious outbreaks in London during Parkinson's lifetime.[67] Most physicians responded by leaving the capital, but the apothecaries tended to stay put. Quartaine and tertian agues or malarial fevers were common. There were also outbreaks of other infectious diseases, which have virtually been eradicated by modern vaccination programmes and antibiotics, and leprosy still occurred. Syphilis was difficult to treat, and mercury became popular despite its known toxicity.

Administering medicines

Parkinson used a much wider range of herbal preparations than most modern herbalists, and had a good grasp of herbal energetics.

Culpeper's translation of the *Pharmacopoeia* gives a further insight into the herbal and other medicinal preparations of the time, but it also shows how wide Parkinson's repertoire was by comparison with the official list. The *Pharmacopoeia* sanctions the use of a number of animals and animal parts, as well as excrements, which were popular medicines but which Parkinson scarcely mentions. It is usually the bizarre that we like to focus on when we think of 16th and 17th century medicine, but it was actually quite sophisticated if one looks at Parkinson's medicine.

Parkinson applied an impressive range of methods of administering herbs. He used simple infusions and decoctions made with water, but also with wine or vinegar. Herbs were brewed to make wine or ale, or simply infused in wine or ale. Only a few tinctures, the mainstay of modern western herbalists, were made.[68] Parkinson distilled herbs in water or in wine or ale, either in an alembic or in a balneum – a glass still set in a bath of boiling water. What we now call essential oils, then called chymical oils, were also distilled from aromatic plants.

He used powdered dried herbs in a variety of ways, including making them into pills, lozenges, electuaries and lohocs, and taking them in wine. He made syrups with sugar or honey, oxymels with sugar or honey and vinegar, and he made pessaries. Herbs were also introduced as glisters (enemas), and suppositories.

Externally herbs were applied as poultices, plaisters and fomentations. Herbs were infused in oils, either in the sun or heated over a fire, and hardened into ointments with beeswax, or they were pounded with soft animal fat. Herbal baths were applied, sometimes as sitz-baths where the patient sits in a basin of water, or else the affected part was bathed in a basin, sometimes using a sponge. Parkinson also suggested that people sit over the steam of a decoction, or the smoke of herbs placed on coals in a 'close stool' or closed commode.

Parkinson was very knowledgeable about gynaecology, and frequently mentions herbal treatments for menstrual problems and childbirth.[69]

He respected the classical and Arab authors, engaging with them vigorously in his 'Names' sections, but also listened to country people and their cures. He was eager to dispel superstitions, relying on common sense and his own extensive experience.[70]

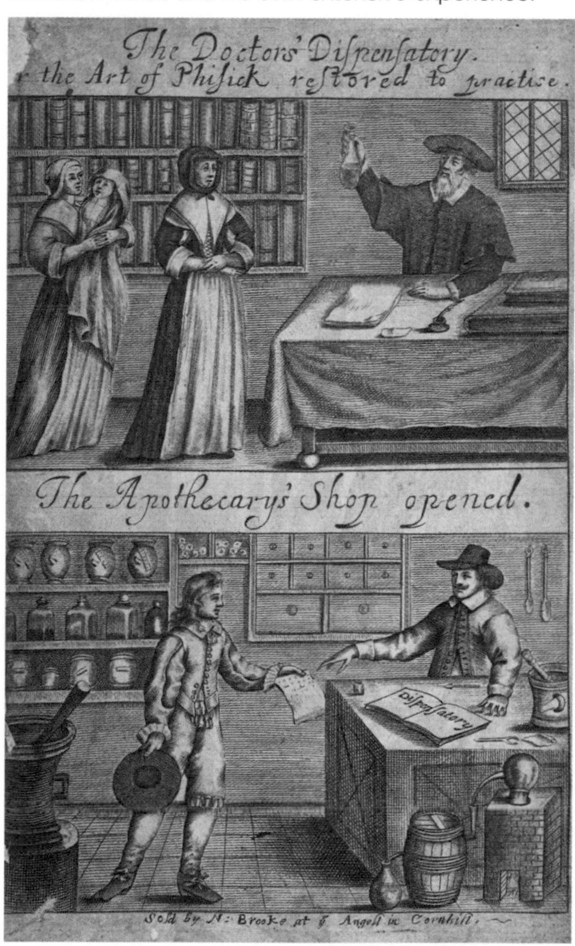

In the medical marketplace, 1650s: the physician (top) examines a patient's urine; he has no medicines, but many scholarly books; the apothecary's shop (below) has a still, pestles and mortars, bottles and jars of remedies; he examines the prescription and consults his *Dispensatory* (frontispiece of Peter Morellus, *The Expert Doctor's Dispensatory*, 1657)

A Note to the Reader

The 1,788 pages of John Parkinson's *Theatrum Botanicum* cover an intimidating 3,800 plants. How have we made **our selection** of 75 chapters, containing (with multiple species in some chapters) nearly 100 plants? We use three broad criteria:

- Herbs well known to Parkinson that continue to be medicinally popular today, sometimes with different uses. He recommended hawthorn for the stone, but didn't know it as the heart tonic of modern herbalism; he used St John's wort as a wound herb, but not for treating depression or seasonal affective disorder. Comparisons over time can be more than tangentially interesting.
- Herbs known and used medicinally in Parkinson's time but which have since dropped out of common practice – in other words, 'lost herbs' that we think deserve a second look. We include, among others, bugle, figwort, ground ivy, houseleek, mistletoe, sanicle, tribulus and weld.
- Herbs 'new' to Parkinson from either European herbal knowledge or as part of the explosion of plant samples or seeds then arriving in England from North and South America, China, the Indies (West and East), India and the Middle East. These were often sent by Parkinson's friends overseas direct to him for his renowned garden at Long Acre. Read him on chilis, coca, corn, love apples (tomatoes), sassafras and tobacco, and share the excitement towards the end of his book, when plants arrive pell-mell on the page, in his 'unordered tribe' and 'exotics' chapters.

Overall we have tried to give a balanced choice from Parkinson's huge coverage. There is enough material for several selections such as this one, and further volumes are anticipated.

The **organization of Parkinson's plants** in this book is alphabetical by common modern English name (on right-hand pages); scientific names are added, while Parkinson's common and scientific names are given (left-hand pages), along with the reference to his 'tribe' (genera) and page number.

Our focus is on the medicinal uses of plants, so we unavoidably by-pass Parkinson's detailed exposition of plant names and his descriptions. His classificatory scholarship is dense but informed by long experience and good sense, and merits its own study.

For the selected plant we print Parkinson's **'vertues'** complete as a transcript on the left-hand page, with **our commentary** on the facing page. The original has long and convoluted sentences, with a wide text measure: you really need a ruler to read his lines comfortably. For ease of reading we adopt a shorter line width, and split his text into paragraphs at colons, semicolons or sometimes commas. We add short headings, and often follow these in our commentary.

Parkinson's text is laid out in a serif typeface on a sepia-toned page while our commentary is in a sans-serif face on white paper; this should reinforce visually the contrasting older and modern presentations.

His **spelling and punctuation** have been retained, with the exceptions noted below. Otherwise these are Parkinson's 'vertues' as he wrote them, and will prove useful source material for present-day readers.

Words that may be unfamiliar, including older medical terms like imposthume, king's evil, quinsy and tertian fever, and personal and place names, are **glossarized** on Parkinson's page; the more significant of the personal names are expanded in the Brief Biographies at the back of the book.

We reproduce Parkinson's original **woodcut illustration**, or the main one if he has several. It took heroic efforts by Julie to clean these up for reproduction: woodcuts are inherently messy and accumulate blobs of ink. Our **modern photographs** of the same plant, almost all taken by Julie, appear on the right; text boxes on various matters of interest, including some recipes, are added.

Dates: In Parkinson's lifetime old-style dates applied, with the new year beginning on 25 March – when Elizabeth I died on 24 March 1603, this was the last day of the old year. To avoid confusion the year has been updated, so that 1 January 1600 is given here as 1 January 1601, unless otherwise noted.

Apothecary weights: Parkinson uses these surprisingly rarely – 1 grain: 1/480 ounce; 1 scruple: 20 grains; 1 dram/drachm: 60 grains or 1/8 ounce.

Spelling: his &c. is etc.; we use i or j as he has it (both laundies and Jaundies occur); we substitute s for his long f-like s, and u for his v (as in Vrine).

Capitals: City means the district of the City of London; Apothecary is capitalized for a member of The Society of Apothecaries and in that connection.

Names: A vernacular form is preferred to a Latinate – de l'Obel rather than Lobelius, Morris not Mauritius – but a few escape: Camerarius it was and still remains.

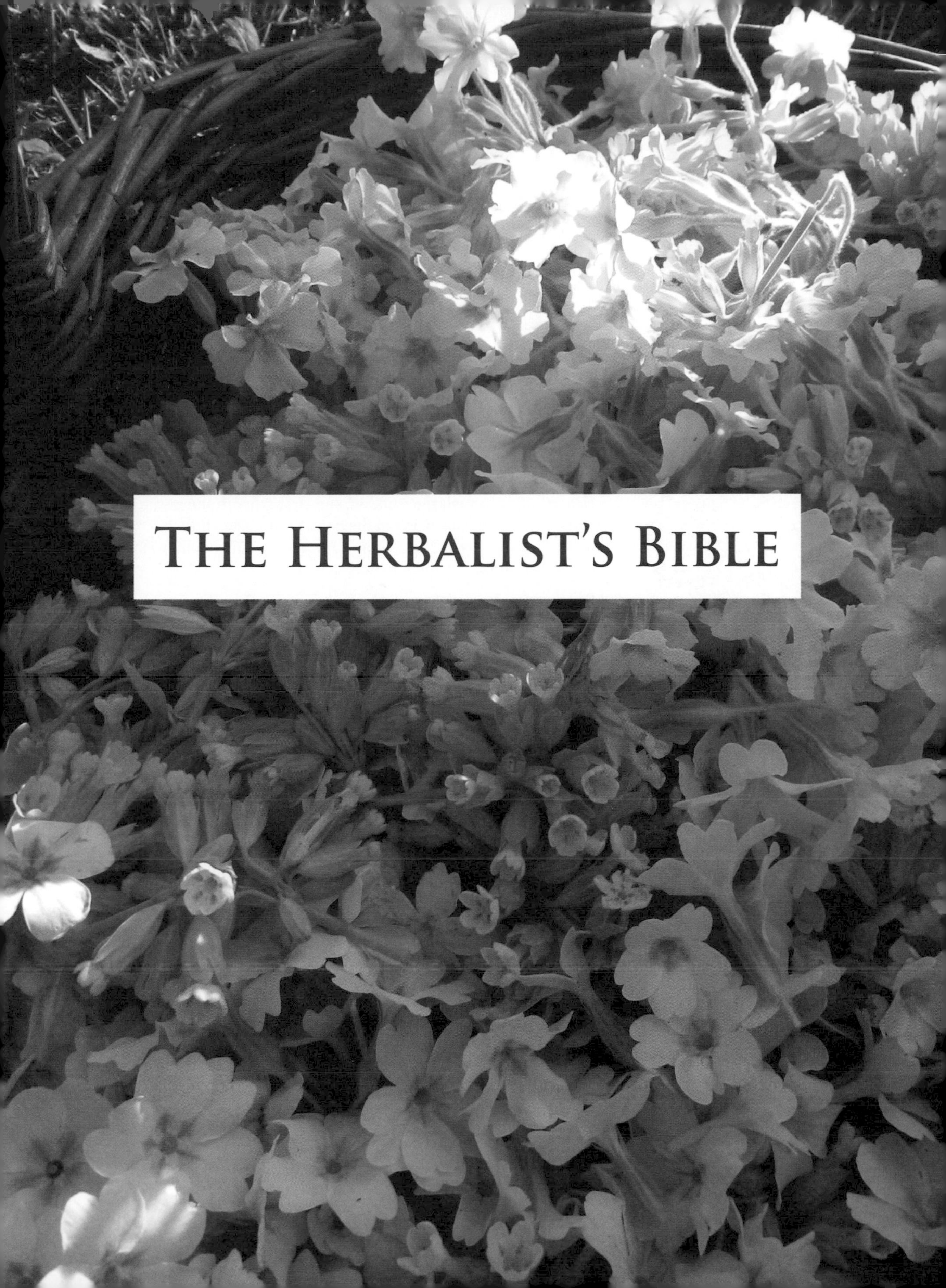
THE HERBALIST'S BIBLE

Agrimonie

Theatrum Botanicum

Tribe 5, Chapter 60, pp594–97

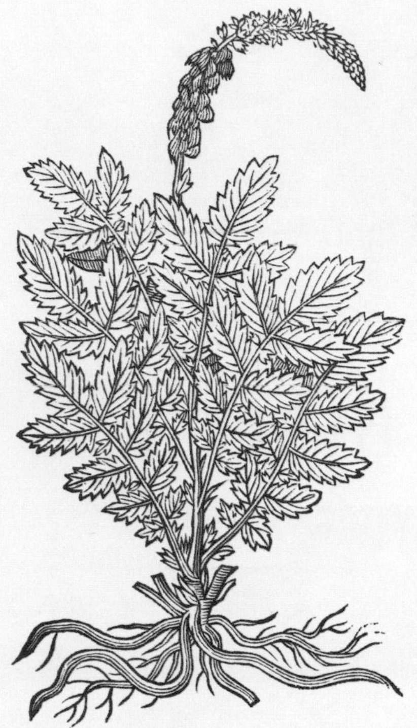

sweete Agrimony: *Agrimonia odorata* (now *A. procera*)
divers: various people
Serapio: probably Serapion the Younger, 12th century author
Galen: Claudius Galen (AD130–200), Roman physician and author
distemperatures: disorderings
foule, or troubled and bloody waters: various urinary problems
strangury: painful, scanty urination
quartain/tertian ague: four- or three-day malarial-type fever
Dioscorides: Greek-speaking Roman physician (mid-first century AD)
Pliny: Pliny the Elder (AD23–79), Roman naturalist
bloody flixe: dysentery
stamped: beaten in a mortar
nayles: nails
members: limbs
impostumed: abscessed

The Vertues

Agrimonia

Agrimony

The sweete *Agrimony* is held by divers to be more excellent in all the properties of *Agrimony*; but because we cannot have it in that quantity, that may serve all mens continuall uses, our ordinary sort will serve sufficiently well and effectually.

Serapio saith, it is hot and dry in the first degree, and as *Galen* saith, it is of thinne parts, and hath a clensing and cutting faculty, without any manifest heate; it is also moderately drying and binding;

Liver & bowels: it openeth the obstructions of the Liver, and clenseth it; it helpeth the jaundise, and strengthneth the inward parts, and is very beneficiall to the bowels, and healeth their inward woundings and bruises or hurts, and qualifieth all inward distemperatures, that grow therein:

Snakebite: the decoction of the herbe, made with wine and drunke, is good against the sting, and bitings of Serpents,

Urinary system: and helpeth them that have foule, or troubled and bloody waters; it is good for the strangury, and helpeth them to make water currantly, and helpeth also the collicke;

Coughs & fevers: it clenseth the brest, and helpeth the cough: it is accounted also a good helpe to ridde a *quartaine* as well as a *tertian* ague, by taking a draught of the decoction warme before the fit, which by altering them, will in time ridde them:

Dysentery & sores: the leaves and seede saith *Dioscorides*, the seede saith *Pliny*, stayeth the bloody flixe, being taken in wine: outwardly applyed it helpeth old sores, cancers, and ulcers that are of hard curation, being stamped with old Swines grease and applyed, for it clenseth and afterwards healeth them:

Splinters: in the same manner also applyed, it doth draw forth the thornes or splinters of wood, nayles, or any other such thing, that is gotten into the flesh,

Joints: and helpeth to strengthen members that be out of joynt:

Ears: it helpeth also foule impostumed eares, being bruised and applyed, or the juyce dropped into them:

Distilled water: the distilled water of the herbe, is good to all the purposes aforesaide; either inward or outward.

Agrimony & hemp agrimony

Rosaceae

These two plants are not related botanically, but were traditionally classed together, as in Parkinson, because of their similar uses. Both are good wound-healing herbs, and are used for liver and urinary problems as well as coughs and fevers.

Agrimony is mainly used to stop bleeding, to treat diarrhoea and as a digestive tonic.

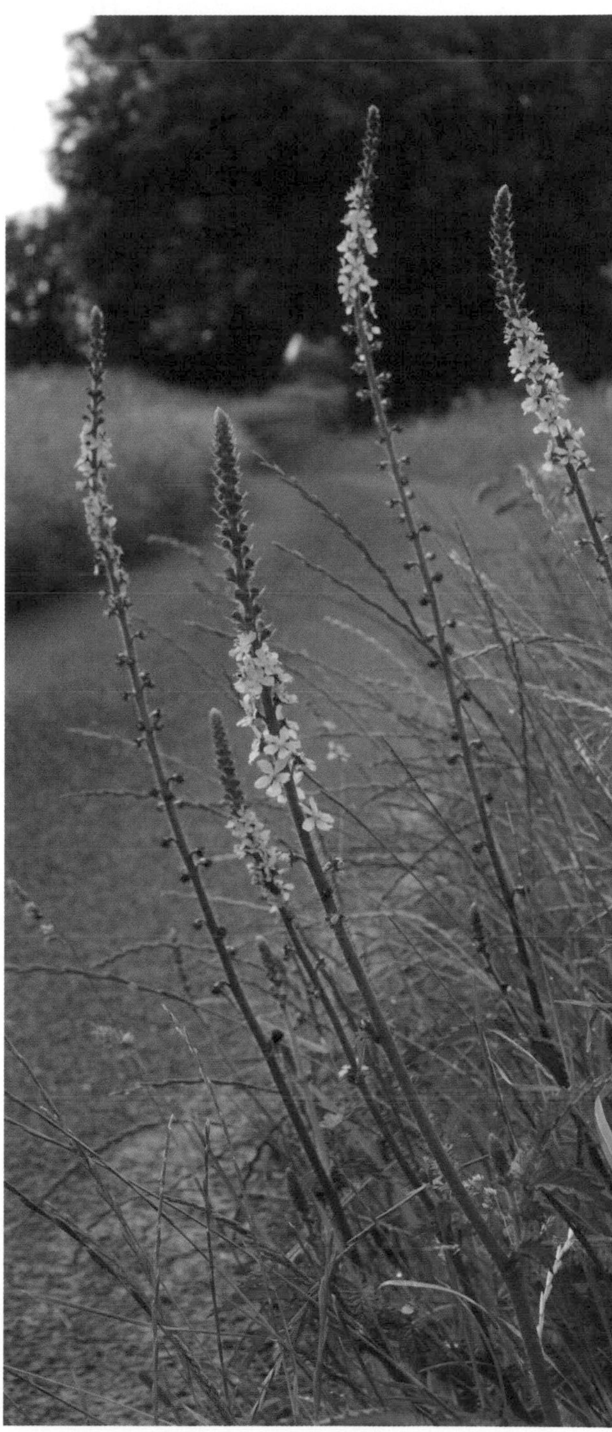

Agrimony *Agrimonia eupatorium, A. procera*

Agrimony is a member of the Rosaceae, and various species are found across Europe, Asia and North America. In western Europe, *A. eupatorium* is the common species, with *A. procera* being the sweet agrimony that Parkinson refers to. In North America, it is hairy agrimony (*A. gryposepala*) that is most common, while in Chinese medicine *A. pilosa* is used, under the name *xian he cao.*

Liver & bowels: Agrimony can treat jaundice and various liver problems, and is good at releasing tension held in the liver and other organs. It helps heal and tone the bowels, and is used for diarrhoea and irritable bowel syndrome.

Urinary system: Agrimony is still used to treat chronic cystitis and irritable bladder, and eases the pain of kidney stones. It can be helpful to reduce bed-wetting in children and incontinence in the elderly.

Coughs & fevers: This herb thins mucus and helps clear it from the body, just as Parkinson says. It is of most use where the phlegm is thick and sticky, and coughing makes the ribs feel bruised.

Bleeding, wounds & ulcers: Agrimony is an excellent healing herb because it first cleans the wound, and then its gentle astringency helps heal it. Parkinson relates the old use for drawing up splinters. In China, agrimony is used in surgery and trauma treatment to stop bleeding.

Agrimony tea, once cooled, is also used as an eyewash for gritty eyes and conjunctivitis, and as a mouthwash. It can help with sprains and strains, by bathing the affected area or applying it as a fomentation or poultice.

Other uses: Agrimony has been found effective in treating vaginal infections caused by *Trichomonas*, and can repel tapeworms. There is little call for it in snakebite treatment any more, but it may be useful to remember it for domestic emergencies, and for summer insect bites and stings. The distilled water has the same properties, as Parkinson says.

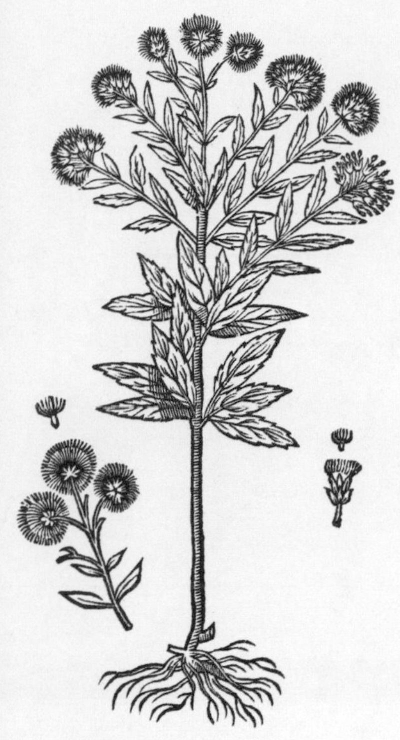

humors: bodily fluids, temperaments
dropsie: oedema, water retention
Iaundise: jaundice
fulnesse: extreme
evill disposition or habit: tendency to illness
impostumes: purulent abscesses
without: external
agues: malarial-like fevers with chills
courses: menstruation
Fumiterry: common fumitory, *Fumaria officinalis*
anointeth: anointed
scruple: apothecary's weight, 20 grains or 1/25 oz or 1.3 gm
steeped: soaked
greene: fresh
Deare: deer

Eupatorium cannabinum

Hemp Agrimony

The Hempelike *Agrimony,* or *Eupatorium Cannabinum,* is of the same temperature of heate and dryeth, for it also openeth, clenseth, cutteth and maketh thinne those humors that are thicke and tough, and therefore is very effectuall for the dropsie, yellow Iaundise, obstructions of the Liver, and hardnesse of the Spleene, fulnesse of humors, and the evill disposition or habit of the body:

Juice: the juyce hereof drunke, is commended much against the imposthumes that come of a cold cause within the body, and for those that are without, the herbe bruised and applied outwardly:

Decoction: the decoction thereof taken before the fits of long and lingring agues, doth helpe much to free any from them: the same also provoketh urine, and womens naturall courses; and boyled with Fumiterry in whey and drunke, helpeth scabbes, and the itch, which proceede of salt and sharpe humours;

Juice: but the juyce mixed with vinegar, and annointed cureth it outwardly; and cureth the Leprosie also, if it be taken in the beginning, but the juyce being drunke, is held to be more effectuall: the juyce being clarified and dryed, and the weight of a scruple taken in pills, killeth the wormes of the belly, and the leaves steeped in drinke, and given to children doth the same.

For animals: The leaves are often given by the Country people, to their cattle, and other beasts, troubled with coughes, and when they are broken winded, or have griping paines within them, all which it helpeth;

Flowers: the flowers chiefely are used to heale both greene and old sores, but the herbe it selfe will doe so likewise; it is sayd that hunters have observed, that Deare being wounded, by the eating of this herbe have beene healed of their hurts:

Smoke: the dryed herbe being burned, driveth away by the smoake and smell thereof, all flies, waspes, and the like, and all other hurtfull and venemous creatures.

Pyrrolizidine alkaloids (PAs)
This group of over 200 plant alkaloids contains several shown to cause toxic reactions in humans, primarily veno-occlusive liver disease. Most reports of human toxicity come from contamination of grain crops by toxic weeds during drought conditions. There are a handful of cases of toxicity from herbal remedies, some from adulteration. It is wise to err on the side of caution and only use plants with harmful PAs externally, or if internally for a short time. Pregnant and breastfeeding women, and children, should avoid internal use.

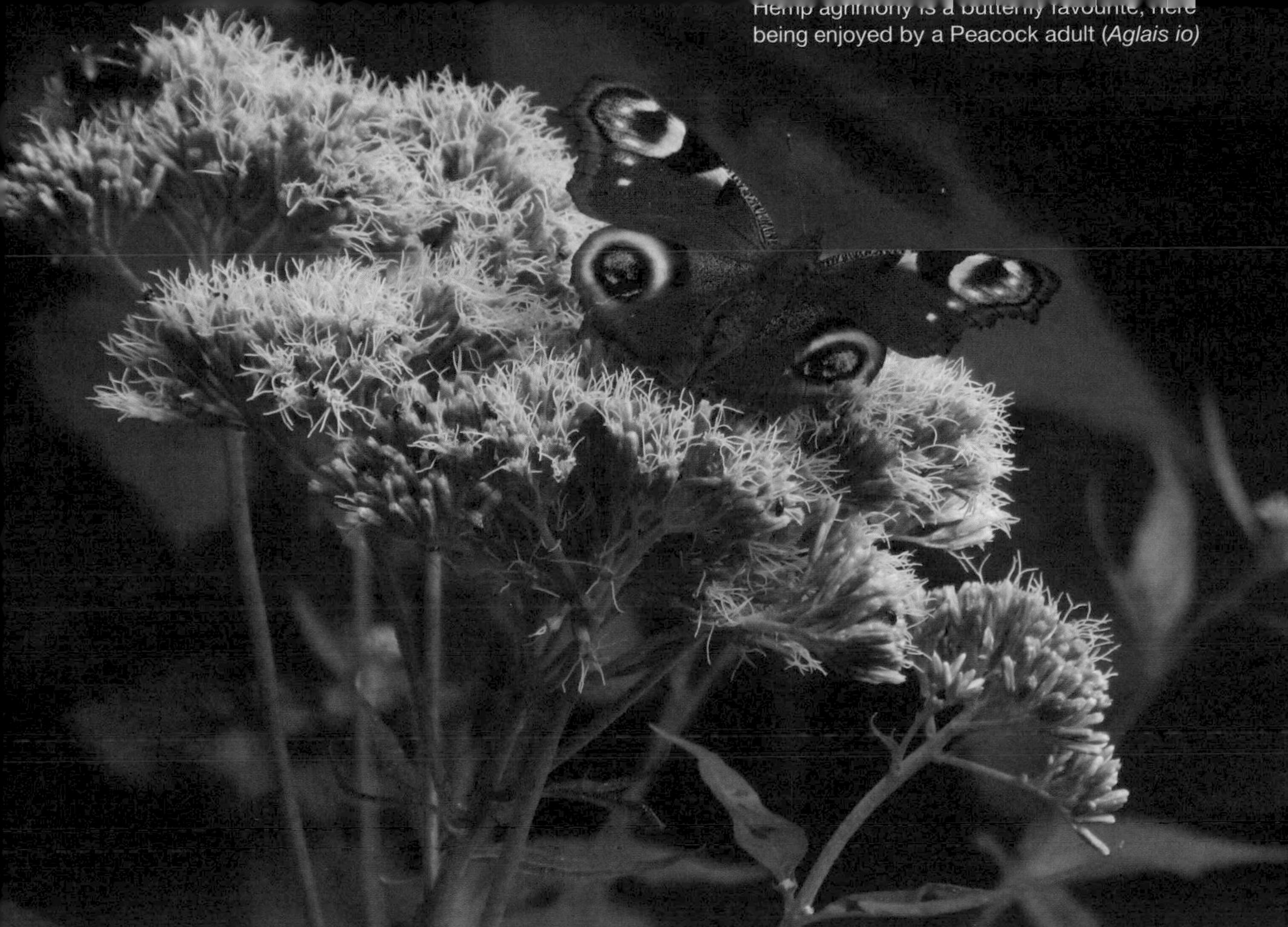

Hemp agrimony is a butterfly favourite, here being enjoyed by a Peacock adult (*Aglais io*)

Hemp agrimony *Eupatorium cannabinum* — Asteraceae

This plant in the Asteraceae family is not used so much today in western herbal medicine, but it is still widely favoured in India and China. It is perhaps the discovery of pyrrolizidine alkaloids in hemp agrimony that has discouraged its use. However, the many different alkaloids in this class vary greatly in their effect, and the chemistry of the whole plant needs to be taken into account. The alkaloids found in hemp agrimony are damaging to the liver in isolation, but on the other hand research has shown a water extract of the herb to have liver-protective properties.

Like its North American relatives, boneset (*Eupatorium perfoliatum*) and gravel root (*E. purpureum)*, hemp agrimony has antiviral properties and is useful for colds, flu and fevers, where it helps detoxify the body and return digestion to normal. Hemp agrimony also has immunomodulating properties, increasing spleen weight, antibody levels and antibacterial activity.

It is a tall, stately plant, and the flowers are adored by butterflies for their rich supplies of nectar. Hemp agrimony and gravel root are often grown in gardens.

The leaves, picked before the plants flower, and the flower heads, are taken as infusions or made into a tincture. The roots are normally decocted gently before use. The bitter infusion has a tonic effect and promotes digestion and appetite, but larger doses are emetic. Take it for biliousness and for constipation.

Externally, hemp agrimony has a good reputation as a wound herb, applied as a poultice or as an ointment made from the leaves and flowers, just as in Parkinson's day. He recommends using the smoke of the dried herb as an insect repellent.

Also, the leaves and flowers can be distilled to obtain an essential oil that is high in monoterpenes and sesquiterpenoids.

Archangell

Theatrum Botanicum

Tribe 5, Chapter 65, pp604–07

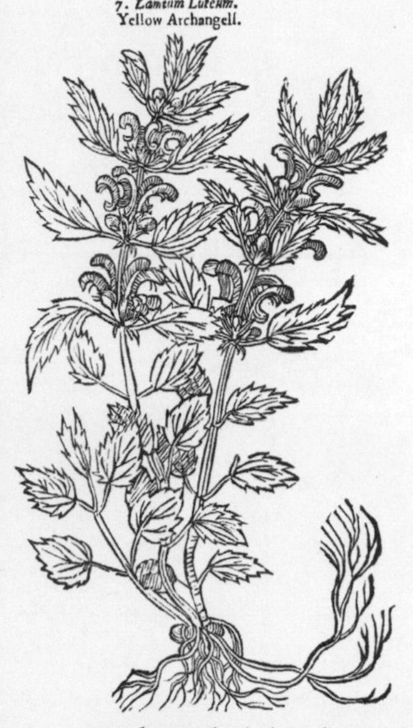

Lamium

The Vertues

The Archangells are somewhat hotter and drier then the stinging Nettles, and are more appropriate, and with better successe used for the obstructions and hardnesse of the spleene then they, to be used inwardly by drinking the decoction of the herbe in wine, and afterwards applying the herbe hot, or the decoction unto the region of the spleene, as a cataplasme or fomentation with spunges.

White deadnettle: The flowers of the white Archangells are preserved or conserved daily to be used, or the distilled water of them is used to stay the whites,

Red deadnettle: and those of the red to stay the reds in women, and is thought good to make the heart merry, to drive away melancholly, and to quicken the spirits.

Fevers: It is commended also against quartaine agues.

Bleeding: It stancheth bleedings also at the mouth or nose; if the herbe be stamped and applyed to the nape of the necke:

Tumours & swellings: the herbe also bruised and with some salt and vinegar, or with *Auxungia* that is, Hogs Lard laid upon any hard tumour or swelling, and that in the neck or throate, which is called the Kings Evill doth helpe to dissolve, or discusse them;

Aches & pains: in the like manner applyed to the Goute, Sciatica or other joynt aches or of the sinewes, doth very much allay the paines, and give ease.

Inflammation, wounds & ulcers: It is also very effectuall for all inflammations, as a repercussive, and to heale all greene wounds, by drying and closing up the lippes of the wounds, and for old Ulcers also to stay their malignitie of fretting, and corroding or spreading, thereby causing them to heale the more speedily:

Splinters: it draweth forth splinters, or other such like things gotten into the flesh.

Yellow archangel: *Pliny* highly commendeth it for many other things, as for bruises and burnings: but the Archangell with yellow flowers is most commended, for old filthy and corrupt sores or corrupt Ulcers, yea although they grow to be fistulous or hollow, and to dissolve tumors.

cataplasme: herbal poultice
fomentation: poultice of warm liquid
spunges: sponges
stay the whites: stop leucorrhoea
stay the reds: stop menses
stamped: crushed
Auxungia: lard or other soft fat
quartaine agues: four-day fevers
Kings Evill: scrofula
discusse: disperse
joynt: joint
repercussive: drives out infection
greene: fresh
malignitie of fretting: seeping
fistulous: hollow, tube-like
Pliny: Pliny the Elder (AD23–79), Roman naturalist

Lamium album leaf

Archangels & deadnettles

Lamiaceae

Lamium spp.

This genus of Old World plants has spread to many other temperate regions, and some are grown in gardens as ornamental ground cover. Deadnettles are still used by herbalists and homeopaths, but are no longer considered major remedies. Perhaps it's time we had another look at them, based on their traditional uses and modern research.

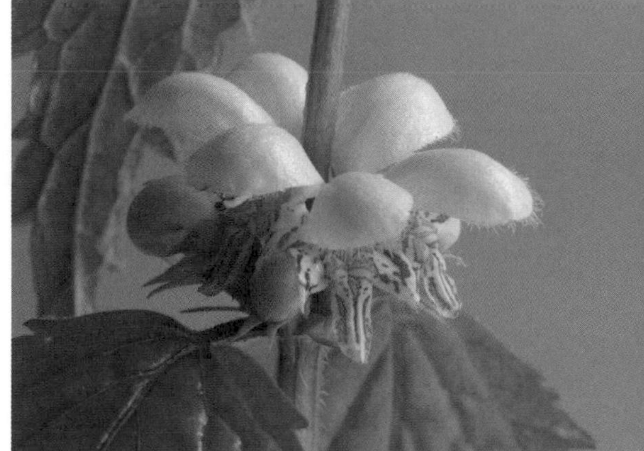

Yellow archangel, *Lamium galeobdolon*, above, Red deadnettle, *L. purpureum*, below

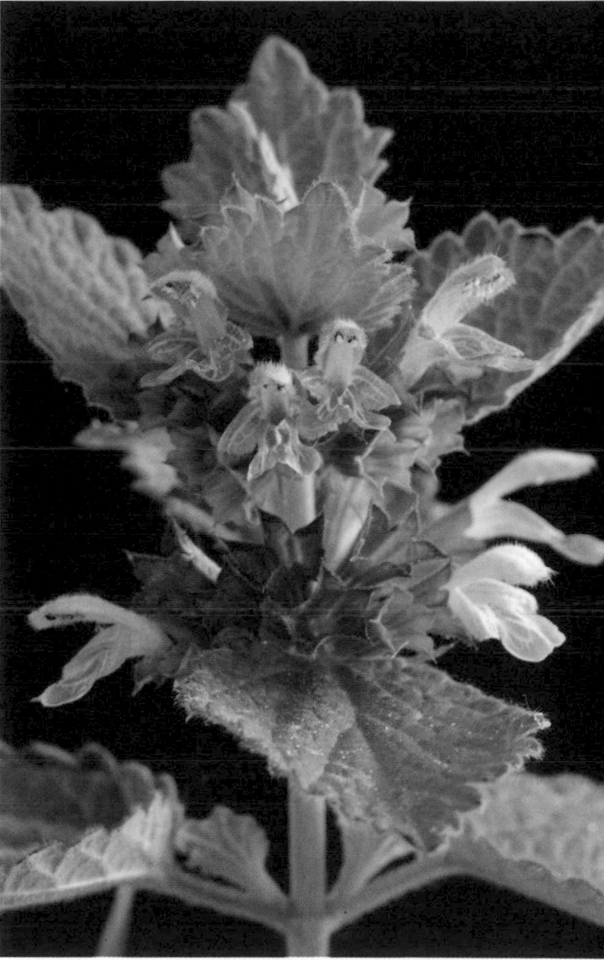

These plants, especially the white deadnettle, look like nettles when they aren't flowering, but they have no sting. The flowers are very beautiful up close, resembling miniature orchids. White and red deadnettles can be found in flower almost all year round, but yellow archangel only flowers in early summer. The other common European species is the henbit deadnettle, which has purple flowers.

White deadnettle is still used by herbalists to treat leucorrhoea or vaginal discharges. It is also useful for heavy menstruation and painful periods. Parkinson's use of the white species to stop the whites, and the red to stop the reds, is one of the few examples in his book where he follows the doctrine of signatures, the colour or form of the flower indicating the use. In practice, the two are interchangeable.

As the deadnettles and archangels are common weeds, they are often available for first-aid use for cuts, splinters and burns. Simply pick a few flowering tops, scrunch them up or chew them, then apply to the affected area. Whether they are as effective for the spleen, tumours and swellings as Parkinson writes deserves further investigation.

All the deadnettles are edible, but we prefer the white to eat as the leaves are succulent and mild-tasting. The flowers and young leaves can be eaten in salads or the leaves cooked like spinach. Children love to suck the sweet nectar from the blossoms. Red deadnettle is slightly aromatic, but the smell tends towards the musty and unpleasant.

Recent research has shown that the seeds of Lamium species contain phytoecdysteroids. These substances are produced by plants to protect themselves from insect attack, but they have interesting beneficial effects in humans. They increase strength and muscle mass, protect the liver and immune systems, lower blood sugar levels and guard cells against oxidative damage. Phytoecdysteroids are found in many adaptogenic herbs. It would be well worth taking a fresh look at deadnettle seeds in herbal practice.

Baulme & Motherwort

Theatrum Botanicum

Tribe 1, Chapter 16, pp40–44

1. *Melissa vulgaris.* The common garden Baulme.

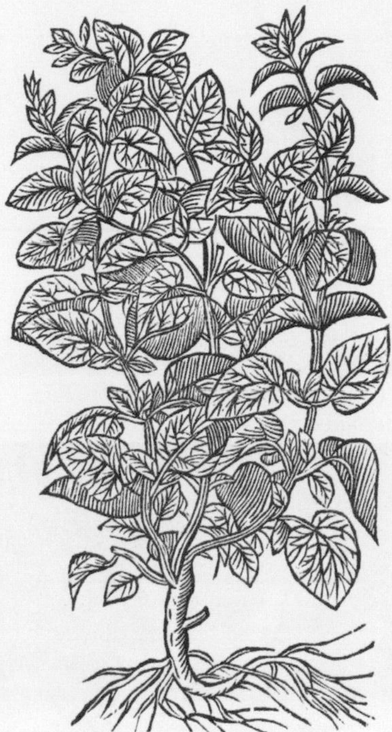

Serapio: probably Serapion the Younger, a 12th century author
swounings: faintings
melancholly: sadness, depression
burnt flegme: hot phlegm
Avicen: Avicenna, Persian physician (980–1037)
Dioscorides: Greek-speaking Roman physician (mid-first century AD)
Phalangium: venomous spider
bloody flixe: dysentery
niter: saltpeter
surfet: surfeit, too many
Mushroms: mushrooms
Lohoc or licking Electuary: linctus or ground herb with honey
wennes: cysts
kernels: hard swellings
foule sores: infected sores
gowt: gout
Galen: Claudius Galen (AD 130–200), Roman physician
Pliny: Pliny the Elder (AD23–79), Roman naturalist

Melissa & Cardiaca

The Vertues

Balm:

Heart & Mind: The Arabian Physicians have extolled the vertues of Baulme, for the passions of the heart in a wonderfull maner, which the Greekes have not remembred: for *Serapio* saith, it is the property of Baulme, to cause the minde and heart to become merry, to revive the fainting heart falling into swounings, to strengthen the weaknesse of the spirits and heart, and to comfort them, especially such who are overtaken in their sleepe, therewith taking away all motion of the pulse, to drive away all troublesome cares and thoughts out of the minde, whether those passions rise from melancholly or black choller, or burnt flegme, which *Avicen* confirmeth in his book of medicines proper for the heart, where he saith that it is hot and dry in the second degree, that it maketh the heart merry, and strengthneth the vitall spirits, both by the sweetnesse of smell, austerity of taste, and tenuity of parts, with which qualities it is helpfull also to the rest of the inward parts and bowels.

It is to good purpose used for a cold stomack to helpe digestion, and to open the obstruction of the braine. It hath a purging quality therein also saith *Avicen*, and that not so weake, but that it is of force to expell those melancholly vapours from the spirits, and from the blood, which are in the heart and arteries, although it cannot doe so in the other parts of the body.

Dioscorides: *Dioscorides* saith that the leaves drunke in wine and laid to, is a remedy against the sting of Scorpions, and the poison of the *Phalangium*, or venemous Spider, as also against the bytings of Dogges, and commendeth the decoction thereof, for women to bathe or sit in to procure their courses, and that it is good to wash the teeth therewith when they are full of paine, and that it is profitable for those that have the bloody flixe.

Leaves: The leaves also with a little *Niter* are taken in drinke against a surfet of *Mushroms*, it helpeth the griping paines of the belly, and is good for them that cannot take their breath, unlesse they hold their necks upright, being taken in a Lohoc or licking Electuary:

With salt: used with salt it taketh away wennes, kernels, or hard swellings in the flesh or throate, it clenseth foule sores, and is an helpe to ease the paines of the gowt.

Galen & Pliny: *Galen* saith in his seventh Booke of Simples, that Baulme is like unto Horehound in qualities, but weaker by much, and therefore few will use Baulme when Horehound is so plentifull, and

Balm & motherwort

Lamiaceae

Parkinson includes motherwort with balm 'for the vertues' sake'. Both lemon balm and motherwort lift the spirits, calm the heart and ease tension. Both are used in the treatment of over-active thyroid, and can be used to aid digestion.

Both plants are easily grown in gardens, and will happily self-seed and spread their virtues.

Balm *Melissa officinalis*

Balm is often called lemon balm because of its strong lemony fragrance. Just smelling it is enough to lift the spirits, and it is delicious as a fresh herbal infusion to be drunk hot or cold. The flavour can also be used in sorbets and other desserts, or to lift the flavour of herbal formulas.

Balm is best used fresh, as the dried leaves lose much of the lemony taste and aroma. If you have it in the garden, keep cutting back the flowering tops so that you have a supply of fresh leaves all summer. In milder areas, it will stay green all winter and can still be harvested in the cold weather.

Heart & mind: Balm is a remedy for mind and heart, just as Parkinson says. It lifts the spirits, reduces anxiety and calms the heart. It is useful for mild depression as well as restlessness and irritability.

Wounds, boils & stings: Traditionally used to treat wounds and boils, balm is also useful for bee and wasp stings and insect bites.

Viral infections: Because balm is antiviral, it can be used against a range of viral infections including flu, chicken pox and shingles. Balm relieves cold sores and reduces the chance of their recurrence if used regularly. Hot balm tea encourages sweating, so it can help control fevers.

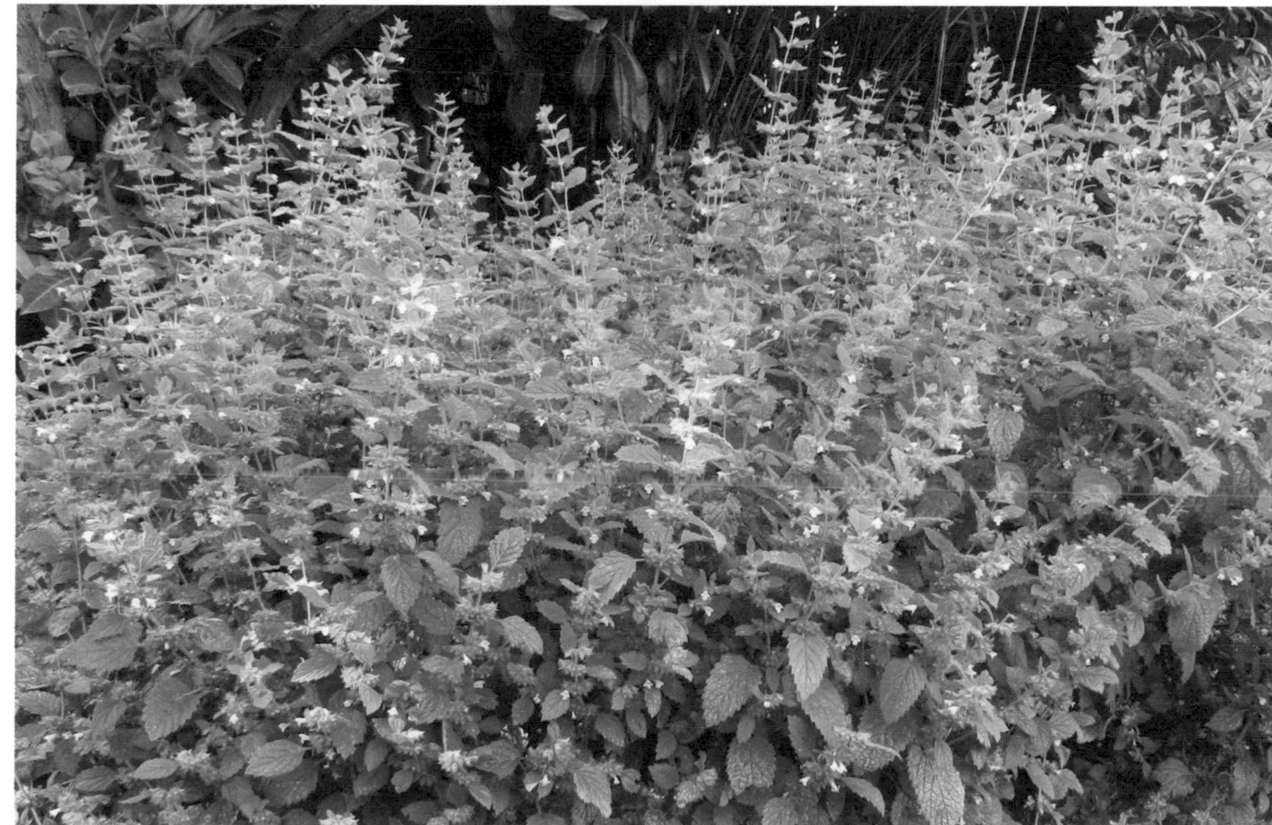

Apium risus: *Sardinian herba*, laughing or Sardinian parsley
Apuleius: Roman writer (AD125–180)
Apiastellum: *Bryonia*, bryony
Apiastrum: *A. angustifolium*, mock parsley
Tansie or Caudle: egg pudding or warm drink
avoided: voided
sore travels: hard labour
comfortable: soothing
Bile: boil
Aqua-vitae: water of life
receit: recipe
morter: mortar
Limbeck: alembic still
Cubebes: cubeb pepper, *Piper cubeba*
Galanga: galangal, *Alpina galanga*
sacke: dry white wine
moneth: month
swounings: faintings
availeable: effective
salve: ointment
greene: fresh

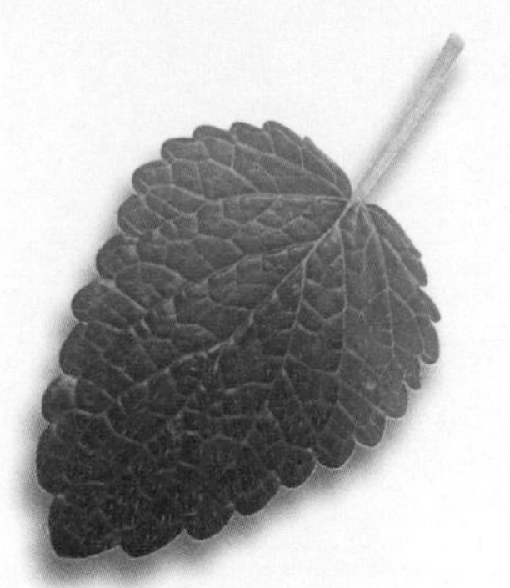

neere at hand to be had every where. *Pliny* saith in *lib*. 20 *cap*. 11. that in *Sardinia* it is poyson, wherein it is very probable that he was much mistaken, and for *Sardonia herba*, which is called of some *Apium risus*, and of *Apuleius Apiastellum*, he tooke this *Apiastrum* or Baulme:

Eyes: the juyce thereof used with a little honey is a singular remedy for the dimnesse of the sight, and to take away the mistinesse of the eyes.

Plague, liver & spleen: It is of especiall use among other things, for the plague or pestilence, and the water thereof is used for the same purposes. It is also good for the liver and spleene.

Birth: A Tansie or Caudle made with egges, and the juyce thereof while it is young, putting some Sugar and Rosewater unto it, is often given to women in child-bed, when the afterbirth is not thoroughly avoided, and for their faintings upon, or after their sore travels.

Aches & boils: It is used in bathings among other warme and comfortable hearbes for mens bodies or legges in the Summer time, to comfort the joynts and sinews, which our former age had in much more use than now-adayes. The hearbe bruised and boyled in a little wine and oyle, and laid warme on a Bile will ripen and breake it.

Aqua-vitae: There is an ordinary *Aqua-vitae* or strong water stilled, and called Baulme water used generally in all the Land, which because it hath nothing but the simple hearbe in it which is too simple, I will commend a better receit unto you.

Recipe: Take two pound of Baulme while it is young and tender, of Mints and Sage, of each one pound, bruise them well in a stone-morter, and put them into a pot or Limbeck, and put thereto of Aniseeds foure ounces; of Cloves, of Nutmegs, of Cinamon, of Ginger, of Cubebes, and of Galanga, of each one ounce, being all a little bruised and put into two gallons of good Sacke if you will have it excellent good, or else into foure gallons of Ale, and so still it as *Aqua-vitae* is distilled, and let it distill as long as you shall finde any strength in the water, yet so that the latter water bee not so weake, to make all the reste white: whereupon put a pound of Sugar, shaking it well before you set it away, and after it hath rested so one moneth, you may use of it as occasion shall require: for it is of especiall use in all passions of the heart, swounings and faintings of the spirits, and for many other purposes, whereunto the hearbe is here declared to be availeable.

Oils & ointments: The hearbe is often put into oyles or salves to heale greene wounds, and it is very probable the name of Baulme, was given to this hearbe, from the knowledge of the healing properties of the true and naturall Baulme.

Bees: It is also an hearbe wherein Bees doe much delight, both to have their Hives rubbed therewith to keep them together, and draw others, and for them to suck and feed upon; and it is a remedy against the stinging of them.

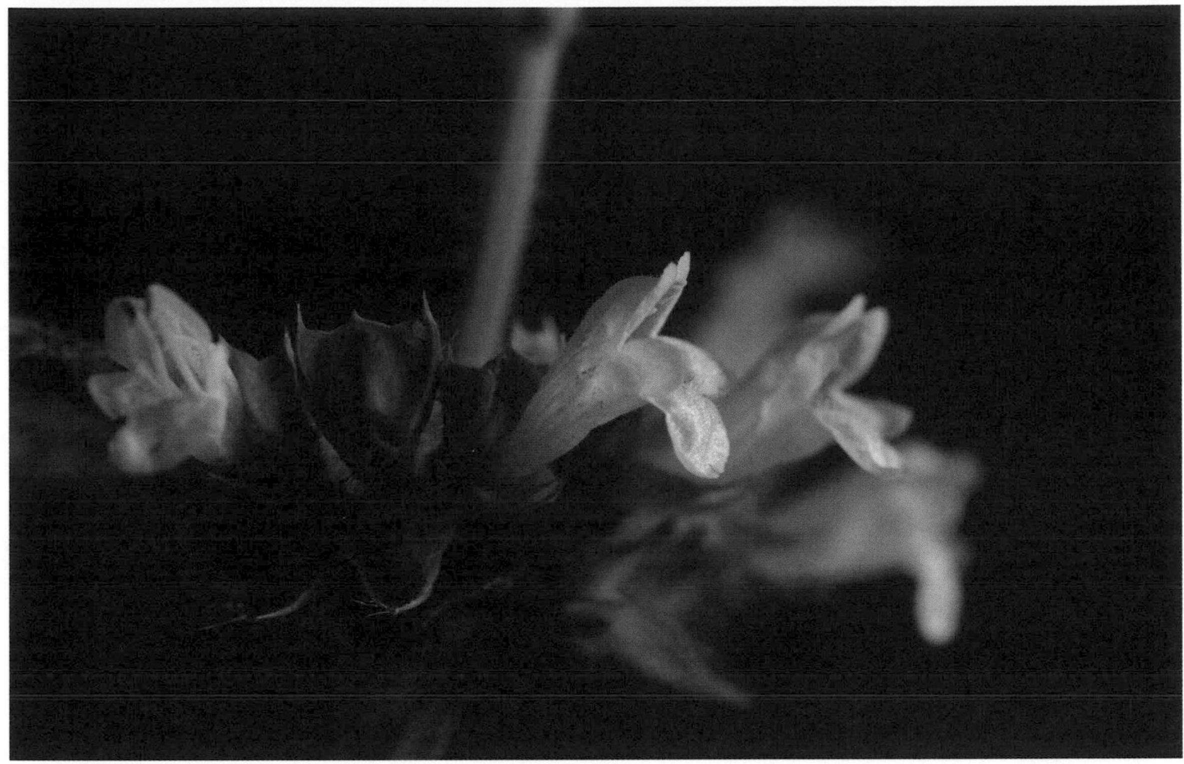

Parkinson's aqua-vitae recipe

We have reduced the quantities in our version of Parkinson's 'better receit' (opposite).

½ pound (225g) of young balm leaves
¼ pound (110g) of mint leaves
¼ pound (110g) of sage leaves
1 ounce (28g) aniseed
¼ ounce (7g) cloves
¼ ounce (7g) nutmegs
¼ ounce (7g) cinnamon
¼ ounce (7g) ginger (powder)
¼ ounce (7g) cubeb pepper or black peppercorns
¼ ounce (7g) galangal
½ imperial gallon (2.25 litres or 0.6 US gallon) of dry white wine or 1 gallon (4.5 litres or 1.2 US gallon) of ale

Distill it gently until the distillate starts to lose flavour and fragrance – there will be little water left.

Add ¼ pound (110g) of sugar, and shake until well mixed. Put the bottle away for a month before using. Drink as an elixir or take before meals as an apéritif.

Thyroid: Balm, like motherwort, is used for treating overactive thyroid. It calms the palpitations and overactivity associated with this condition, and reduces the activity of the thyroid gland. For this reason, people with an under-active thyroid should not use too much balm.

Digestion: Balm's volatile oils, which give it its fragrance, are strongly antispasmodic, so will help with tension anywhere in the digestive tract. The herb also helps with gas and griping pains. The simple distilled aromatic water or a tea of the fresh leaves work well for digestive upsets.

Parkinson's aqua-vitae recipe (left) adds other aromatic herbs and spices to the formula in an alcohol base of wine or ale, for a recipe that is guaranteed to aid the digestion and lift the spirits.

Other uses: Research indicates that balm may help improve cognitive function and decrease agitation in people with Alzheimer's disease. Balm is helpful for children with ADHD. It has also been shown to have antibacterial activity.

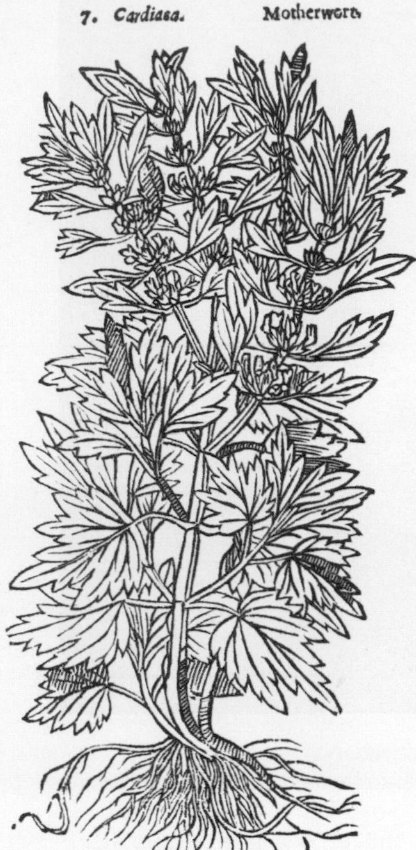

The Turkey Baulme is of as good effect to all the purposes aforesaid, as is the ordinary.

The Assirian Baulme is of excellent vertue to expell any poison or venome, as also against the plague or pestilence used inwardly and outwardly, it killeth the wormes, and helpeth the jaundise, and the paines of the Mother, for it openeth obstructions, warmeth the cold parts, rarifyeth and clenseth.

Motherwort

Heart: Motherwort is held of the later Writers, to bee of much use for the trembling of the heart, and in faintings and swounings, from whence it tooke the name *Cardiaca*:

Women's tonic: the powder thereof to the quantity of a spoonefull drunke in wine, is a wonderfull helpe to women in their sore travels, as also for the suffocations or risings of the Mother, and from these effects it is likely it tooke the name of Motherwort with us.

Other uses: It also provoketh urine and procureth the feminine courses, clenseth the chest of cold flegme oppressing it, and killeth the wormes of the belly.

Warming & relaxing: It is of good use to warme and dry up the cold humours, to digest and disperse them that are settled in the veines, joynts, and sinewes of the body, and to helpe crampes and convulsions, &c.

Turkey balm: Parkinson's *Melissa turcica* is now *Cedronella canariensis*
Assirian Baulme: Parkinson has *Melissa Molucca laevis, sive Syriaca laevis*
the Mother: the uterus
rarefyeth: thins
swounings: faintings
sore travels: difficult labours
provoketh urine: diuretic action
procureth the femine courses: causes menstruation
cold flegme: cold mucus
cold humours: cold bodily fluids
digest: dissolve

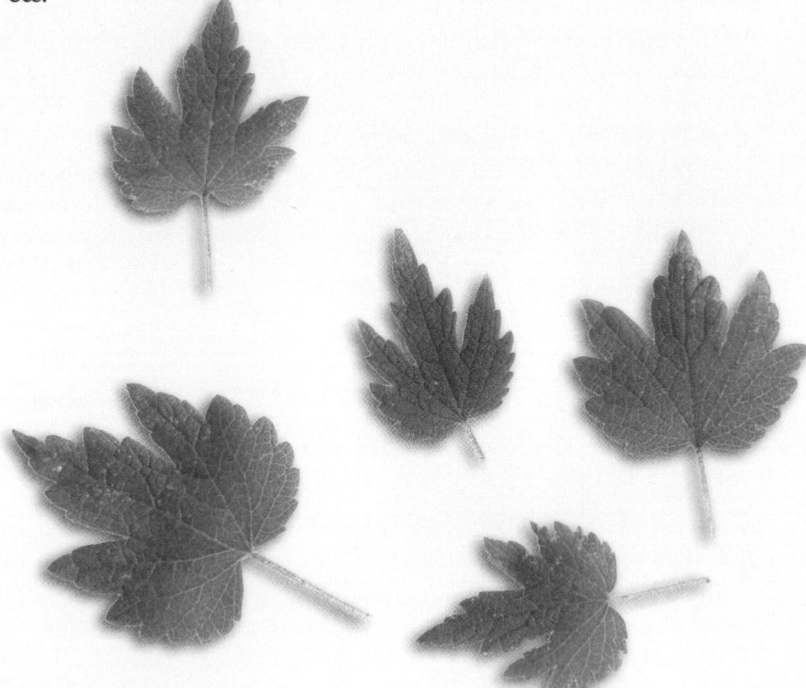

Motherwort *Leonurus cardiaca*

Motherwort is a tall plant, growing to over 6 feet (2 metres) in our garden. As a tea, it is very bitter, so acts as a digestive stimulant. The tincture is less bitter, more full-bodied, aromatic and palatable.

Heart: Motherwort is still used for heart problems, especially in cases of palpitations and rapid heart beat, such as those caused by anxiety or an overactive thyroid. It strengthens a weak heart.

Woman's herb: Motherwort, as the name suggests, is useful for women at all stages of the reproductive cycle. Motherwort tea helps with anxiety and restlessness in pregnancy, while a motherwort powder can help strengthen and promote labour, and help birth the placenta.

The alkaloids responsible are not water-soluble, so a tea would not work in this case, but the powder in wine, just as Parkinson says, would be effective, as would a modern alcohol-based tincture. For the same reason, motherwort tincture or glycerite should not be used during pregnancy as they can stimulate uterine contractions.

Motherwort is also best avoided in cases of heavy menstrual bleeding, but will also promote menstrual bleeding where it is scanty or non-existent. It is very effective for post-partum depression and anxiety.

Motherwort is also useful for the stress and anxiety of the various phases of parenthood, and is useful in treating menopausal symptoms.

In traditional Chinese medicine the Asian variety, *Leonurus japonicus*, is used for menstrual problems and post-partum pain, and is considered a herb that invigorates the blood.

Warming & relaxing: Motherwort is useful for anxiety and tension, for people who just can't relax. It helps relax tense muscles, whether from mental stress and anxiety, or the cold, or spinal problems. It is particularly useful where the tension is lodged in the chest, around the heart. Motherwort relaxes without causing drowsiness, which is a very useful property.

As Parkinson says, motherwort warms and dries up cold humours, making it effective for rheumatism and stiff cold joints and sinews. It promotes the flow of blood, and relaxes tight muscles, relieving attendant pain.

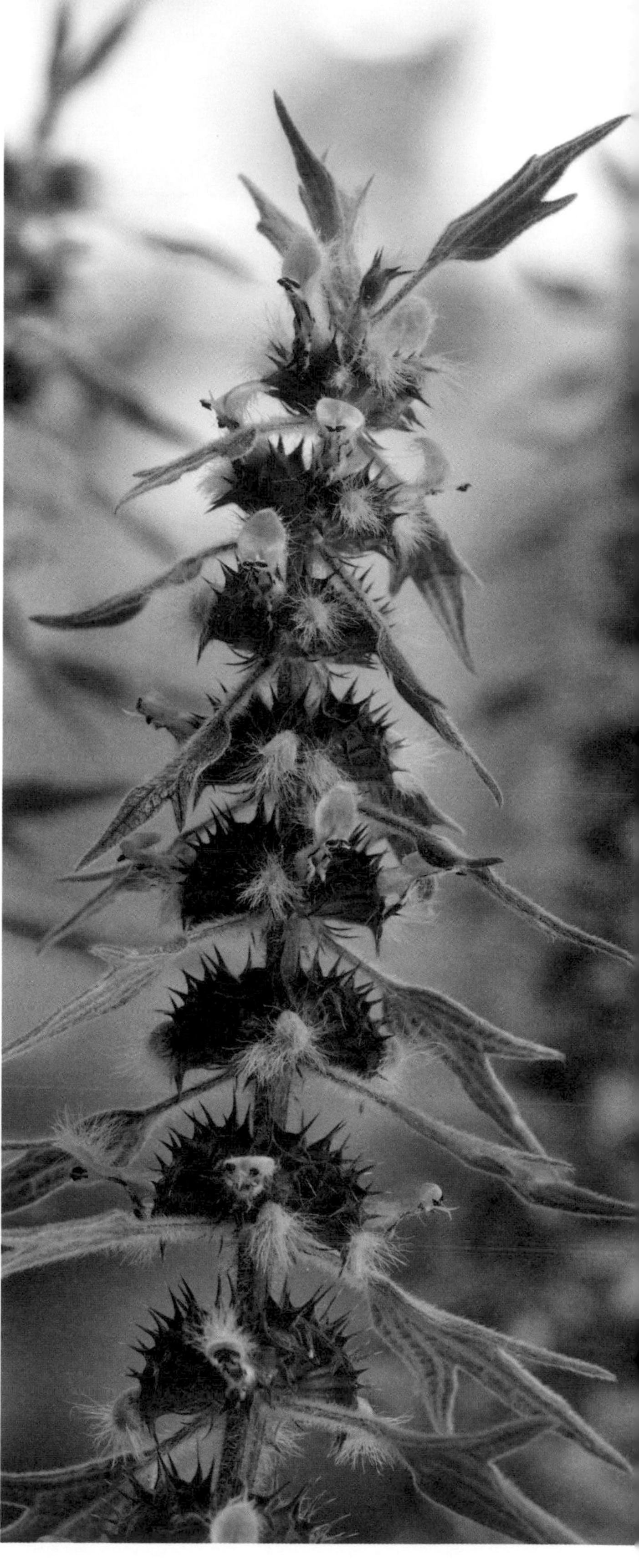

Betonie

Theatrum Botanicum

Tribe 5, Chapter 69, pp614–16

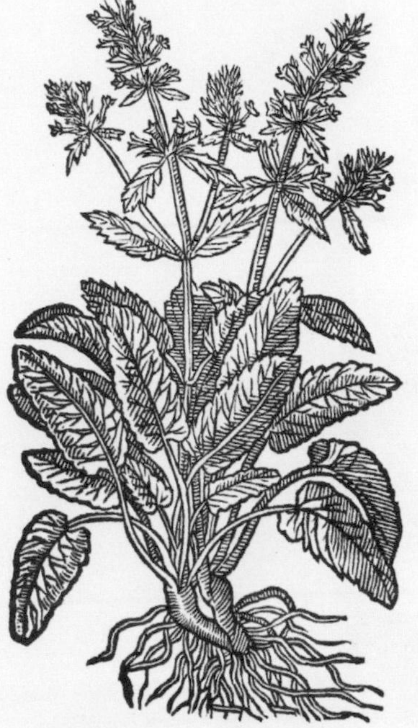
1. *Betonica vulgaris flore purpureo.* Common Wood Betony.

Pliny: Pliny the Elder (AD23–79), Roman naturalist
ante cunctas Laudatissima: most praiseworthy of all
Antonius Musa: physician
Emperour Augustus: Roman emperor (27BC–AD14)
physition: physician
Dioscorides: Greek-speaking Roman physician (mid-first century AD)
Matthiolus: Pierandrea Mattioli (1501–77), physician and author
risings in the stomacke: reflux
in brothe drunke: drunk in broth
falling sicknesse: epilepsy
palsie: paralysis, tremor
dropsies: oedema
Mede: mead
pennyroyall: *Mentha pulegium*
putride agues: foul-smelling fevers
quotidiane, tertian or quartane: one-, three- or four-day fevers
wind Collick: gas pains
purge the belly: empty the belly
the mother: womb

Betonica

The Vertues

Betonie is hot and dry, almost in the second degree: it is saith *Pliny ante cunctas Laudatissima*, and so have others also set it forth, with admirable (and yet not undeserved) praises: *Antonius Musa*, the Emperour *Augustus* his Physition, who wrote a peculiar booke hereof, saith of it, that it preserveth the lives and bodies of men, free from the danger of diseases, and from witchcrafts also;

Digestion: but it is found by dayly experience, as *Dioscorides* formerly wrote thereof, to be good for innumerable diseases, as *Matthiolus* termeth it, for it helpeth those that either loath or cannot digest their meate, those that have weak stomackes, or have sower belchings, or continuall risings in their stomacke, if they use it familiarly, either greene or dry, either the herbe, the roote, or the flowers, in broth drunke, or meate, made into conserve, syrupe, electuary, water, or powder, as every one may best frame themselves unto, or as the time or season requireth, taken any of the foresayd wayes:

Other uses: it helpeth the jaundise, falling sickenesse, the palsie, convulsions or shrinking of the sinewes, the goute, and those that are enclining to dropsies, as also those that have continuall paines in their heads, yea although it turn to frensie:

Electuary: it is no lesse availeable the powder mixed with pure honey, for all sorts, of coughes or colds, wheesing and shortnesse of breath, distillations of thinne rheume upon the lungs, which causeth consumptions, the decoction made with Mede and a little Pennyroyall added thereunto, is good for those that are troubled with putride agues, whether *quotidiane*, *tertian*, or *quartane*, that rise from the stomack: and to draw down and evacuate the blood and humors, that by falling into the eyes, do hinder the sight:

Worms: the decoction thereof made in wine & taken, killeth the wormes in the belly;

Abdominal pain: is good to open the obstructions, both of liver & spleene, & for stitches or other paines in the sides or back, the torments also & griping paines of the bowels, and the wind Collick, and with honey helpeth to purge the belly:

Uterus: the same also helpeth to bring down womens courses, and is of especiall use for those that are troubled, with the falling downe and paines of the mother, and to cause an easie and speedy delivery for those in travaile of childbirth:

Other uses: it helpeth also to breake and expell the stone, either in the Kidnies or bladder; the decoction with wine gargled easeth the

Betony *Stachys officinalis*

Lamiaceae

Betony, or wood betony as it is often known, was one of the most important medicinal herbs in times past. As Parkinson points out, Antonius Musa, the physician to Roman Emperor Augustus, wrote a whole book on the virtues of betony. Does it deserve its old reputation as a panacea? We think that maybe it does.

It is tonic to the whole body, especially to the nervous system and digestion, and promotes the circulation of energy around the body. Betony relaxes tension, relieves headaches, calms the mind and improves memory and concentration.

From Roman times to the Middle Ages and beyond, betony was a vital herb for protection against witchcraft and various evil influences. This translates into modern use in post-traumatic stress disorder and drug addiction, and protection from environmental pollution and electromagnetic sensitivity.

Betony is warming and invigorating, gently increasing physical and mental resilience. By relaxing tension, betony improves circulation. It is a very useful herb to take during exams or whenever we really need to be able to focus and concentrate, and it can help with insomnia and bad dreams.

Head remedy: It is a superb remedy for headaches of all sorts, including migraines, and can also help with head pain resulting from injuries. Betony is perfect for when you are mentally obsessing, with scattered thoughts going round and round. It calms and focuses, and helps us reconnect with our gut instincts. For treating tension, it is combined with motherwort.

Digestion: By working on the solar plexus and improving digestion, betony helps the whole body. It is particularly good for those with weak digestion, or for people who have lost weight from a long illness. As Parkinson says, the flowers, leaves or root can all be used, in all sorts of preparations, but the root is less pleasant to take and is little used today.

Electuary: Mixing the powdered herb with honey as an electuary is still a good remedy for treating coughs and colds.

Abdominal pain: Betony will relieve gas and griping pains and abdominal cramping. It is useful in treating IBS and liver congestion.

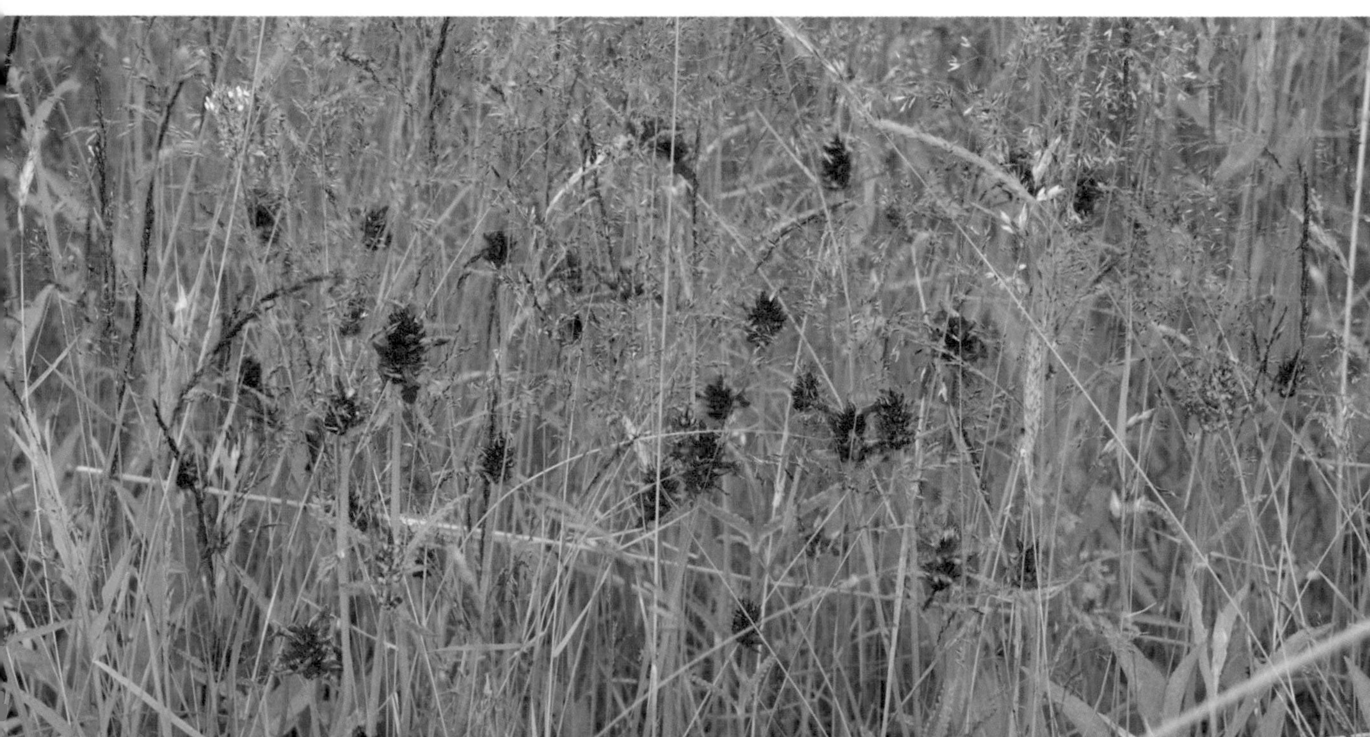

travaile: labour
dramme: ⅛ oz apothecary weight, 3.89 gm or 3 scruples or 60 grains
pisse: urinate
bursten: have a rupture
greene wound: fresh wound
profitable: effective
fistulous: hollow
Hogges Lard: pig fat
biles: boils
pushes: skin eruptions
loathing: rejection of food
meate: food

toothach: it is commended against the sting or biting of venemous Serpents, and mad dogs, both used inwardly, and applyed outwardly also to the hurt place: it is sayd also to hinder drunkenesse, being taken before hand, and quickely to expell it afterwards:

Weariness: a dramme of the powder of Betonie taken with a little honey, in some Vinegar, doth wonderfully refresh those that are overwearied by travaile:

Bleeding: it stayeth bleedings at the mouth or nose, as also those that spit or pisse blood: it helpeth those that are bursten and have a rupture, and is good for those that are bruised by any fall or otherwise: the greene herbe bruised, or the juyce applyed, to any inward hurt, or outward greene wound, in the head or body, will quickely heale it and close it up, as also any veines or sinewes that are cut, and will also draw forth any broken bone, or any splinter, thorne, or such other thing, gotten into the flesh:

Sores: it is no lesse profitable for old filthy sores, and ulcers, yea though they be fistulous and hollow; but some doe advise to put a little salt thereto for this purpose: being applyed with a little Hogges Lard, it helpeth a Plague sore and other biles, and pushes: the fumes of the decoction while it is warme, received by a funnell into the eares, easeth the paines of them, destroyeth the wormes, and cureth the running sores in them; the juyce dropped into them, doth the same likewise:

Root: the roote of Betony is found to be of much differing quality from the leaves and flowers, as being much displeasing both to the taste and stomacke, procuring loathing, vomitings, and belchings; whereas the leaves and flowers, by their sweete and spicie taste, are comfortable both in meate and medicine.

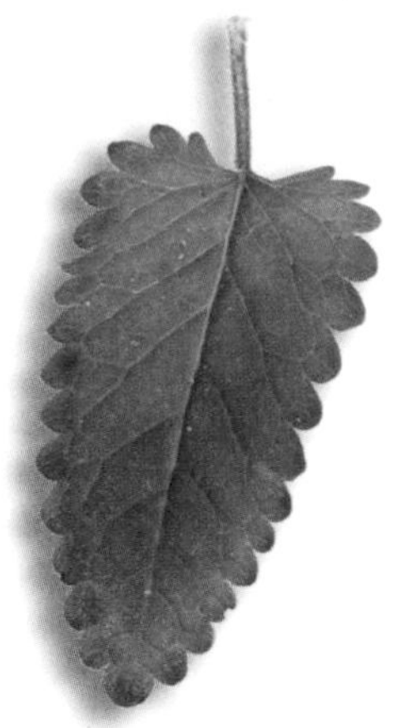

Emmenagogue effects: Betony increases circulation to the pelvic area, encouraging menstruation. It has relaxing and astringent effects, which help with cramps and prolapse. It stimulates the uterus to facilitate childbirth, but should not be taken earlier in pregnancy.

Weariness: Parkinson suggests an oxymel, mixing betony powder with honey and vinegar, for exhaustion. Today we might also consider a tea or a tincture, as betony is still valued for its restorative properties. Being a tonic, its benefits are best experienced by taking it regularly.

Bleeding & sores: Fresh or dried betony can be used to stop bleeding, and to help wounds heal. Luckily plague sores are a thing of the past, but is useful to remember betony for boils and ulcers, as well as for drawing out splinters.

Note: Betony is no longer used for snake bites and the bites of mad dogs, something the classical writers seemed to encounter frequently.

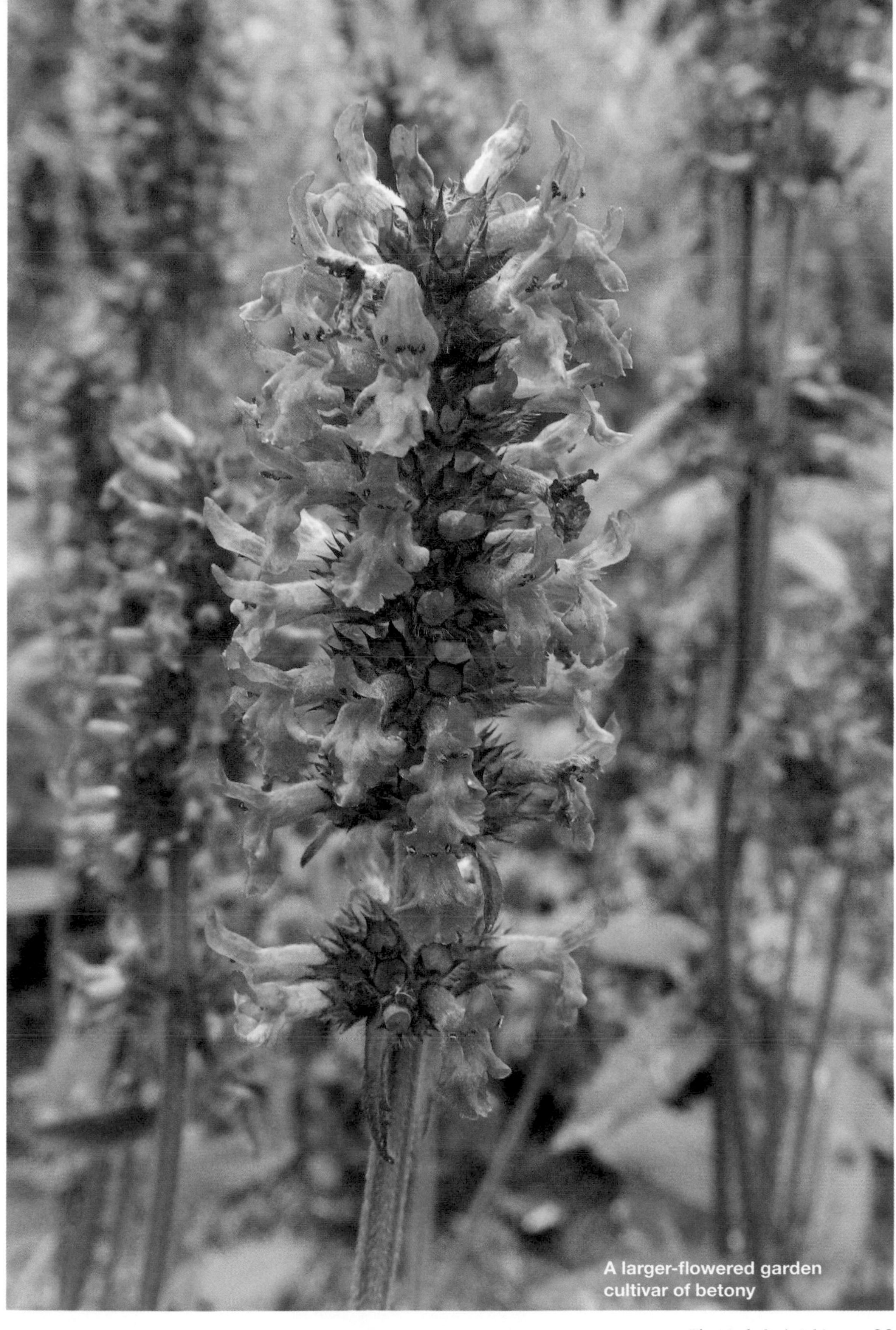
A larger-flowered garden cultivar of betony

Blacke Thorne

Theatrum Botanicum

Tribe 9, Chapter 32, pp1033–34

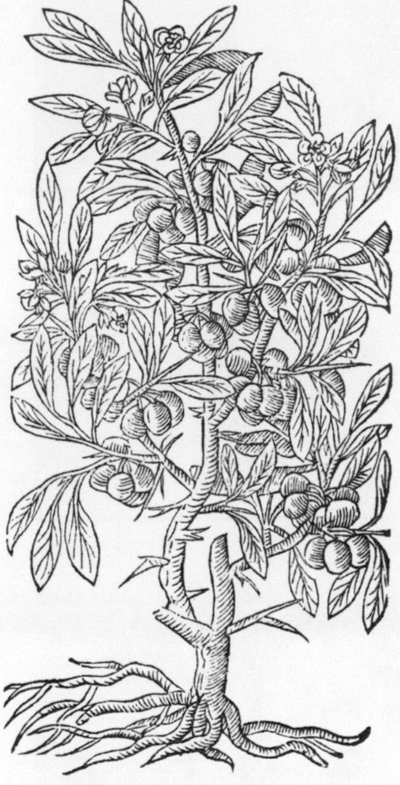

Prunus sylvestris

The Vertues

All the parts of the Sloe bush are binding, cooling and drying, and all are effectuall to stay bleedings at the nose or mouth or any other place, the Laske of the belly or stomack or the Bloody flux, the abundance of womens courses, and helpeth to ease the paine in the sides, bowells and guts, that come by overmuch scowring, to drinke the decoction of the barke of the roote, or more usually the decoction of the berries eyther fresh or dryed.

Conserve: The Conserve likewise is of very great use and most familiarly taken for the purposes aforesaid:

Distilled in alcohol: but the distilled water of the flowers first steeped in Sacke for a night, and drawne therefrom by the heate of a *Balneum*, is a most certain remedy tryed and approoved, to ease all manner of gnawings in the stomacke, the sides heart or bowells, or any other griping paines in any of them, to drinke a small quantitie when the extremities of paine are upon them:

Leaves: the leaves also are good to make lotions, to gargle and wash the mouth and throate, wherein is swellings, sores or kernells, and to stay the defluxions of rheume to the eyes or other parts, as also to coole the heate and inflammations in them, and to ease the hot paines of the head, to bathe the forehead and temples therewith.

Distilled water & condensed juice of sloes: The simple destilled water of the flowers is very effectuall also for the said purposes, and so is the condensate or thickned juice of the Sloes: the distilled water of the greene berries before they be ripe is used also for the said effects of cooling binding and staying the flux of blood and humours, and some other purposes *que studio praetereo.*

Substitutions: The juice of the fruit of Sloes is taken as a substitute for the juice of *Acacia* in all our Apothecarie shoppes, which substitution although it bee not much to be misliked, as having one and but one qualitie of the *Acacia* in it which is the binding, yet is it deeper in the degree of cooling: but divers learned men in sundry places, and namely the Physitians of *Padoa* and *Naples*, have accunted the condensate juyce of Sumach or of Mirtles, to be a better substitute answering to the qualities of the *Acacia*, in more than the juyce of Sloes doth:

for substitutes had neede of much consideration and judgement, not onely to be alike in the first qualities, that is a roote for a roote, a seede for a seede, a juyce or gum, for a juyce or gum, &c. and not a juyce or gumme in steede of a roote or seede, or contrariwise: but in the second qualities also of a substitute, that is in heate and cold, that contraries

stay: stop
laske: diarrhoea
bloody flux: dysentery
courses: menstruation
scowring: cleansing
Conserve: preserve or jam
Sacke: white dry wine
Balneum: a hot water bath, bain Marie
extremities: extremes
kernells: hard swellings
defluxions of rheume: flow of watery mucus
destilled: distilled
que studio praetereo: which we shall pass over
Acacia: wattle or thorntree
physitians: physicians
accunted: accounted

Blackthorn *Prunus spinosa*

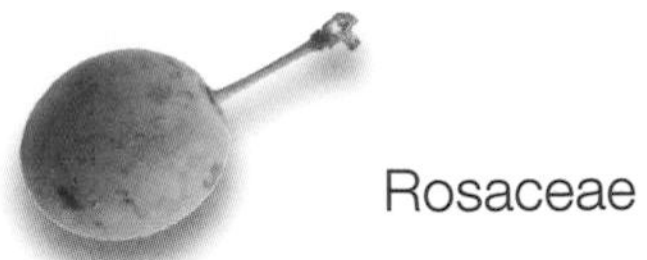

Rosaceae

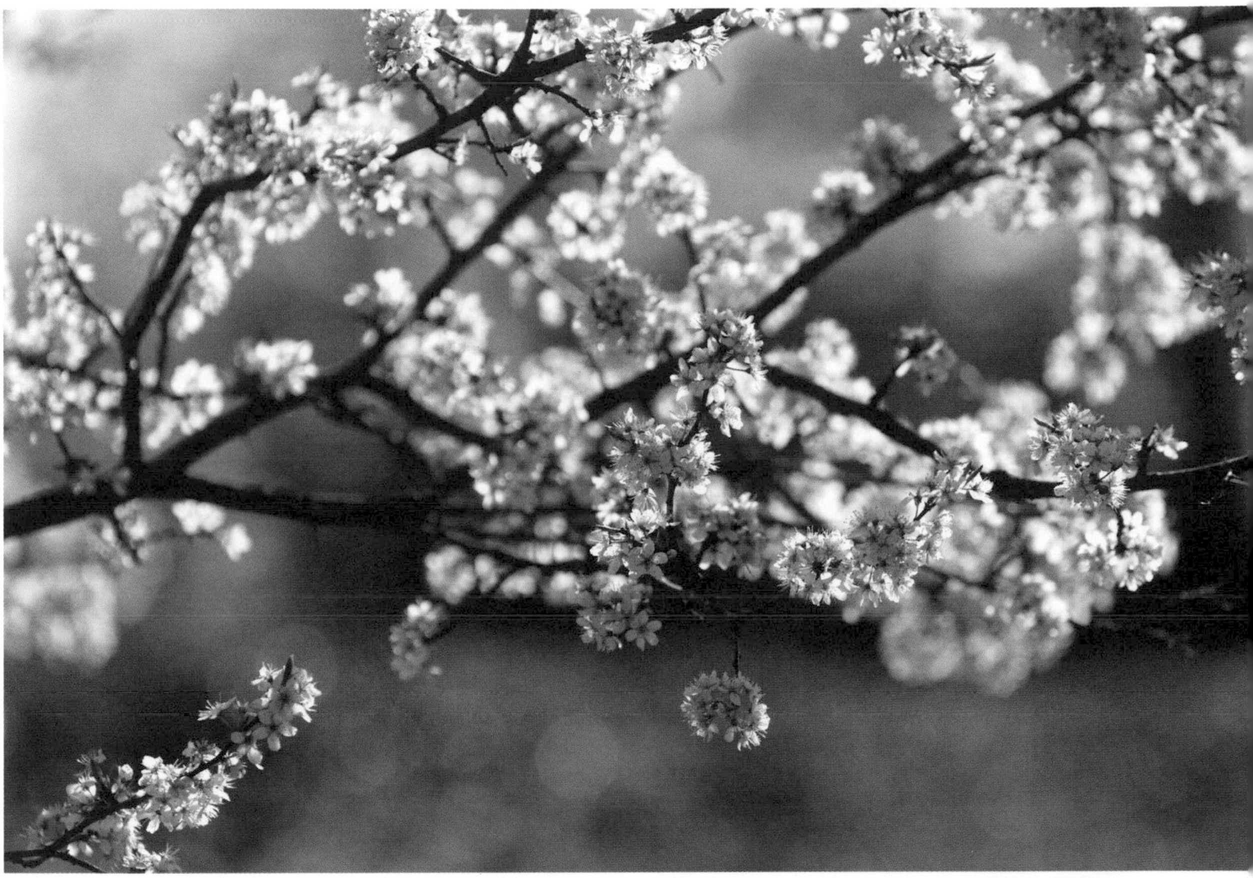

One of the earliest flowers of spring and the latest fruits of fall, blackthorn is ancient (archaeologists have found dried sloe berries in human sites dating back 10,000 years) and complex. It is a pioneer bush/tree that is native to most of Europe and the Middle East to Iran, and has been introduced into North America, where it is known in some northern states on the east and west coasts.

The delicate, musky, white flowers contrast sharply with the plant's fearsome, black protective spines and a blue-black fruit that transforms from the sourest of plums in summer into an almost palatable fruit after the first frost of winter.

Astringency: The astringency of sloes is legendary. The effect, the early 19th century journalist William Cobbett once wrote, is to stick the tongue to the roof of your mouth. Cobbett's contemporary, John Hill, noted in his *Family Herbal* (1812 edn, p314) that it was 'a little plum of a very austere taste when unripe, but pleasant when mellow'.

But it also does wonderful things medicinally, as Parkinson states. In France it has been called 'the regulator of the stomach', whose flowers loosen the bowels while its fruits bind them, a dual action that exemplifies blackthorn's complex chemistry, mythic history and potential therapeutic value.

Parkinson notes that all parts of the bush share astringency, cooling and drying qualities, with the bark or root being even stronger; his decoction of either would be hard to swallow without some sweetening. The effects, now and in Parkinson's time, include stopping bleeding, settling the stomach, reducing diarrhoea and dysentery, and easing all manner of internal pain.

Conserve: The conserve or jam, he says, works similarly and would be easier to take.

Sumach: sumac, shrub of Rhus family
Mirtles: myrtle, evergreen shrub
Galen: Claudius Galen (AD130–200), Roman physician and author
cassia: *Cinnamonum cassia*
Cinamon: cinnamon, *Cinnamonum*
Quintus: Roman anatomist, one of whose pupils taught Galen
cast into his dish: be sick over food
antidotes: i.e. to poisons
Michradatium: Mithridatium: named for Emperor Mithridates VI
Theriaco Andromachi: lit. treacle of Andromachus, Nero's physician
Canella alba: white cinnamon tree
Cortex Winterani: a South American tree
Costus: tropical plant family, the 'spiral gingers'
Simple: herb used alone in medicine
scant: scarce
aromaticall rosine: aromatic resin
rules of Art: skill of the apothecary
drugges: vegetable medicinals
hola: hello, oh dear!

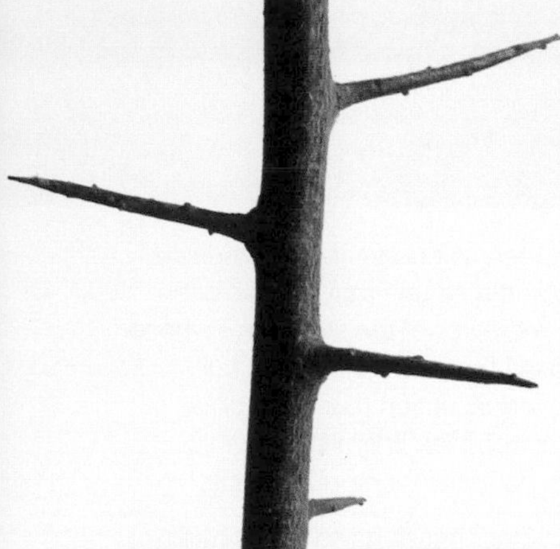

be not admitted, either of cold for hot, or hot for cold; yea and in the third quality likewise, that they may answere as neere as may be possible, the same degrees that they neither want nor abound in any degree.

And although *Galen* did appoint the double quantity of *Cassia* in the stead of *Cinamon* which made *Quintus* to cast into his dish, that by the same rule he might take double the quantity of course bread, in the stead of so much fine, as was appointed to make a medicine; yet *Galens* answere to him standeth good, that the respect of substitutes, standeth not in taking twice so much, of that which is worse in stead of that which is good, but as in the actions of men, when the strength of one man is not sufficient to beare, lift, or move, a stone or engine, we put two or more to doe it:

but there are other substitutes admitted among our Apothecaries, into these two great Antidotes of *Michradatium* and *Theriaca Andromachi*, which are no way to be allowed or tollerated, nor ever would be in any of the famous Citties of *Italy*, which is to suffer the *Canella alba* (falsly called *Cortex Winterani*) which is the barke of a tree, to be the substitute for *Costus* which is a roote, in one mans dispensation when as the like was never seene before, and to deny a genuine and right Simple, to be put into another mans composition, because the thing was scant, and not for every one easily to obtaine, nor the price low, that every man might have cheape, and therefore in steade of an aromaticall rosine, use an unctuous or fat Oyle, quite contrary to the rules of Art, the rule of substitutes, and the course of other famous and worthy professours in other Countries, who by sparing no cost to obtaine such genuine drugges as are rare, scarcely to be had, and yet of especialle use, have made themselves and their compositions famous through the whole world:

whereas others by being too greedy of gaine, and too envious of any others better proceedings than their owne, have used, and still doe, farre meaner things than they should: but *hola*, what hath just anger against the errours in my profession drawne me to utter? it is rather in hope that all will amend being forewarned, than to touch any in particular, that it will hereby take himselfe to be taxed, for thereby he shall shew himself guilty of the crime, although none doe accuse him.

A thorn in the flesh

Parkinson does not mention blackthorn spines here as a specific problem. These were the longest, cruellest and most painful of thorns, common in fields and gardens, with the reputation of puncturing leather shoes or jerkins and causing wounds that never heal. Some now say the thorn tip breaks off deep inside the skin and carries algal or fungal contamination. Crippling sinovitis and granuloma from infected blackthorn spines, often with fever, can be the result.

The folklore of blackthorn wounds was so prevalent by Parkinson's time that it is thought the translators of the King James Bible (1611) had blackthorn in mind when they wrote of the 'thorn in the flesh', which was the 'messenger of Satan' (II Cor. 12.7).

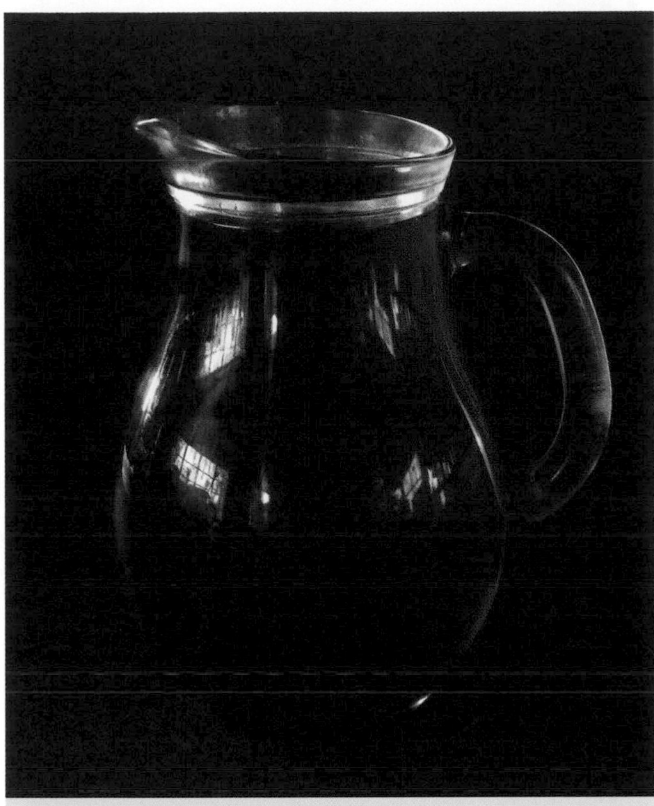

A quick recipe for sloe syrup

There are numerous sloe gin formulas, but this is our simple take on sloe syrup (above). We gathered a bag of sloes in autumn and put them in the freezer for some weeks. Then we transferred them into a large jar and covered them with vegetable glycerine. We stoppered the jar and put it on a sunny windowsill for about two months.

It appeared after this time that the sloes had given their strength to the glycerine, which had become a warm red, and we drained off the depleted berries, put the extract into a fresh clean bottle, stoppered and labelled it. It is ready for use but tastes more mellow if left even longer.

The usual advice to leave sloes on the tree as long as possible can be thwarted in practice: our most recent English winter saw the sloes more or less eaten by birds and squirrels (or picked by human sloe gin makers) by November.

The way around this is to pick the sloes when they reach full size in autumn and then freeze them in your domestic fridge, using them at your leisure. They may not be as flavoursome but you will have something to work with rather than nothing at all.

Distilled flowers in alcohol: This alternative method receives Parkinson's strong endorsement as 'a most certain remedy tryed and approved'. His graphic phrase, 'to ease all manner of gnawings in the stomacke', can be borne out by Julie. She was recovering slowly from appendicitis, and a German friend gave her a recipe for a thrice-decocted sloe syrup to settle the whole abdominal region, which it did within a few days.

Blackthorn, a giver of pain through its thorns, contrary-wise, is here a soother of pain within.

Leaves: Skin lotions, gargles, mouthwashes and eyebaths made from a decoction of the leaves (or flowers, we can add) and used externally can cool and ease the pain of various swellings or inflammations and running mucus of the head and upper body.

The tea is drunk to relieve constipation, bladder and kidney disorders, and is favoured as a remedy for children with diarrhoea.

Distilled water & condensed juice of sloes: Parkinson confirms that the distilled or aromatic water of the flowers, with its almond taste, and the condensed juice of the berries, work in the same manner.

Substitutions: Parkinson mentions the substitution of blackthorn juice for the more expensive imported acacia in the apothecary shops of his time, and this practice angers him sufficiently to launch a tirade about the principle of substitution in general.

This leads him to the already ancient problem of counterfeitng cassia for cinnamon, noted by Galen 1,400 years before, and the contemporary vexed matter of the Antidotes of Mithridatium and Theriaca Andromachi. These were complex mixtures of herbs and spices, long regarded as panaceas for most conditions, including plague. Hence they were contested territory for ownership, as between Venice (whence 'Venice treacle', or theriaca was imported) and London (where many attempts were made to produce a 'London treacle'), and apothecaries and grocers.

Parkinson had battled with this issue in 1618 when helping revise the *London Pharmacopoeia*, and was still upset in 1640.

Bugle

Theatrum Botanicum

Tribe 5, Chapter 25, pp524–26

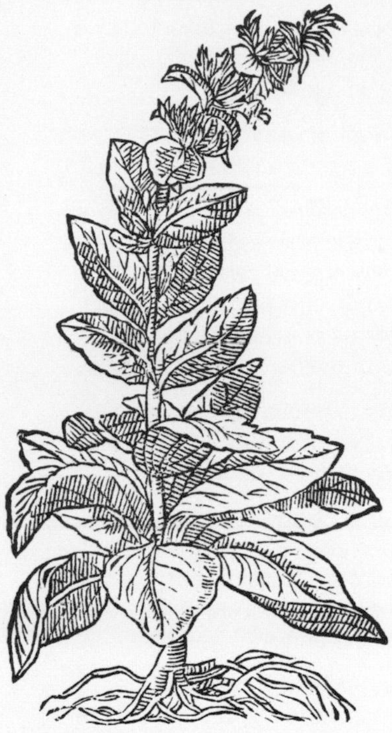

Liver growne: congestion and swelling of the liver
fistulaes: deep narrow ulcers or sores
Hony of roses: rose petals steeped in honey
allome: alum, a double sulphate salt often containing aluminium
Scabious: *Scabiosa* sp.
Sanicle: *Sanicula europea*
Axungia: a soft animal fat, often goose fat
Physition: physician
Chirurgion: surgeon

Bugula vulgaris

The Vertues

Bugle is temperate in heate, but drying moderately, and is somewhat astringent.

Bruises: It is of excellent use for those that have caught any fall, or are inwardly bruised, for it dissolveth the congealed blood, and disperseth it by taking the decoction of the leaves and flowers made in wine;

Wounds: the same is no lesse effectuall for any inward, wounds, thrusts or stabbes into the body or bowels, and is an especall helpe in all wound drinkes,

Liver: as also for those that are Liver growne as they call it, whose inward griefes and paines arise from the obstructions of the Liver, and gall, and strengthening the parts afterwards;

Ulcers & sores: it is wonderfull in curing all manner of ulcers and sores, whether they be new and fresh, or old and inveterate, yea gangrenes and fistulaes also, either the leaves bruised and applyed, or their juice used to wash and bathe the places; and the same made into a lotion with some hony of roses and allome cureth all sores of the mouth or gums, be they never so foule or of long continuance, it worketh no lesse powerfully and effectually, for such ulcers and sores as happen in the secret parts of men or women;

Broken bones & dislocations: it helpeth those also that have broken any bone of their body, or have any dislocation of a joynt, both used inwardly, and applyed outwardly;

A singular good ointment: an ointment made with the leaves of Bugle, Scabious, and Sanicle, bruised and boyled in *Axungia* untill the herbes be dry, and then strained forth and kept in a pot, for such occasions as shall require it, is found so singular good for all sorts of hurts in the body, or any part thereof, that I would not wish any good Gentlewoman in the land, that would do good either to her owne family, or other her poore neighbors, that want helpe and means to procure it, to be without this ointment alwayes at hand by them, it hath done and would doe so much good, for beyond the Sea in *France* and *Germany*, it is a common proverbe amongst them, that they neede neither Physition to cure their inward diseases, nor Chirurgion to helpe them of any wound or sore that have this Bugle (or the *Prunella* Selfeheale, for with them they are accounted but one herbe, as I said before) and Sanicle at hand by them to use.

Bugle *Ajuga reptans* Lamiaceae

Bugle is a perennial wild member of the mint family, growing in colonies to about 10 inches (25 cm) high in damp wooded areas, and is a favourite garden ornamental. It is a lost herb in the sense that it is little used these days, and there is not much modern information about it. Its old reputation was so strong, however, that it warrants a new appraisal of its virtues. The use of bugle for aligning bones, ligaments and tendons is particularly interesting – appropriate research may well show bugle to be as useful as North American boneset, *Eupatorium perfoliatum*.

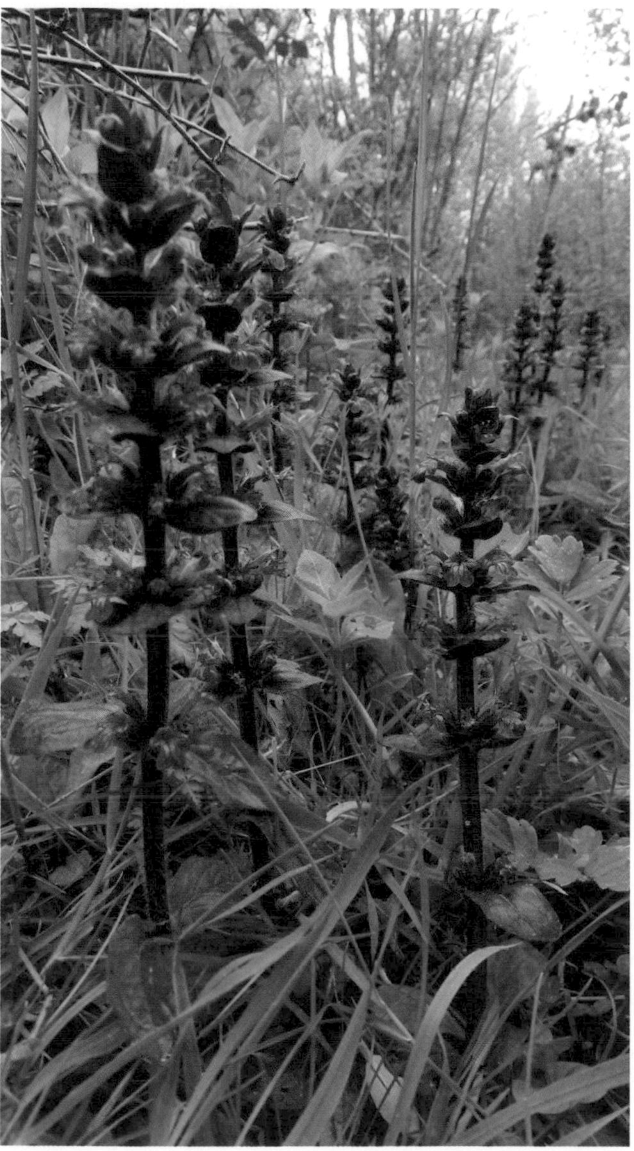

For bruising: For Parkinson's recipe, take a handful of flowering bugle, chop it coarsely and simmer gently in enough wine to cover. When the leaves and flowers start to lose their colour – after about 10 or 15 minutes – strain the liquid out and drink it while warm. The dosage would be a small wineglassful twice daily as needed.

For wounds: The moist plant matter that has been strained out could be applied as a poultice over wounds or bruises. A fresh poultice of crushed bugle is also effective. Parkinson suggests that wound drinks were a popular treatment in his day – try mixing bugle with selfheal, yarrow or St John's wort as tea used for wounds. The cold tea can also be applied as a wound wash.

For liver & gallbladder congestion: Drink 50 ml of the decocted wine twice daily. Apply a poultice of the crushed fresh leaves over the liver, covering with a cloth and keeping it warm with a hot water bottle. Leave in place for half an hour, or overnight if possible.

For ulcers & sores: Apply the bruised leaves or the juice of the plant directly to the ulcer or sore. Hold in place with a gauze dressing.

For dislocations & broken bones: For modern use, we made a tincture of bugle by filling a jar with the chopped leaves and flowers, and pouring in enough vodka or grain alcohol to cover. Leave in a cool dark place for a month, then strain and bottle.

To use, soak a cotton wool ball or a gauze pad in the tincture and apply over the problem area. Keep in place for half an hour, or longer if possible. Or, use a poultice of the leaves and drink the wine decoction above.

A mixed ointment: Take roughly equal amounts of bugle, sanicle and scabious, and chop or crush in a mortar and pestle. Put in a saucepan with melted ghee, coconut oil or goosefat and cook gently until the herbs are dry and crispy. Strain, and pour the fat into a clean jar.

Use for all sorts of sores, pain and minor wounds.

Burre Docke

Theatrum Botanicum

Tribe 14, Chapter 9, pp1222-23

4. *Xanthium ſive Bardana minor.*
The leſſer Burre.

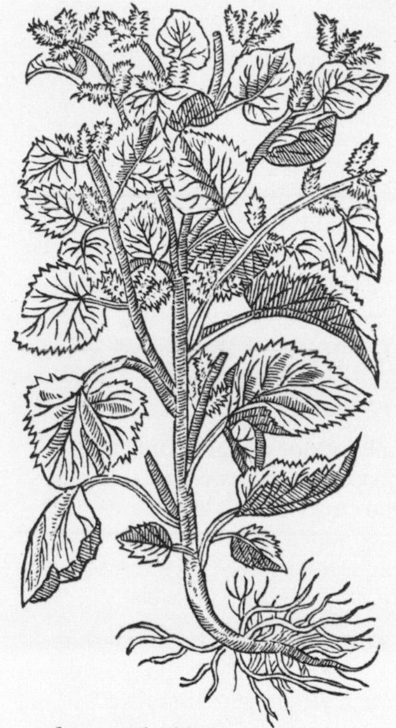

Lappa sive Bardana

The Vertues

Leaves: The Burre leaves are cooling, and drying moderately, and discusseth withall as *Galen* saith, whereby it is good to heale old Ulcers and sores:

Roots: a dramme of the rootes taken with Pine kernels, doth helpe them that spit foule mattery and bloody flegme:

Leaves: The leaves applyed on the places troubled with the shrinking of the sinewes or arteries give much ease:

the juyce of the leaves, or the rootes rather themselves, given to drinke with old wine doth wonderfully helpe the bitings of any serpents, as also of a mad dogge, and if the roote be beaten with a little salt and laid on the place, it will suddenly ease the patient of the paine:

Urinary problems: the juyce of the leaves taken with hony provoketh urine, and remedieth the paines of the bladder:

Seed: the seede being drunke with wine, forty dayes together doth wonderfully helpe the Sciatica:

Burns: the leaves being bruised with the white of an egge, and laid on any place burnt with fire, doth take out the fire, giveth suddaine ease, and healeth it up afterwards,

Leaf decoction: the decoction of them fomented on any fretting sore or cancker, stayeth the torroding quality, which after must be annointed with an ointment made with the said liquor *Axungia*, niter and vinegar boiled together.

Roots & seeds: The rootes may be preserved with Sugar and taken fasting, or at other times for the said purposes, and for Consumptions, as also for those that are troubled by the stone or laske: the seede is much commended to breake the stone, and cause it to be expelled by Urine, and is often used with other seedes and things for that purpose:

Lesser burdock: The lesser burre seedes as *Galen* saith have a digesting quality in them, and are hot and dry, and thereby good to asswage tumours, the seede or the roote bruised and often imposed on kernels or hard knots in the flesh doth dissolve them:

Decoction: the decoction also of the rootes made with wine, helpeth to consume the hardnesse of the spleene, being fomented warme on the place:

Hair: the burres being gathered before they be ripe, bruised and laid to steepe in warme water or wine, and the haires moistened therewith, after they have been rubbed with a little niter doth make them yellow.

discusseth: dilutes
dramme: ⅛ oz apothecary weight, 3.89 gm or 3 scruples or 60 grains
Galen: Claudius Galen (AD130–200), Roman physician and author
provoketh urine: diuretic effect
suddaine ease: fast relief
fomented: applied hot and wet
fretting: eroded
canker: cancer
stayeth: stops
torroding: corroding
annointed: covered
axungia: soft animal fat, often goose
niter: saltpetre
taken fasting: on an empty stomach
Consumptions: wasting conditions
laske: diarrhoea
digesting quality: breaking down
asswage: soothe or relieve
kernels: hard swellings
hardnesse of the spleen: swelling of spleen due to infection

Burdock *Arctium lappa, A. minus* Asteraceae

Burdock is a big bold plant with powerful medicinal effects, traditionally paired with dandelion, both in medicines and to make the temperance drink dandelion and burdock, a European root beer.

Burdock is a wonderful cleansing tonic, which gently works on the liver and kidneys to 'cleanse the blood' or gently clear congestion and toxins from the body.

The roots, leaves and seeds can all be used, and greater or lesser burdock are interchangeable. Burdock root is a popular vegetable in Japan, where it is called gobo. The young leaf stalks and flower stems can also be peeled and cooked.

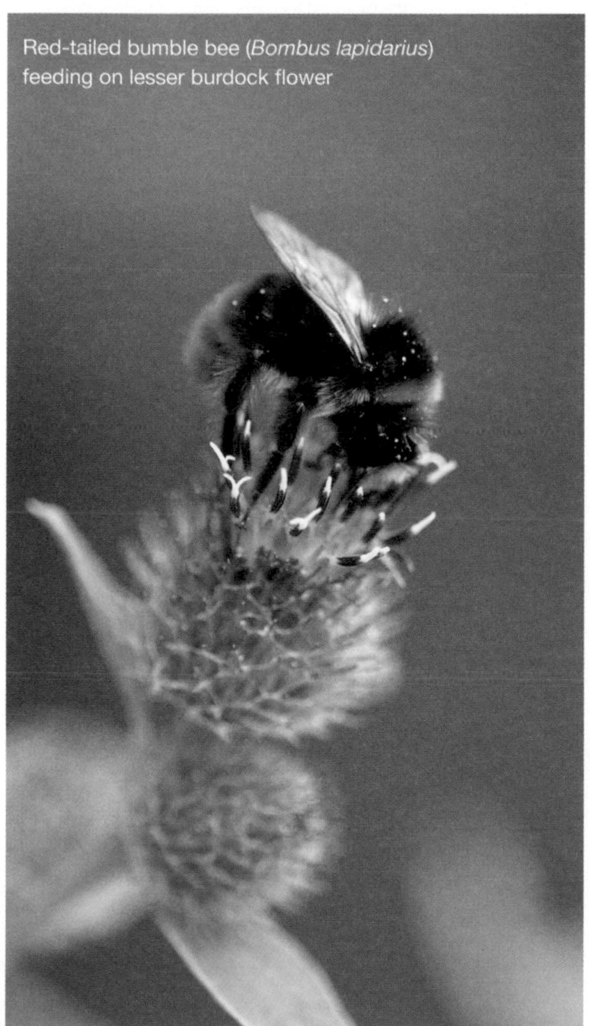

Red-tailed bumble bee (*Bombus lapidarius*) feeding on lesser burdock flower

The benefit of burdock will be most noticeable if it is taken over a period of time, though it can also provide quick relief.

Burdock is used for a range of skin problems from eczema and acne to psoriasis. By its action on the liver and kidneys it can clear the skin, as well as restoring either dry or greasy skin to normal.

Roots: Burdock is a biennial, so the roots should be harvested in the autumn of the first year or the following spring, before the plant flowers. Parkinson's woodcut, unusually, shows the wrong root: it has a long, straight taproot.

Leaves: The leaves are very bitter, stimulating appetite and digestion; they are strongly diuretic.

Parkinson suggests burdock leaf for 'shrinking of the sinewes', and it is always worth trying it for Dupuytren's contracture, where the connective tissue in the hands tightens the fingers towards the palm – today treated solely by surgery.

The leaves are used externally for skin problems, often in combination with taking the root internally.

Seeds: The seeds are effective for much the same issues as the root, but are also beneficial for kidney stones and strong, dark, gritty urine.

Greater burdock seeds are used in Chinese medicine to relieve hot conditions from red sore throats and fevers to rashes and boils, especially where toxicity is an issue. It is interesting that Parkinson says that the seeds of lesser burdock are heating.

Urinary problems: Burdock leaf is diuretic, increasing the flow of urine and helping cleanse the bladder.

Burns: Parkinson's burns remedy of crushed burdock leaf and egg white is still used today.

Cancer: Burdock has been used in cancer treatments since the early Middle Ages. Twelfth-century German Abbess Hildegard von Bingen used it, and burdock is an ingredient in the Hoxsey cancer formula and in Essiac.

Hair: We haven't tried Parkinson's recommendation for making the hair yellow, but burdock leaf infused oil is used as a scalp rub for hair loss.

Burnet *Pimpinella sive sanguisorba*

Theatrum Botanicum
Tribe 5, Chapter 55, pp582–84

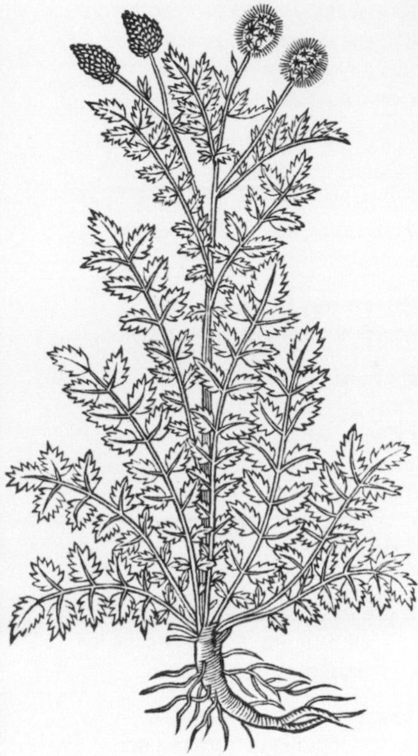

The Vertues

Both the greater and the lesser Burnet are accounted to be of one property, but the lesser, because it is quicker and more aromaticall, is more effectuall being both hot and dry in the second degree, especially the lesser (yet some say it is cold in the second degree) which is a friend to the Heart, Liver, and other the principall parts of a mans body;

In wine: two or three of the stalkes with leaves put into a cup of wine, especially Claret, as all know give a wonderfull fine rellish to it, and besides is a great meanes to quicken the spirits, refresh the heart, and make it merry, driving away melancholly: it is a speciall helpe to defend the heart from noysome vapours, and from the infection of the Plague or Pestilence, and all other contagious diseases, for which purpose it is of great effect, the juice thereof being taken in some drinke, and they either layd to sweate thereupon, or wrapped and kept very warme.

They have a drying and astringent quality also, whereby they are availeable in all manner of fluxes of blood, or humours, to stench bleeding inward or outward, Laskes or Scowrings, the Blooddy flix, womens too abundant courses, and the whites also, and the chollericke belchings, and castings of the stomake, and is also a singular good Woundherbe, for all sorts of wounds, both of the head and body, either inward or outward, for all old Ulcers, or running Cancers and moyst sores, which are of hard curation, to bee used eyther by the juice or decoction of the herbe, or by the pouder of the herbe or roote, or the water of the distilled herbe; or else made into oyle, or oyntment by it selfe, or with other things to be kept: the seede also is no lesse effectuall, both to stay fluxes and to dry up moyst sores, to be taken in pouder inwardly in steeled water or wine, that is wherein hot gadds of steele have beene quenched, or the pouder of the seede mixed with their oyntments, or injections.

friend to: assists
noysome vapours: offensive smells
availeable: effectively treat
fluxes: irregular flows
stench: stop, staunch
Laskes: diarrhoea
Scowrings: cleansing
the Blooddy flix: dysentery
courses: menstruation
the whites: leucorrhoea
chollericke belchings: upset stomach
castings: vomiting
pouder: powder
stay fluxes: stop flow of liquid
hot gadds: heated small bars
quenched: extinguished

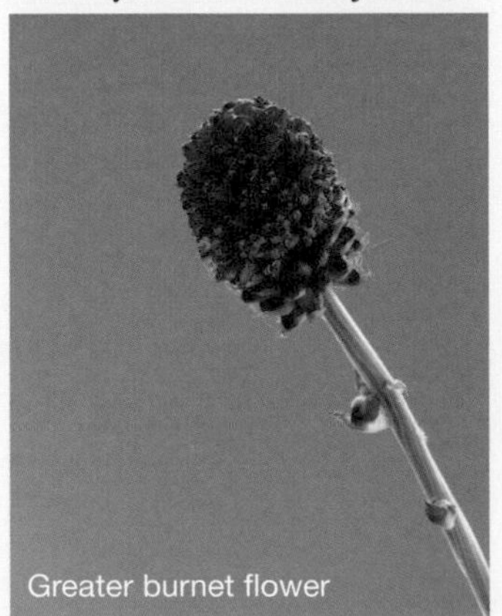
Greater burnet flower

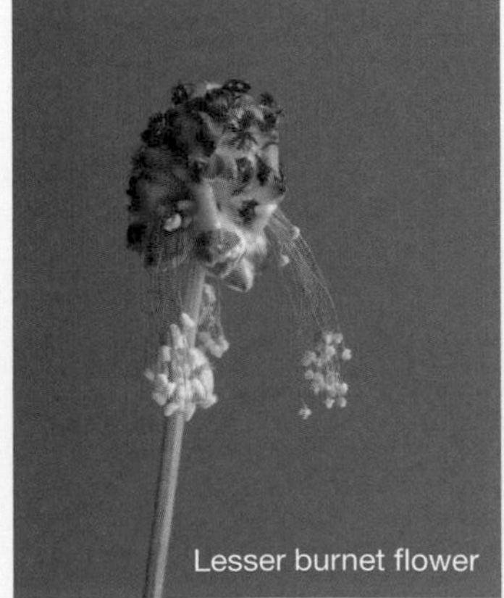
Lesser burnet flower

Burnet *Sanguisorba officinalis, S. minor* Rosaceae

Burnet is an attractive slender plant, with sets of toothed leaves. The greater burnet stands some three to four feet high, with a red-brown elongated flower (the colours possibly relate to the French 'brunette'), while the lesser is about half as tall, with much more humble yellow-red flowers. Both are drying and astringent.

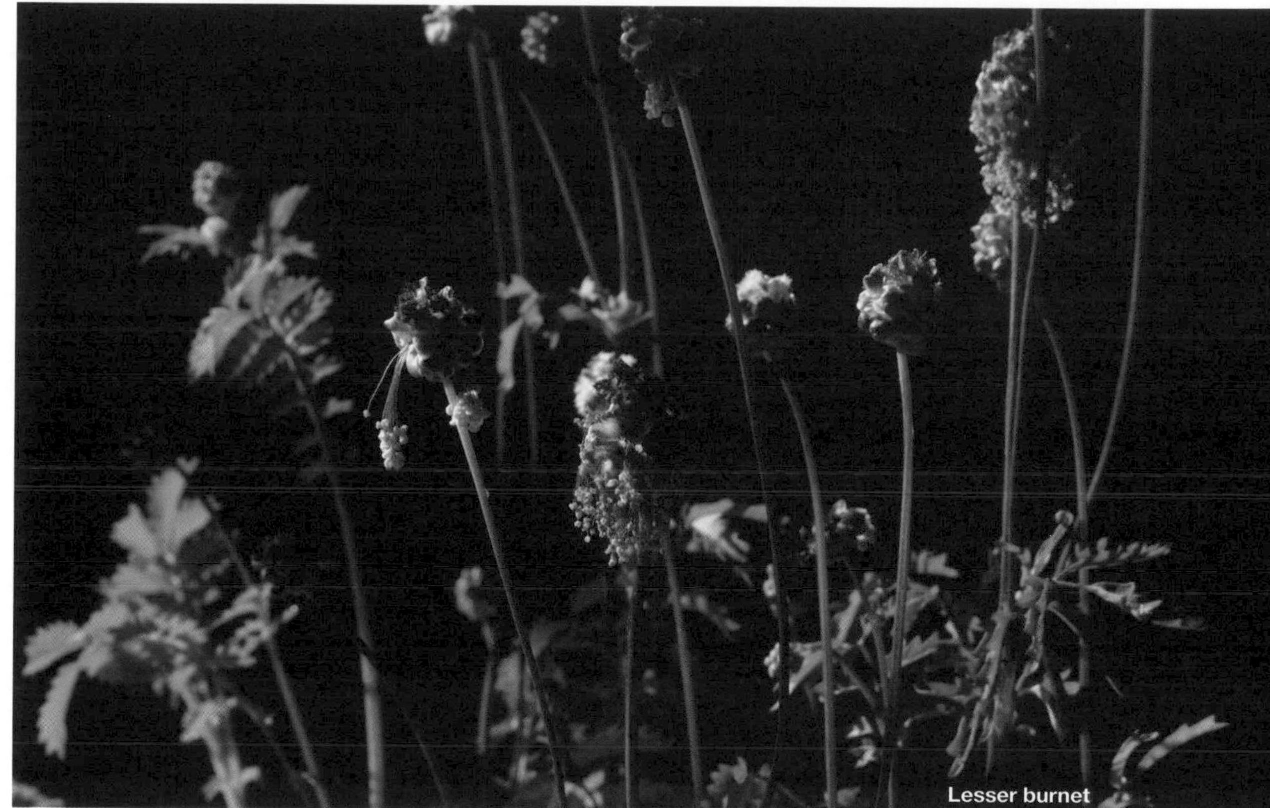

Lesser burnet

It is interesting that Parkinson prefers the lesser burnet medicinally, 'because it is quicker and more aromaticall', and a 'friend' to the major organs of the body. Modern-day nomenclature gives the description *officinalis*, or 'official medicinal' to the greater burnet, but, as Parkinson says, the properties are very similar.

Another noteworthy point is how Parkinson gives primacy to burnet soaked in wine as a heart tonic, which not only drives away melancholy but defends the person against contagious diseases, taken either as a drink or compress. The germ theory of disease would not be known for another two centuries and more, but it is clear here that the concept and terminology of contagious disease were accepted by 1640.

Modern herbalism, and Chinese medicine, both old and new, stress the blood-absorbing qualities (the literal meaning of *sanguisorba*) as burnet's principal use. Its drying and astringency capacity, as Parkinson identified, enables it to stop 'all manner of fluxes of blood', externally and internally. It remains valuable in the conditions he names, with the added value of being a wound-healer as well. It also has the ability to dry and heal damp discharges of various sorts, especially where there is bleeding.

He outlines a wide range of means of using all parts of the plant herbally. An infusion makes a tangy digestive tonic, and the leaves of lesser burnet are traditional in salads (salad burnet is now seen as a subspecies of lesser burnet, and makes a fine perennial garden plant), though perhaps the most pleasant option would be the 'fine rellish' of the leaves in a glass of claret!

Burnet Saxifrage

Theatrum Botanicum

Tribe 8, Chapter 41, pp946–48

Saxifraga Pimpinella

The Vertues

These sorts of Saxifrages are hotter than any the former kindes of *Apia* Parslies, and as hot as Pepper, and as *Tragus* saith, more wholesome, by his often experience: it hath the same properties that the Parslyes have, but in provoking Urine, and easing the paines thereof, or of the Wind and Collicke is much more effectuall, the rootes or seede being used either in powder or in decoction or any other way, and likewise helpeth the windie paines of the Mother, and to procure their courses,

Kidney stones: to breake and avoyde the stone in the Kidnies, to digest cold viscous and tough flegme in the stomacke; and is a most speciall remedy against all kinde of venome.

Cramps: *Castoreum* being boyled in the distilled water hereof, is singuler good to be given to those that are troubled with Crampes and Convulsions:

Comfits: some doe use to make the seede into Comfits, as they doe Caraway seede, which is effectuall to all the purposes afore sayd,

Distilled water: and some doe distill the water that the more tender stomackes may take it, being a little sweetened with Sugar:

Head wounds: the juyce of the herbe being dropped into the most grievous wounds of the head, doth dry up their moysture and healeth them quickely: the experiment is taken from Hennes whose combes and head being pierced through, so as the braine was not hurt, were soone helped hereby:

Skin: some women also use the distilled water to take away freckles, or other spots in the skinne or face, and to make it the more cleere and smooth.

1. *Pimpinella Saxifraga Hircina major.* Great *Germane* Burnet Saxifrage.

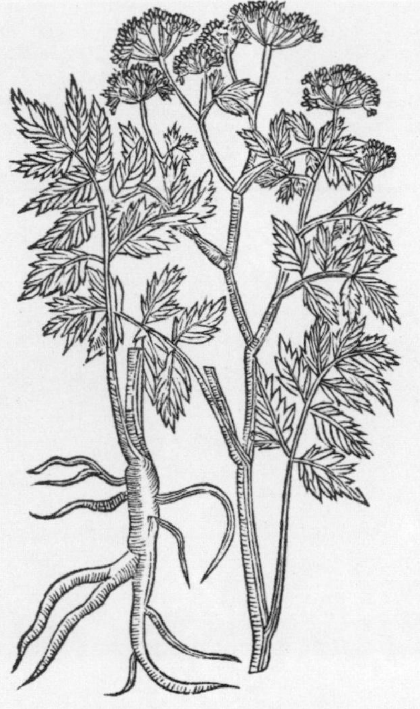

Apia parslies/parslyes: parsleys
Tragus: Hieronymus Bock (1498–1554), physician, priest and author
windie paines: cramps
procure their courses: bring on menses
Castoreum: exudate from the scent glands of beavers, still used as a food additive and in perfumery
Comfits: sweets
Caraway: *Carum carvi*
Hennes: hens

In his introduction Parkinson discusses cochineal, which he correctly asserts is not derived from grains on the roots of burnet saxifrage, as stated by other authors, but rather comes from an insect on prickly pear cactus as farmed in Peru (pictured right)

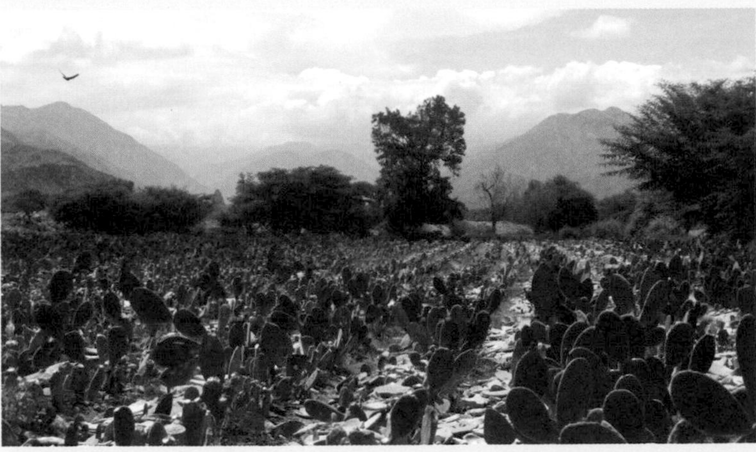

Burnet saxifrage *Pimpinella saxifraga, P. major*

Apiaceae

Unrelated either to burnet or saxifrage, this umbellifer has leaves that look a little like burnet. Saxifrage means 'stone-breaker', and refers to this herb's ability to help dissolve kidney stones. Burnet saxifrage is closely related to aniseed, *Pimpinella anisum*. A native of Europe and the Middle East, burnet saxifrage has been introduced to North America, and is found in the East. It is little used in herbal medicine today, but we think it deserves another look. The leaves can be eaten in salads, but the seeds are quite bitter and spicy.

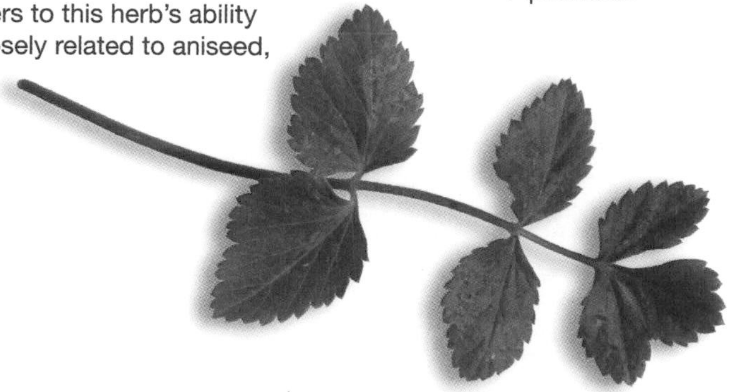

Digestion: For medicinal purposes, the root is used more than the leaves as it is stronger. It can be taken as a tea before meals to increase the appetite, and help relieve cramps; the seeds have the same effect of soothing wind and colic, especially in nursing mothers.

Urinary system: Burnet saxifrage is a diuretic and urinary antiseptic, useful for cystitis and other urinary problems, including the old use of dissolving kidney stones. Its antispasmodic action helps relieve spasms, and it can be helpful for treating gout.

Other uses: Burnet saxifrage is also used to treat coughs and throat infections, to increase lactation, and to heal weak gums and minor wounds. Its under-appreciated versatility extends, as Parkinson says, to drying up head wounds (at least of chickens, in his account), and as a distilled water for clearing and smoothing the complexion. He suggests a comfit or sweet from the juice, or a distilled water, to make the bitterness more palatable.

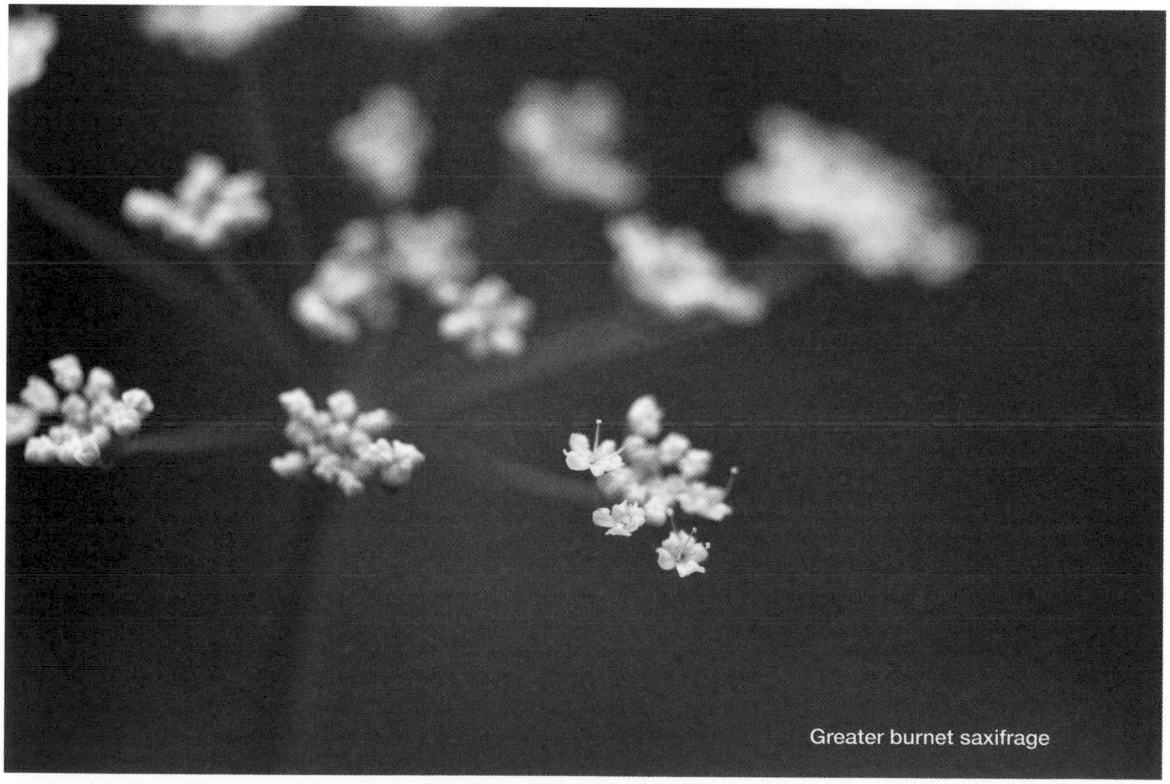

Greater burnet saxifrage

Celandine

Theatrum Botanicum

Tribe 5, Chapter 70, pp616–19

Chelidonium

The Vertues

Greater Celandine

The greater Celandine is hot and dry in the third degree, and of a clensing facultie;

Liver & gallbladder: It openeth the obstructions of the Liver and Gall, and thereby helpeth the yellow Iaundies, the herbe or the rootes being boyled in white wine with a few Anneseedes and drunke: *Mattiolus* saith that if the greene herbe be worne in their shooes that have the yellow Iandies, so as their bare feete may tread thereon, it will helpe them of it;

Other uses: the same also taken in the same manner, helpeth those that are inclining to the dropsie, or have it confirmed in them by often using it, as also for those that are troubled with the itch, or have old sores in their Legs, or other parts of their bodies: the juice thereof taken fasting, is held to bee of singular good use against the Plague or Pestilence,

Distilled water: and so is the distilled water also with a little Sugar, but especially if a little good Treackle bee mixed therewith, and they upon the taking layd downe to sweate a little:

Juice: the juice dropped into the eyes doth clense the eyes from filmes and clouds that darken them: but because it is somewhat sharpe, the hardned juice relented with a little breast milke will well allay it: it is to a good purpose used in old filthy or corroding and creeping Ulcers wheresoever, to stay their malignitie of fretting and running, and to cause them to heale the more speedily: the juice often applyed to tetters, ringwormes or other such like spreading Cancers, will quickly kill their sharpenesse and heale them also: the same rubbed often upon warts will take them away:

Pain: the herbe with the rootes bruised, and heated with oyle of Camomill, and applyed to the Navill, taketh away both the griping paine in the belly and bowells, as all the paines of the mother, and applyed to womens breasts that have their courses in two great aboundance stayeth them; the juice or the decoction of the herbe gargled betweene the teeth that ake, taketh away the paine, and the powder of the dryed roote, layd upon an aking, hollow, or loose tooth, will as they say cause it quickly to fall out:

Juice: the juice mixed with some powder of brimstone is not onely good to annoint those places that are troubled with the itch, but taketh away all the discolourings of the skinne whatsoever, be they spots or markes of bruises, stripes or wounds, the Morphew also, sunburning or any the like; and if it chance that in a tender body it cause any itching or inflammation, by bathing the place with a little Vinegar it is soone helped:

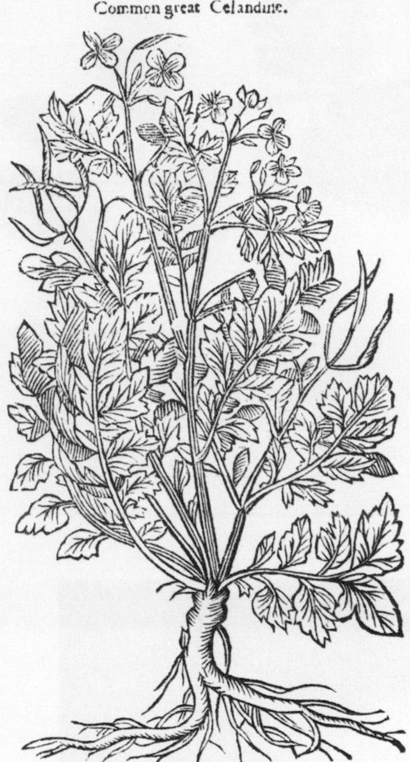

Iaundies: jaundice
Anneseedes: aniseeds
Matthiolus: Pierandrea Mattioli (1501–77), physician and author
dropsie: oedema
the itch: skin irritation
taken fasting: on an empty stomach
Treackle: theriaca, herbal compound
films & clouds: faulty vision
stay their malignitie: stop symptoms
tetters: herpes or eczema
sharpenesse: pain, activity
camomill: Roman chamomile, *Chamaemelum nobile*
navill: belly button
paines of the mother: uterine cramps
courses: flow of milk
ake/aking: ache/aching
brimstone: sulphur
Morphew: skin discolouration

Celandine *Chelidonium majus & Ranunculus ficaria*

Though they are both yellow flowers, greater and lesser celandine are not related. Greater celandine is in the poppy family and lesser celandine is in the buttercup family. Interestingly, even their uses are different. Greater celandine is known for its bright yellowy-orange sap, which can be used to remove warts. Dried, it is a traditional gallbladder remedy. Lesser celandine is also known as pilewort, which reveals its main use for treating haemorrhoids. But, as Parkinson reviews them together, we will follow suit.

Greater celandine *Chelidonium majus* — Papaveraceae

Greater celandine is the only plant in its genus. It is widespread in temperate Europe and Asia, and also found in North Africa and much of North America.

This in an interesting plant in that it is surrounded by contradictions. For example, the orange sap is noted as an irritant that can cause the skin to blister, and yet it has traditionally been dropped in the eyes to improve eyesight. It is perhaps this very 'clensing facultie' that makes it effective for the eyes, and Parkinson does suggest mixing it with milk to soften the effects a little.

Research has mainly been done on isolated alkaloids from greater celandine rather than on the whole plant extract. While isolated alkaloids may be toxic, other research has shown that the whole plant extract protects the liver. Isolated alkaloids from this plant have been shown to have antibacterial action. The alkaloids are better extracted in tinctures than teas.

Warts: The bright orange sap is still considered effective when applied to warts and allowed to dry. Several applications may be needed. The same treatment can be used for ringworm and skin cancers.

Pain: Greater celandine is acknowledged as a pain-relieving herb, and Parkinson's suggestion of combining it with oil of chamomile is intriguing. Today we understand it to be an antispasmodic, for relaxing smooth muscle and alleviating cramping. It can be beneficially used for tooth pain, as in Parkinson's day.

Liver & gallbladder: Greater celandine is one of those herbs that should generally be used in low doses, though in a study of liver-protective effects, it was the highest dose studied that gave the most benefit. It is traditionally and currently used to treat viral liver infections and some forms of cancer.

Cautions: Use only under professional supervision. Do not take during pregnancy. Subject to legal restrictions in some countries.

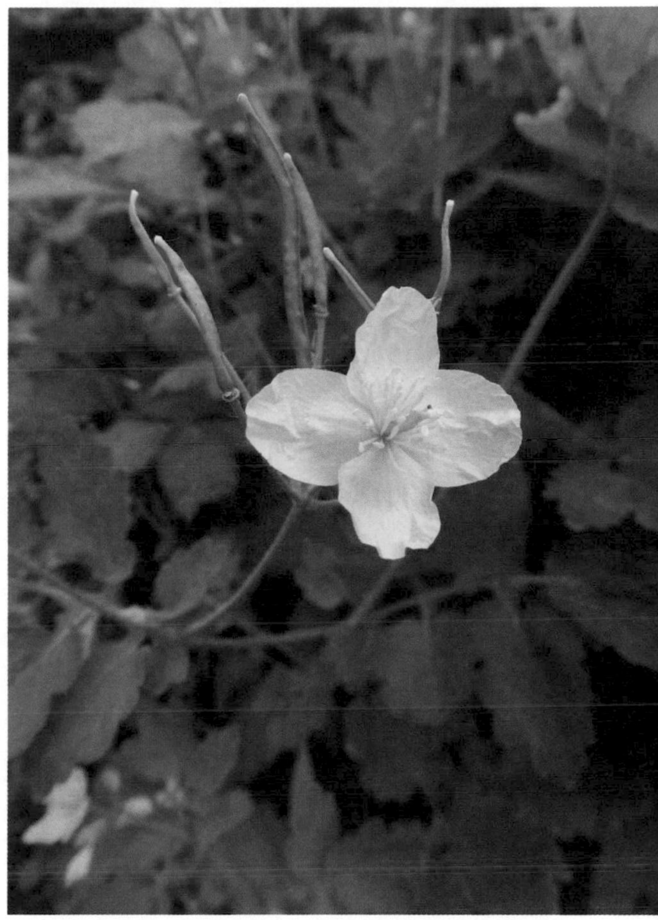

Modern research: Crude extracts of *Chelidonium*, and purified compounds derived from the crude extracts, exhibit antiviral, anti-inflammatory, anti-tumour and anti-microbial properties in vivo and in vitro. Recent in vitro testing has shown cytotoxicity comparable to that in many chemotherapy drugs.

Lesser Celandine

acrimony: bitter, sharp taste
tough humors: persistent, sticky phlegm
offend: cause disease
Dioscorides: Greek-speaking Roman physician (mid-first century AD)
Galen: Claudius Galen (AD130–200), physician and author
kernels: hard swellings
King's evill: scrofula
wennes: cysts

the lesser Celandine, because it hath not that acrimony with us, that it seemeth it hath in Greece, where *Dioscorides* lived, cannot have those properties, they ascribe unto their *Chelidonium minus,* which is, the juice taken from the rootes, and put up into the nose purgeth the head, and a decoction thereof with a little honey put to it and gargled in the mouth, doth the same effectually, and doth purge and cleanse the brest of flegme or any other tough humors that doe offend: it also helpeth a running itch, and those nailes of the fingers and toes that grow deformed, and scabbed: thus farre *Dioscorides* and *Galen*,

Haemorrhoids: but it is certaine by good experience, that the decoction of the leaves and rootes doth wonderfully helpe the piles or hemorrhoides,

Swellings & tumours: as also kernels by the eares and throate, called the Kings Evill, or any other hard wennes or tumors.

3 *Chelidonium minus.*
Small Celandine or Pilewort.

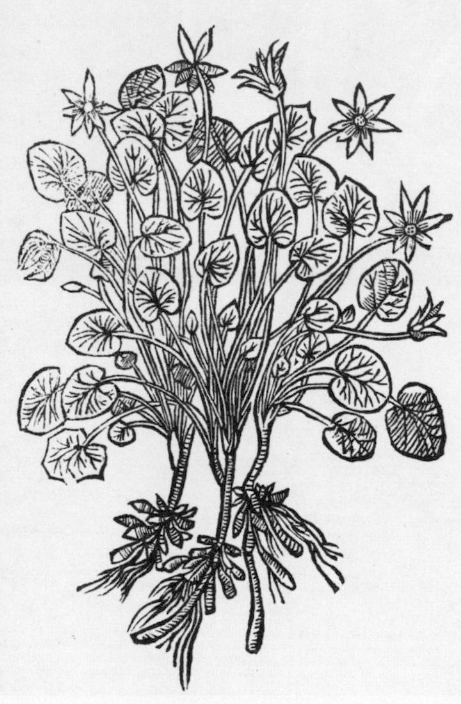

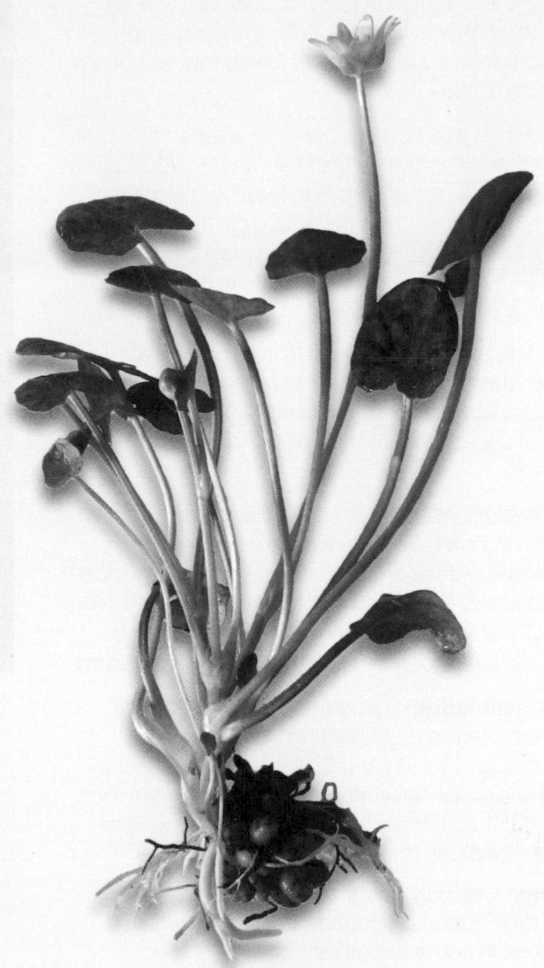

Lesser celandine *Ranunculus ficaria* syn. *Ficaria verna* Ranunculaceae

Lesser celandine is one of the earliest spring flowers to emerge, but it dies back completely in the summer. The flowers are so shiny they seem to be made of glazed porcelain, and are very variable in their petals, which can number anywhere from 7 to 12. Like greater celandine, it is native to Europe, Asia and North Africa but was introduced into North America as an ornamental and is naturalized in many areas.

It is also known as fig buttercup, which is reflected in the Latin name. Figs was an old name for haemorrhoids, and this plant is known as pilewort because it is a popular treatment for haemorroids and piles – but, as Parkinson says, this 'is certain by good experience', rather than because it might accord with the doctrine of signatures (see Figwort, p100).

The fresh or dried root tubers can be used, as can the fresh leaves, and are best gathered before flowering.

The fresh tubers are surprisingly tough and difficult to crush. Make an infused oil by placing the herb in olive oil in a jar in a sunny spot or somewhere warm, or heat gently in a saucepan. We usually make a stronger oil via a double infusion by removing the spent herb from the oil and then adding a fresh batch to repeat the process. For use, the finished infused oil is thickened into an ointment with beeswax.

To make suppositories for internal haemorrhoids, gently heat the herb in melted cocoa butter until the leaves lose their colour, then strain them out. The process can be repeated with a fresh batch of leaves or tubers. Once the herb is finally strained out, pour the liquid into suppository moulds and allow to cool.

Most of us associate the poet William Wordsworth with daffodils, but he claimed lesser celandine as his favourite flower and wrote three poems about it.

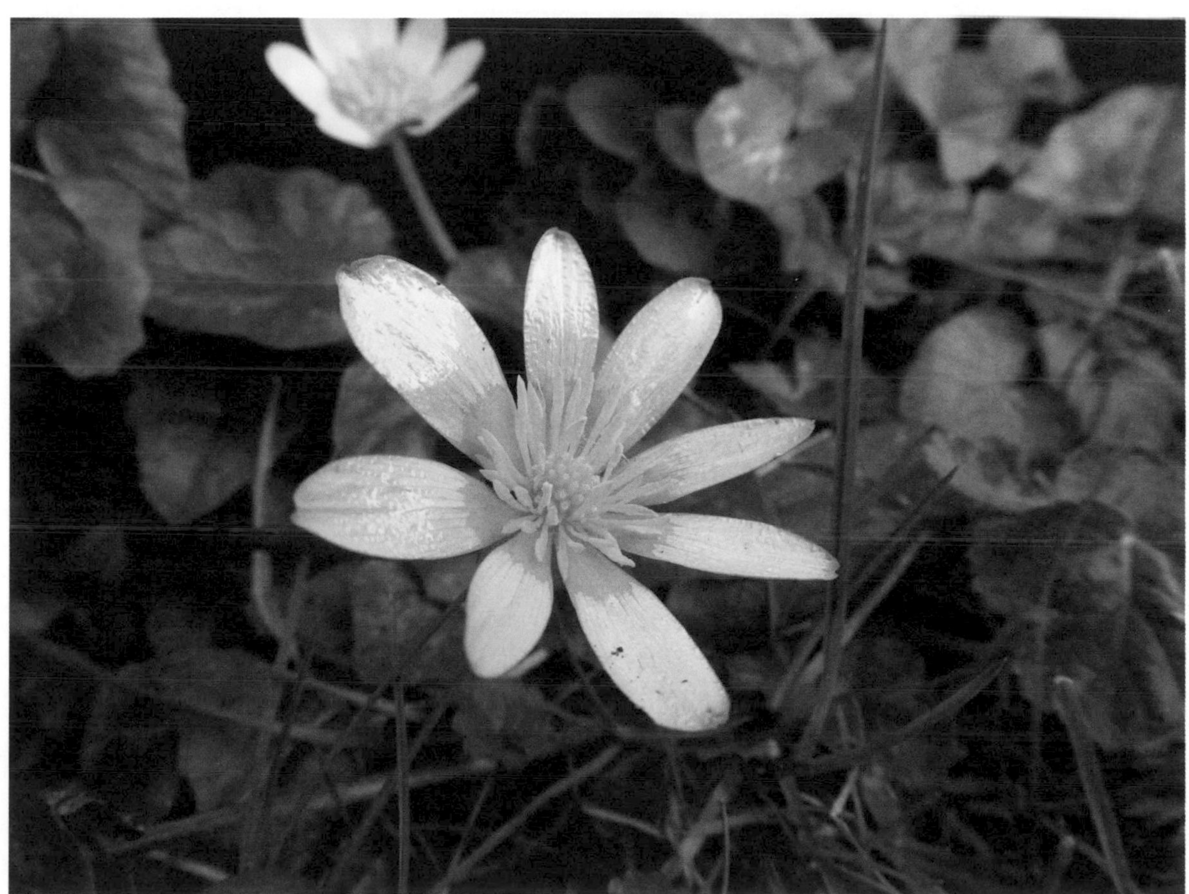

Celandine

The lesser Centory

Theatrum Botanicum

Tribe 2, Chapter 54, pp271–73

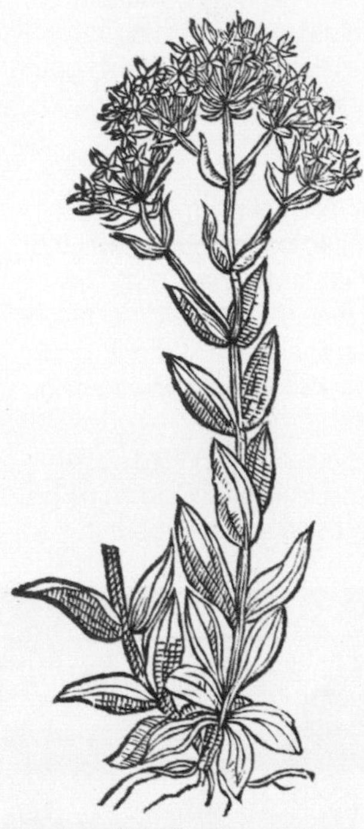
1 *Centaurium minus vulgare.* The ordinary small Centory.

Dioscorides: Greek-speaking Roman physician (mid-1st c. AD)
Pliny: Pliny the Elder (AD23–79), Roman naturalist
Galen: Claudius Galen (AD130–200), Roman physician and author
Mesues: Yuhanna ibn Masawaih, Syriac physician (777–857)
physitions: physicians
chollericke: choleric
Dodonaeus: Rembert Dodoens, Flemish physician and botanist (1517–85)
Gerard: John Gerard, barber-surgeon and herbalist (1545–1612)
agues: fevers
dropsie: oedema
greene sickness: new illness
pouder: powder
rheumes: watery mucus
chollicke: colic
courses: menstruation
fistulous: hollow
laid too: placed on

Centaurium minus

The Vertues

Dioscorides, Pliny, Galen, Mesues, and other *Arabian* Physitions with diverse others doe all agree, that the lesser Centory being boyled and drunke, purgeth chollericke and grosse humors, and helpeth the Sciatica; and yet *Dodonaeus* seemeth to averre that it hath no purging qualitie in it, that he could finde by much experience thereof: which words and saying *Gerard* setteth downe, as if himselfe had made the experience, when as they are the very words of Dodonaeus:

Fevers: it is much used with very good effect to be given in agues, for it openeth the obstructions of the liver, gall and spleene, helping the jaundise and easing the paines in the sides, and hardnesse of the spleene used also outwardly; making thinne both the bloud and humors, by the clensing and bitter qualities therein: it helpeth also those that have the dropsie, or the greene sicknesse as the *Italians* doe affirme, who much use it for that purpose in pouder; it is of much use to be boyled in water and drunke against agues as all know:

it killeth the wormes in the belly found true by daily experience; it helpeth also to drie up rheumes as *Galen* saith, being put with other things for that purpose: the decoction thereof also (the toppes of the stalkes with the leaves and flowers are most used) is good against the chollicke, and to brring downe womens courses, helpeth to avoid the dead birth, and easeth the paines of the mother, and is very effectuall in all old paines of the joynts, as the gout, crampes, or convulsions: a dramme of the pouder thereof taken in wine, is a wonderfull good helpe against the biting and poison of the Adder or Viper:

Juice: the juice of the herbe taken while it is greene, as is used in other herbes, and dried in the Sunne, or by decoction and evaporation by the fire, as was used in ancient times, worketh the same effects: but the distilled water of the herbe, as it is more pleasant to be taken, so it is lesse powerfull, for any the purposes before spoken of, because it wanteth that substance and bitternesse that is in the herbe: the juice thereof with a little hony put to it, is good to cleare the eyes from dimnesse, mistes, or cloudes, that offend and hinder the sight, it is singular good both for greene or fresh wounds, and also for old ulcers and sores, to close up the one, and clense the other, and perfectly to cure them both, although they be hollow or fistulous, the greene herbe especially being bruised or laid too:

the decoction thereof dropped into the eares, clenseth them from wormes, clenseth thc foule ulcers, and spreading scabbes of the head, and taketh away all freckles, spots, and markes in the skinne being washed therewith. The yellow Centory saith *Mesues* worketh the same effects, that the other with the red flowers doth.

Centaury *Centaurium erythraea* Gentianaceae

Centaury is a classic herbal bitter, though not quite so much used currently as its relative the yellow gentian (*Gentiana lutea*). It is also Classical, named for the Centaur Chiron, the exemplar of self-healing who used this plant, and centaury was praised by the standard Greek and Roman authorities. In Parkinson's day it was common, found, he says, 'in fields, pastures, and woods', but its cheery, matt pink, star-like presence is less often seen now because much of its habitat has been lost. It is a protected plant in Britain, but hard to domesticate; it occurs in both eastern and western states of the US.

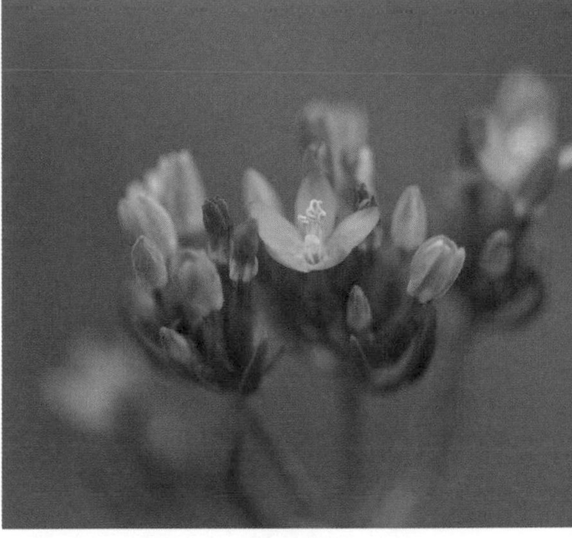

Centaury contains bitter glycosides that have a tonic effect on the liver and gallbladder, accelerating bile flow, which helps improve appetite and the quality of digestion; it also lowers a fever. As Parkinson states, the benefits are multiform, from helping relieve oedema (dropsy), joint pain and sciatica to reducing the severity of jaundice and fevers (agues), drying up mucus (rheum), stimulating menstruation and clearing eyes and ears.

Some of his uses are little tried these days – even if killing worms in the belly with centaury 'is found true by daily experience'; most now will probably ignore his idea of putting centaury powder in wine for snakebite.

It is interesting how varied his medicinal techniques are here: we can benefit from his breadth of approach in looking again at centaury as an infusion or decoction, as the green juice of the herb alone or with honey, as a distilled water, in wine, as a powder. Modern treatments would certainly add an alcoholic tincture, a popular way of concealing the bitterness.

One other point of interest here is how Parkinson criticizes John Gerard for not only copying the earlier writer Dodoens, which might just have been acceptable practice at the time, but certainly not to claim the findings as his own. Parkinson himself suffered wholesale copying, including this text on centaury, by Nicholas Culpeper in *The English Physition* (1652), though the latter has an apt summary for centaury that seems to be original: ''tis very wholesome, but not very toothsome'.

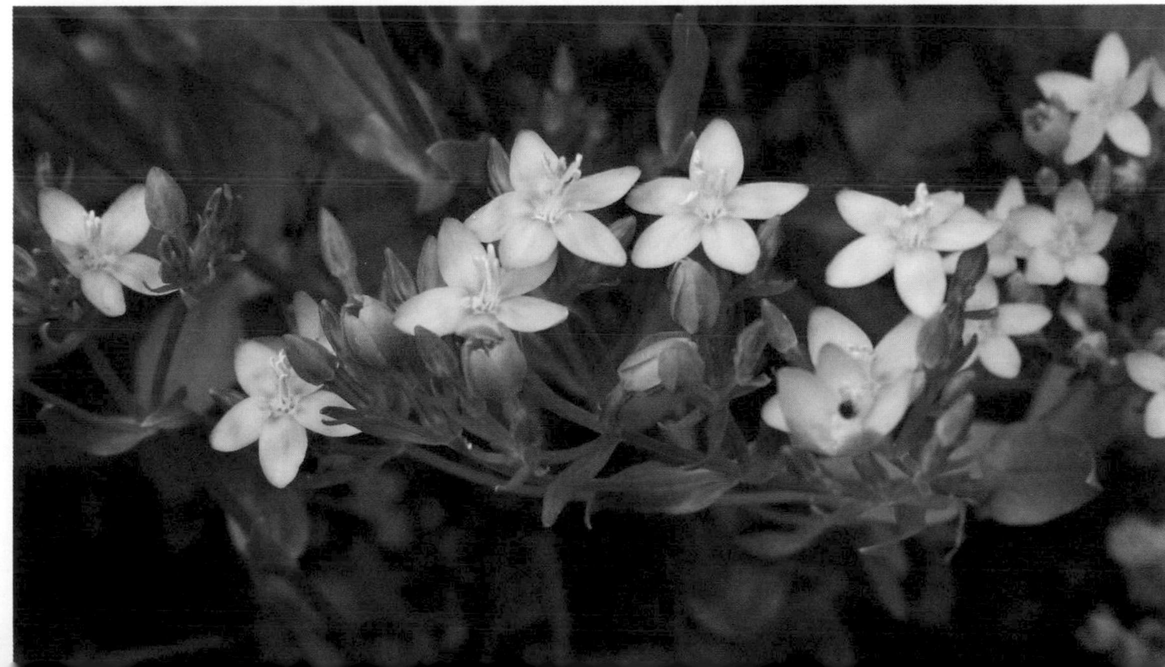

Garden Succory

Theatrum Botanicum

Tribe 6, Chapter 25, pp775–77

2. *Cichorium sylvestre.* Wilde Succory.

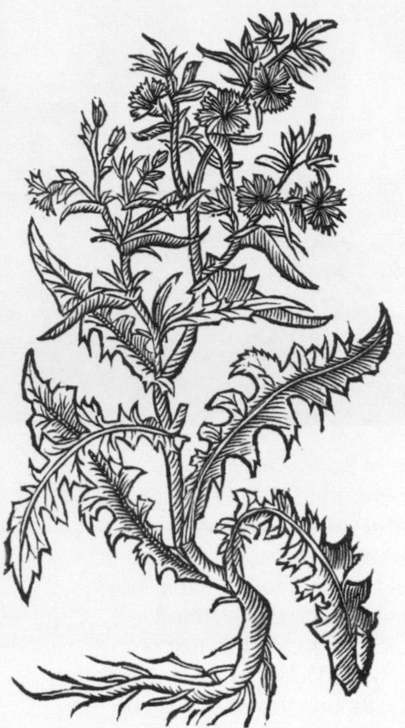

Endive: *Cichorium endivia*, a close relative of chicory
opening: removing blockages
drunke fasting: drunk while abstaining from food
chollericke: hot and dry
flegmaticke: mucus-like
Iaundies: jaundice
reines: kidneys
dropsie: oedema
evill: morbid, disease-producing
cachexia: irreversible loss of bodily mass from chronic illness
agues: fits of fever
dramme: apothecary's weight, ⅛ oz, 3.888g or 3 scruples or 60 grains
pestilentiall: deadly, plague-like
swoundings: swoonings
distemperature: overheating
St Anthonies fire: erysipelas
pushes, wheales: skin eruptions

Cichorium

The Vertues

Garden Chicory: Garden Succory as it is bitter is more dry and lesse cold then Endive, and thereby more opening also.

Leaves & roots: An handfull of the leaves or rootes hereof boyled in wine or water, and a draught thereof drunke fasting driveth forth chollericke and flegmaticke humors: the same also openeth the obstructions of the Liver, Gall, and Spleene, and helpeth the Yellow Iaundies, the heate of the Reines and of the Urine, the Dropsie also, and those that have an evill disposition in their bodies by long sicknesse, evill dyett, &c. which disease the Greekes call καχεξία Cachexia, a decoction thereof made with wine and drunk is very effectual against long lingering Agues;

Seed & distilled water: and a dramme of the seede in powder drunke in wine before the fit of an Ague doth helpe to drive it away, the distilled water of the herbe and flowers performeth the same properties aforesaid, and is especiall good for hot stomacks, and in Agues either pestilentiall or of long continuance, and for swoundings and passions of the heart, for the heate and headach in children, and to temper the distemperature of the blood and Liver: the said water, or the juice or the bruised leaves applyed outwardly allayeth tumors, inflammations, *S. Anthonies* fire, pushes, wheales and pimples, especially used with a little Vinegar, as also to wash pestiferous sores: the said water is very effectuall for sore eyes, that are inflamed or have any rednesse in them, and for Nurses sore breasts that are pained by the aboundance of milke.

Wild Chicory: The wild Succory [*Cichorum sylvestre*] as it is more bitter, so it is more strengthning to the stomack and Liver.

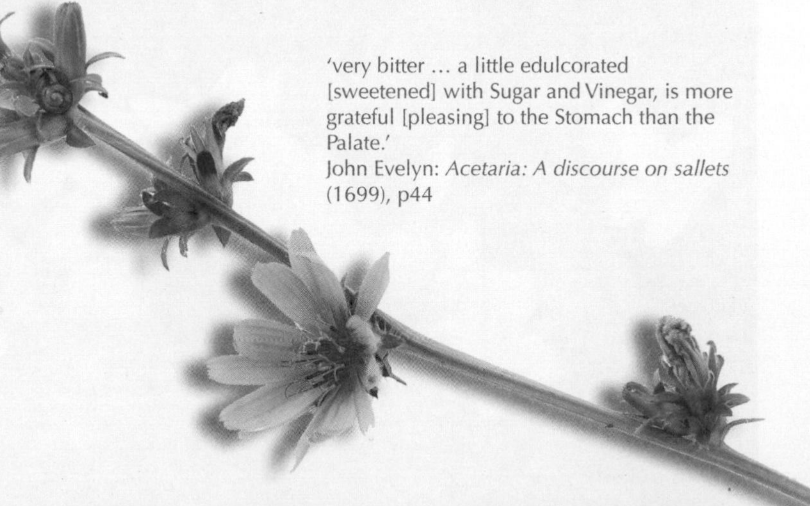

'very bitter … a little edulcorated [sweetened] with Sugar and Vinegar, is more grateful [pleasing] to the Stomach than the Palate.'
John Evelyn: *Acetaria: A discourse on sallets* (1699), p44

Chicory *Cichorium intybus, C. sylvestre* Asteraceae

Chicory is an ancient herbal plant, recorded as cultivated and used medicinally in Egypt, India and China over 4,000 years ago, as it is today. It is one of the 'bitter' herbs mentioned in the Bible (Exodus 12.8), and is still placed on the Seder plate as part of the Passover meal. Its old reputation as a mild bitter tonic and digestive is seldom questioned, and it offers much more than its modern use as a salad ingredient or hot drink. Certainly Parkinson makes full reference to its numerous medicinal virtues.

Chicory is compared here to endive, and some modern herbalists suggest it is also almost interchangeable with dandelion, for treating the liver and urinary issues. In imperial Rome Galen gave a syrup of chicory, rhubarb and oats to patients with liver ailments, and this would make a good recipe today. In both Chinese and Indian healing traditions it is trusted as a liver-cooling herb.

Parkinson also emphaisizes the value of chicory, boiled in wine or water, as a clearing digestive herb and one suitable for 'long sicknesse' and 'long lingering Agues', as well as cachexia.

A good liver herb is always a good herb for the skin, and Parkinson, like many another herbalist, notes how effective chicory is for treating hot skin conditions and eruptions, as well as for soothing sore eyes or breasts of nursing mothers.

Chicory coffee is a favourite in the deep South, in 'Creole coffee'. In his book *Wild Roots* (Rochester, VT, 1995), p73, Southern herbalist Doug Elliott gives his take on this 'un-coffee': cut up roots of chicory and dandelion, simmer with water and carob powder, strain, and add milk and honey. It is 'the most delicious and warming beverage' he can name.

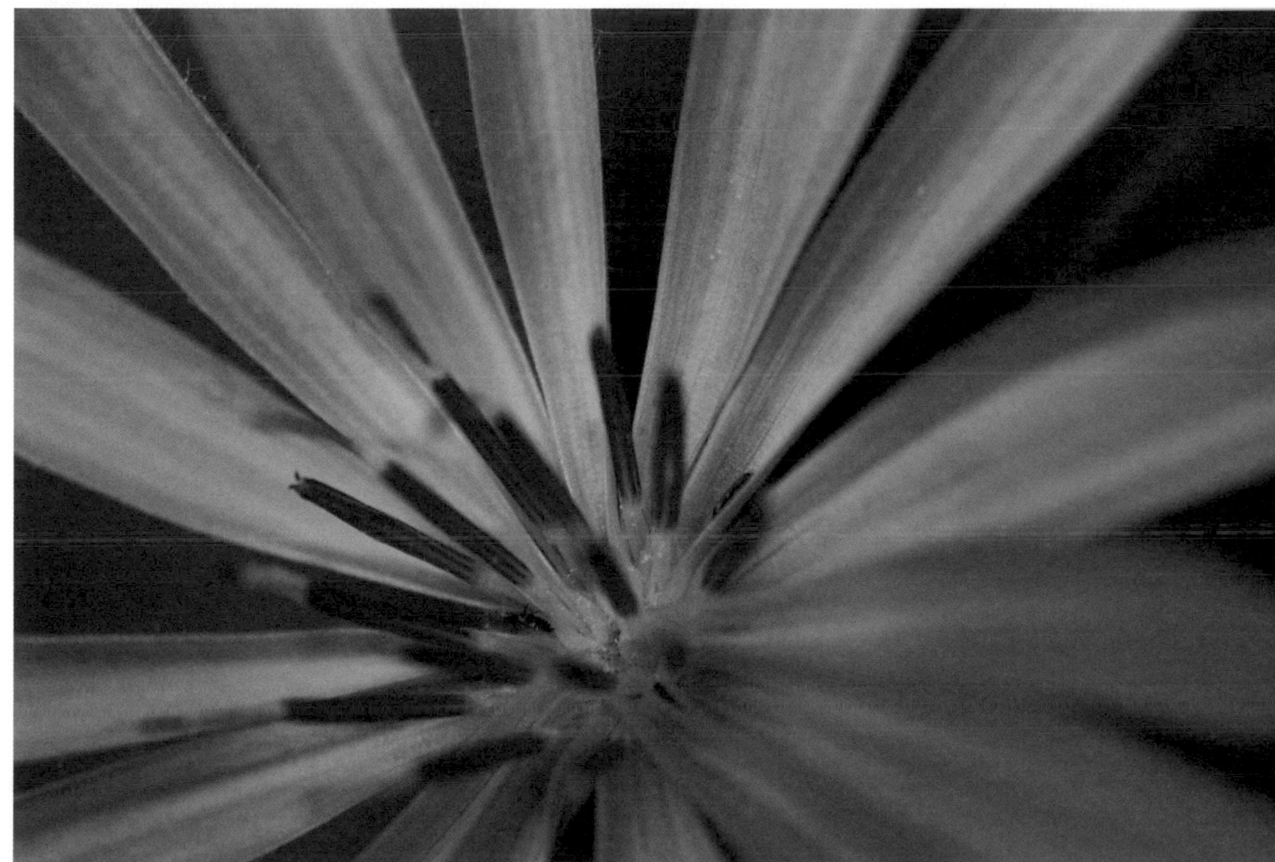

Ginny Pepper

Theatrum Botanicum

Tribe 3, Chapter 11, pp355–59

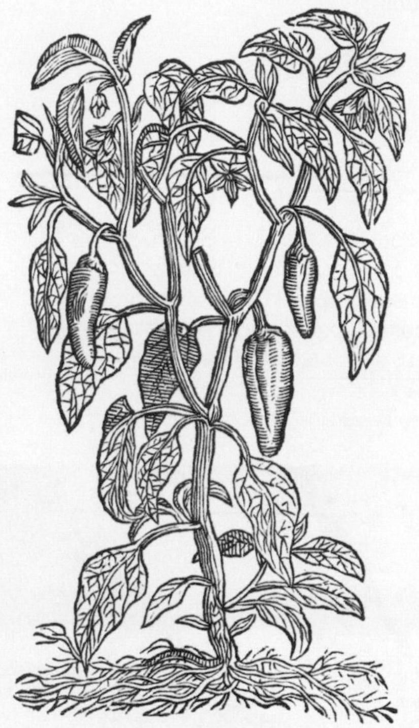

Ginny: Virginia colony
exulcerate: make ulcers
cods: fruit pod
neesings: sneezing
thin rheume: watery mucus
vehemensie: strength
perplexed: disturbed
spoyled: beyond repair
greevous: grievous
casting: another term for vomiting
noysome: offensive
meate: food
Physick: medical treatment
conducible: can be directed
Gregorio de Reggio: Capuchin friar and botanist (d. 1614)
receipt: recipe

Capsicum

The Vertues

The *Ginny* Pepper of all sorts (for herein they are all like) are hot and dry in the fourth degree, and beyond it if there be any beyond it, and are so fiery hot and sharpe biting in tast, that they burne and enflame the mouth and throate so extreamely that it is hardly to be endured;

for if any shall eate thereof unadvisedly, it will bee almost sufficient to choake them, and if it be outwardly applyed to the skin in any place of the body, it will exulcerate it, and raise blisters in the same manner, as if they had been burnt with fire or scalding water: yea the fierce vapours that arise from the huskes or cods, while one doth but open them, to take out the seede, to use or sowe, (especially if they doe mince or beate them into pouder) will so pierce the senses by flying up into the head by the nostrills, that it will procure aboundance of neesings, and draw downe such aboundance of thin rheume, that it is to be admired, forcing teares very plentifully: and passing likewise into the throate, it will provoke a sharpe coughing, and even cause a vomiting in that vehemencie, that all the bowells as well as the stomack, will be much perplexed therewith, and if any shall with their hands touch their face or eyes, it will raise so great an inflammation, both in the face and eyes, that they will thinke themselves utterly spoyled, which will not bee remedyed in a long time, by all the bathing of them with wine or cold water that may be used, but yet will passe away without further harm:

if some hereof be cast into the fire, it raiseth greevous strong and noysome vapours, procuring sneezings very fiercely and coughing, and even vomiting or casting very strongly, to all that be in the roome any thing neare thereunto:

yet marke and observe the goodnesse of our good God, that hath notwithstanding all these evill and noysome qualities, given unto man the knowledge how to tame and maister them, and cause them to be serviceable and profitable for their health: for whereas if it should be taken simply of it selfe, either in pouder or decoction, it were scarse to be endured, although in a small quantitie, and by often taking would prove very dangerous to life, the way here set downe is found to be the safest, both to be taken familiarly and often without offence in meate as well as medicine, as also to worke those good effects in Physick whereunto it is conducible:

How to tame chilies: It is *Gregorio de Reggio* his receipt, for take saith he, of the ripe cods of any sort of *Ginny* Pepper (for as I have sayd before, they are all in propertie alike) and dry them well, first of themselves, and then in an oven, after the bread is taken out, put into a pot or pipkin, with some flower that they may be thoroghly dryed,

Chili, cayenne *Capsicum* spp. Solanaceae

Chilies are now such an important spice around the world that is hard to imagine them as a new discovery. These fiery fruits are a very useful herbal stimulant, improving circulation and bringing heat to the body. They are high in minerals and vitamins, including Vitamin C. Parkinson describes twenty different kinds, saying that they all came originally from America (he uses the name Ginny for Virginia), but they had become quite widely naturalized all over Europe by the time he was writing.

It is easy to see why capsicum seemed so fiery to people who thought that ginger or pepper were the hottest spices. Parkinson wonders if they surpass the hottest degree so far described. His lively description from personal experience certainly brings back memories of the pain caused by a really hot chili – excruciating for several hours, yet, as he says, it 'will passe away without further harm'.

It is interesting that the healing powers of chilies were so well recognized, and that people persevered with the fiery fruits to find a way to moderate the heat but still reap the benefits. Parkinson ascribed this to 'the goodnesse of our good God', but painful human experimentation should also be thanked.

Today, we have a wide range of capsicums available, from the fiery heat of a habañero or naga to the mildest cherry peppers and sweet bell peppers. They also come in a dazzling array of shapes and colours, from green to red, yellow and purple.

People with a hot constitution will find chilies far too heating to bear, but for those with a cold constitution, poor circulation and lots of phlegm they are marvellously beneficial.

Chilies are used internally and externally to promote peripheral circulation. Taking chilies internally, usually as additions to food, helps cold extremities arising from poor circulation, and can be useful for complaints from chilblains to Raynaud's disease. Use chili powder in a hand or footbath for these.

In ointments and salves, chilis bring blood to the skin surface and can also be highly effective for relieving pain. They combine well with mustard and ginger in a hot pain-relieving oil, or are equally valuable on their own.

Some of the American naturopathic herbalists and physicians found chili to be among their favourite herbs. Dr John Christopher (1909–83) used to take a teaspoonful of cayenne pepper in a glass of warm water three times a day. He started using it when he had severe hardening of the arteries in his thirties; ten years later doctors told him he had the circulation of a teenager.

Dr Christopher used cayenne in unlikely ways – in his eyebath formula and to treat stomach ulcers – and with great success. He was a big proponent of chili pepper to treat heart attacks in cases where the patient is conscious and can drink a glass of warm water with a teaspoon of chili powder in it.

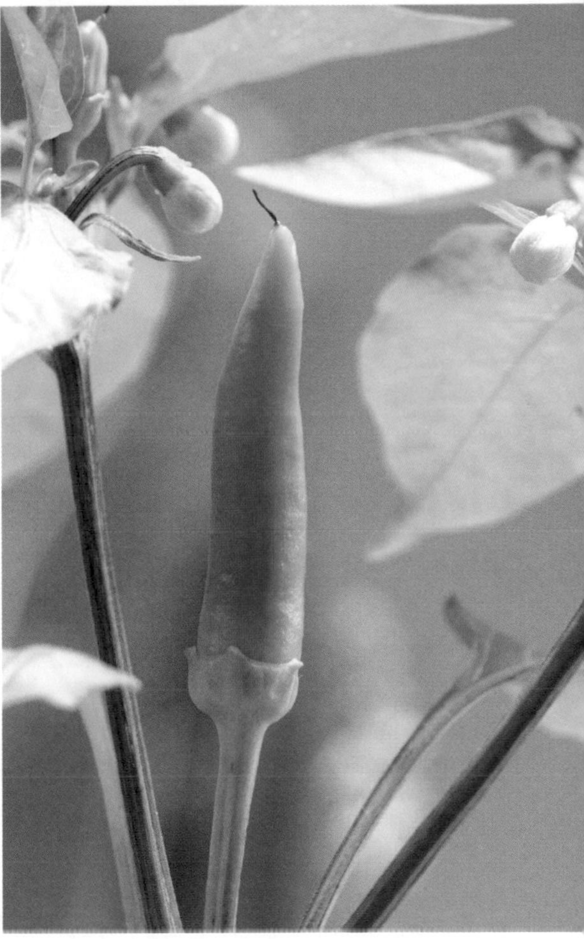

Dr Christopher's student, Dr Richard Schulze, liked capsicum so much as a herb that he earned the nickname 'Cayenne'. He takes the hottest chilies he can find to make a tincture, and uses that as emergency medicine for heart attacks, strokes, and for internal and external bleeding.

Digestion: Chili helps digestion in many ways. It can help repair the stomach, improve acid levels and stimulate peristaltic activity.

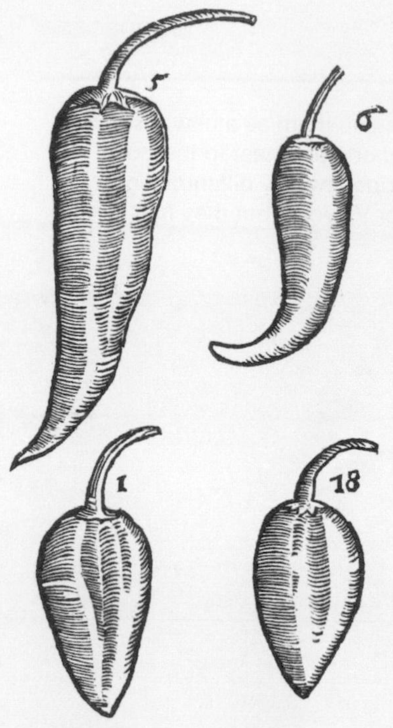

clense them from the flower, and their stalkes if they have any, cut them or clip them very small, both huskes and seedes within them, and to every ounce of them, put a pound of fine wheate flower (the same yee dryed them withall in the oven, may be part if yee will) make them up together into cakes or small loaves with so much leaven, as yee thinke may be convenient for the quantitie you make; bake these as you doe bread of that sise, and being baked cut it againe into smaller parts, and bake it againe, that it may be as dry and hard as bisket, which beaten into fine pouder and sifted, may be kept for any the uses hereafter specified, or may serve in stead of ordinary Pepper, to season meate or broth, or for sauce, or any other purpose the *East Indian* Pepper doth serve:

Digestion: for it not onely giveth as good, but rather a better taste or rellish to the meate or sauce (yea and your wine and other drinke) but it is found to be singular good, to breake and discusse the winde, both in the stomacke and the collicke in the body: it is singular good to be used with such meates as are flatulent or windy, and such as breed much moysture and crudities (whereof fish is reckoned one speciall:) one scruple of the said pouder, taken in a little broth of Veale, or of a Chicken, doth wonderfully comfort a cold stomacke, causing flegme, and such grosse or viscous humours as lye low in the bottome thereof to be avoided, helpeth digestion, for it provoketh an appetite to meate, provoketh urine, and taken with Saxifrage water expelleth the stone in the kidneyes, and the flegme that breedeth them, and taketh away the dimnes or mistinesse of the sight used in meates;

taken with *Pillule Aelephangine* doth helpe the dropsie:

Gynaecological uses: the pouder taken for three dayes together in the decoction of Penyroyall, expelleth the dead birth, but if a peece of the cod or huske, either greene or dry be put into the mother after delivery, it will make them barren for ever after: but the pouder taken for foure or five dayes fasting, with as much Fennell seede, will ease all paines of the mother: the same also made up with a little pouder of Gentian, and oyle of bayes into a pessarie, with some cotten wooll, doth bring downe their courses if they have beene stayed:

Coughs & sore throats: the same mixed with a Lohoc or Electuary for the cough, helpeth an old inveterate cough; being mixed with hony and applyed to the throate, troubled with the squinsie, helpeth it in a short space, and made up with a little pitch or Turpentine, and layd upon any hard knots or kernells in any part of the body, it will resolve them, and not suffer any more to grow there:

Skin: mixed with some niter and used, it taketh away the morphew and all other freckles, spots and markes, and discoulourings of the skin;

Other uses: applyed with Hens grease dissolveth all cold imposthumes and carbuncles, and mixed with sharpe Vinegar, dissolveth the hardnesse of the spleene; if some thereof bee mixed with

pipkin: earthenware cooking pot
flower: flour
leaven: raising agent
sise: size
East Indian Pepper: black pepper
meate: food
discusse: dilute
crudities: rawness
scruple: 20 grains, 1/25 oz, 1.3 gm
flegme: phlegm
viscous humours: thick mucus
avoided: voided
dimnes: dimness
Pillule Aelephangine: small pills for the stomach and digestion
Pennyroyal: *Mentha pulegium*
mother: womb
pouder: powder
fasting: with an empty stomach
oyle of bayes: oil of bay
courses: menstruation
stayed: stopped
lohoc: licking medicine, a thick syrup
electuary: paste of honey and powdered dry herb
inveterate: chronic, unshakeable
squinsie: quinsy
kernells: inflamed glands
niter: saltpetre
morphew: skin discolouration

Taming fire: a simple chili bread

The recipe Parkinson gives from Gregorio de Reggio is designed to moderate the hottest chilies. We bought 1 oz (30g) of the hottest chili powder we could find and mixed it with 1 lb (450g) of wheat flour, 1 teaspoon of yeast and 1½ cups warm water to make a dough. This was kneaded and placed in an oiled loaf tin to rise. This was then baked at 175°C (350°F) for 45 minutes or until done. We ate some fresh, and were amazed to get such a strong chili effect without the expected accompaniment of a hot mouth.

Parkinson then sliced his bread and baked it again until it was crisp, and powdered it. We found the thinly sliced chili melba toast was very tasty, and it can be kept in a jar to stay crisp. We powdered some too, but left it fairly coarse to use in recipes as spicy dry breadcrumbs or to nibble.

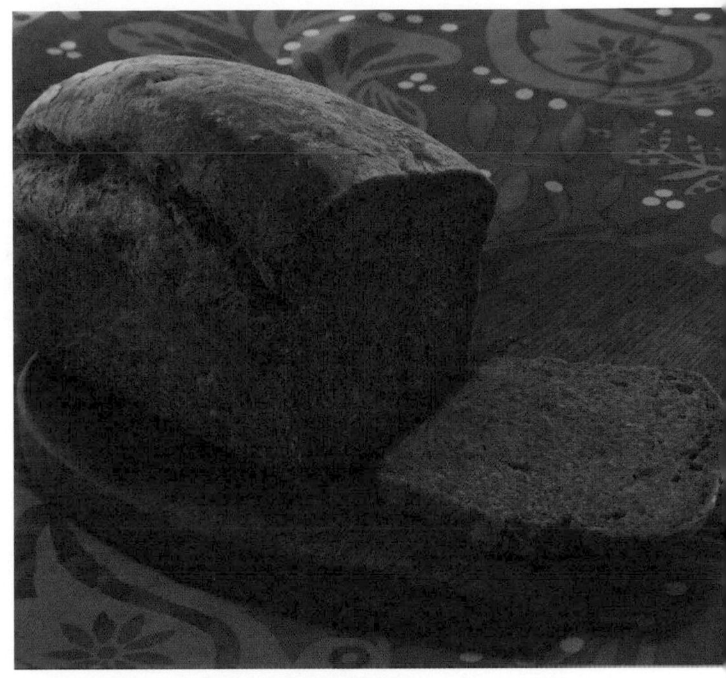

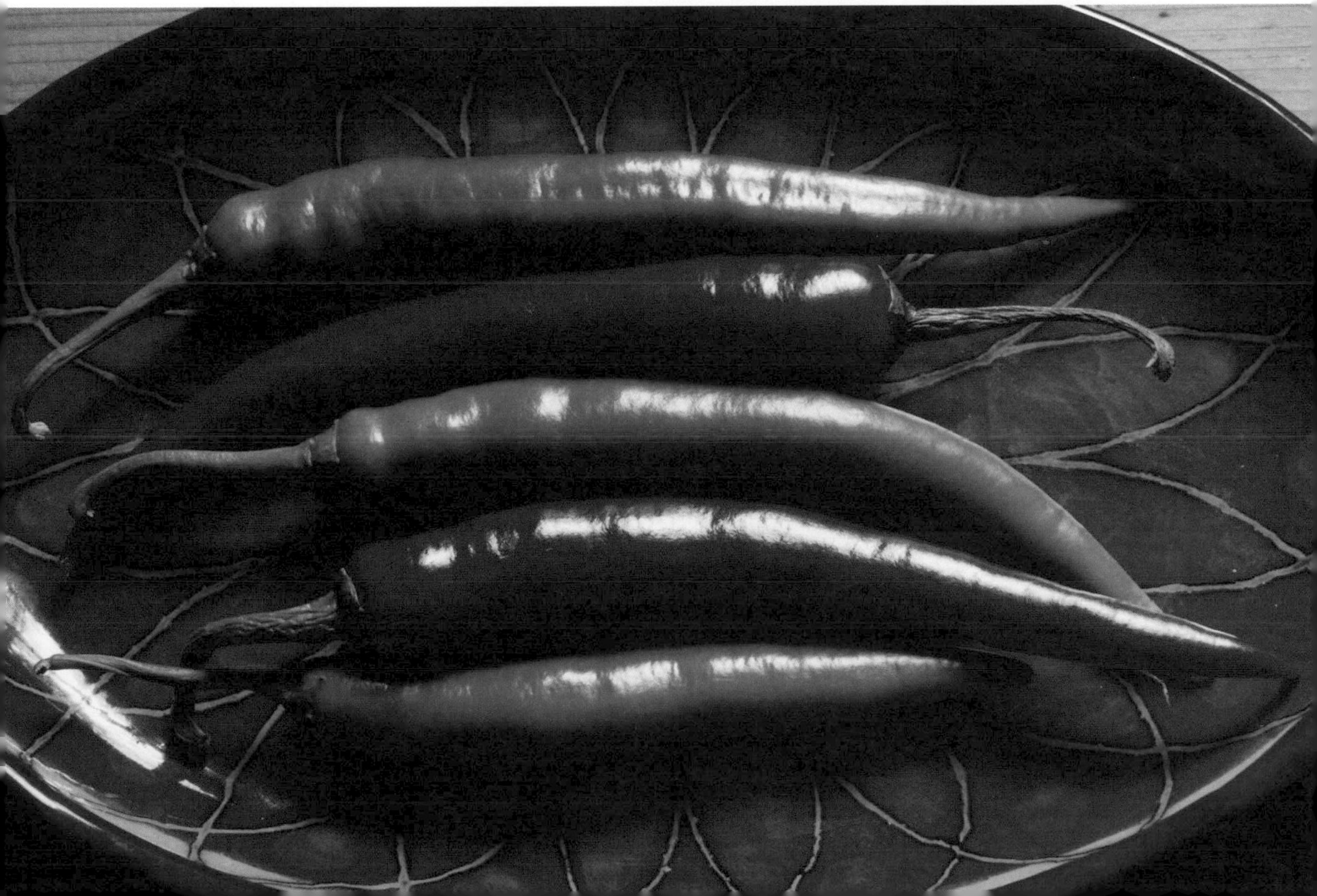

hens grease: chicken fat
imposthumes: abscesses
unguentum de alabastro: ointment made from powdered alabaster, chamomile, rose flowers and oil, with white wax
raines of the backe: kidney area
agues: fevers
plaister: plaster, poultice
rupture that commeth of water: possibly a herniated bladder
steepe: soak
aqua vitae: water of life, herbs distilled in wine
palsie: paralysis
stinch: stench, bad smell
procured of: arises from

unguentum de alabastro, and the raines of the backe anointed therewith, it will take away the shaking fits of Agues:

WITH TOBACCO: a plaister made thereof, and the leaves of Tabacco, will heale the sting or biting of any venemous beast:

TEETH: the decoction of the huskes themselves made with water, and the mouth gargled therewith easeth the toothach, and preserveth them from rottennesse: the ashes of them being rubbed on the teeth, will cleanse them and make them grow white that were blacke:

DECOCTION: the decoction of them with wine helpeth the Rupture that commeth of water, if it be applyed warme, morning and evening;

PALSY: if they put it to steepe for three dayes together in *aqua vitae*, and the place affected with the palsie bathed therewith, will give a great deale of ease;

BAD BREATH: and steeped for a day in wine, and two spoonefull thereof drunke every day fasting, will helpe a stinking breath, although it hath continued long; and snuft up into the nostrills, will correct and helpe the stinch of them, which is procured of flegme corrupted therein.

Gynaecology: Chilies are still used by herbalists to treat heavy menstrual bleeding. Because chilies improve the blood supply to the uterus, they can help with period pain and improve a variety of complaints.

Coughs & sore throats: Chilies are very useful for helping prevent and treat a range of respiratory problems. A hot broth with ginger, garlic and chilies will often chase away a cold and will help you endure the flu. Spicy food helps keep lungs and mucus membranes healthy, even in polluted environments.

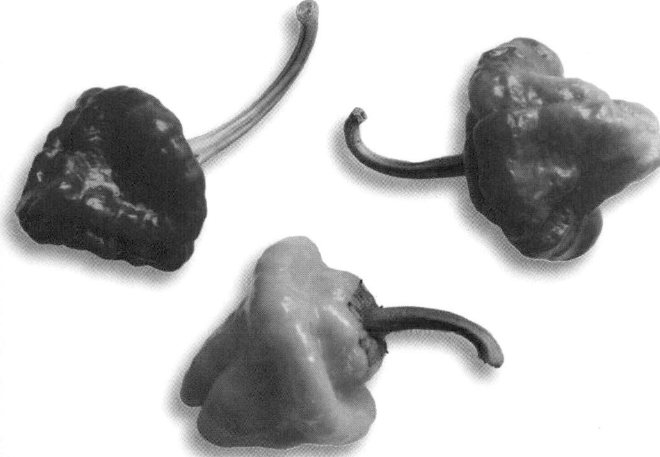

With tobacco: As a poultice for insect bites and stings this is very effective, but we have not had a chance to try it on the bites of any more venomous beasts! To use, crush a leaf of wild tobacco (*Nicotiana rustica*), mix the juice with a little hot chili powder and place it on the bite or sting. If you are using ordinary dried tobacco, chew it first to moisten or mix with a little water. See p210 below.

Teeth: We haven't tried chili ash to whiten the teeth, but it would be a gentle abrasive to clean the teeth, and charcoal whitens teeth – it is often used in commercial tooth powders. We have found that eating a slice of Parkinson's chili bread was enough to cure bleeding gums, making them strong again. The effect lasted several weeks before more chili was needed.

Bad breath: We haven't tried having chili wine for breakfast, but the fact that chili is so beneficial for the stomach and digestion suggests that it would help halitosis.

We have used herbal snuff mixtures containing chili. Assuming that your nasal passages are not too blocked to snuff it up, they are eye-wateringly effective in clearing phlegm.

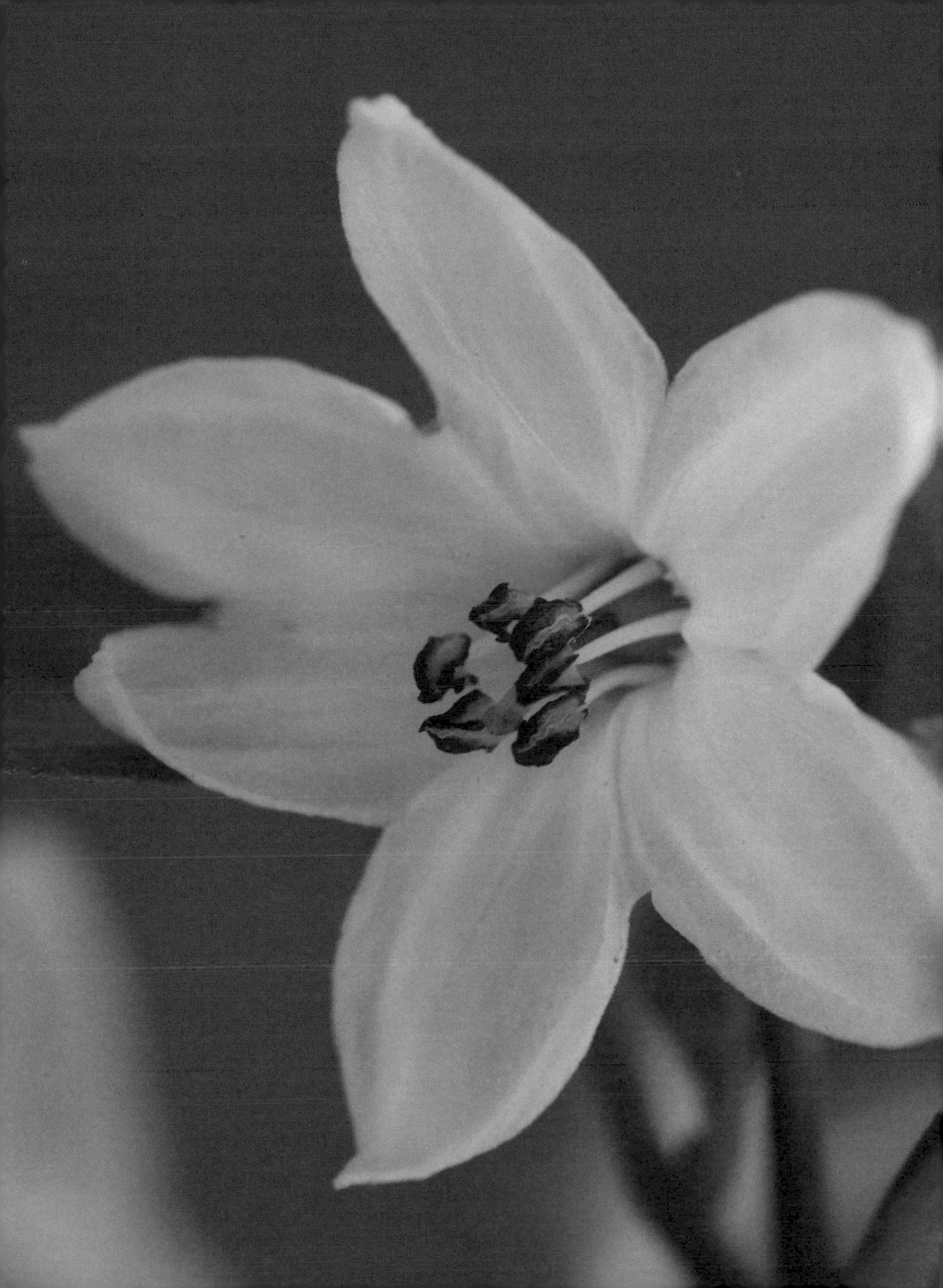

Goosegrasse, Clevers

Theatrum Botanicum

Tribe 5, Chapter 47, pp567–68

Aparine

1. *Aparine Vulgaris.* Common Clevers.

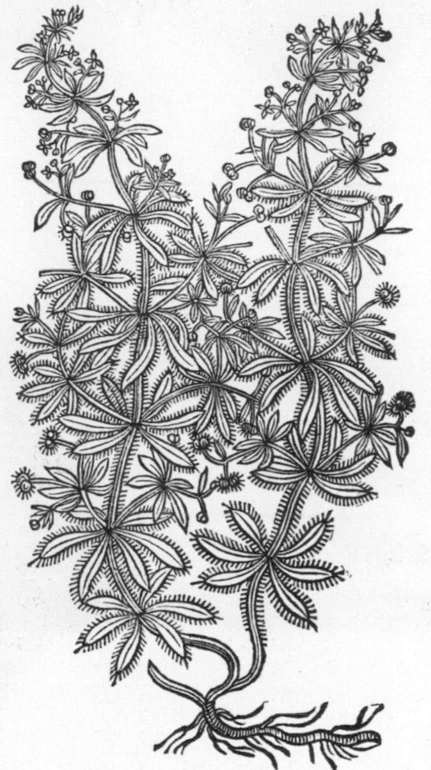

Dioscorides: Greek-speaking Roman physician (mid-first century AD)
Pliny: Pliny the Elder (AD23–79), Roman naturalist
Phalangium: venomous spider
Galen: Claudius Galen (AD130–200), Roman physician and author
Tragus: Hieronymus Bock (1498–1554), physician, priest and author
Iaundies: jaundice
laskes: diarrhoea
bloody flixes: dysentery
Matthiolus: Pierandrea Mattioli (1501–77), physician and author
pouder: powder
Axungia: soft animal fat, often goose
kernells: hard swellings

The Vertues

Clevers are hot and dry, *Dioscorides* saith and *Pliny* from him, that the juice of the herbe and seede together taken in wine, helpeth those that are bitten with Vipers, or the great Spider *Phalangium*, by preserving the heart from the venome;

Weight control: *Galen* saith it clenseth meanely and dryeth, and is of subtill parts: it is familiarly taken in broth to keepe them leane and lanke, that are apt to grow fat.

Distilled water: *Tragus* saith, that the distilled water drunke twice a day helpeth the yellow Iaundies,

Decoction: and the decoction of the herbe is found by daily experience to doe the same, and stayeth Laskes and Bloody flixes;

Bleeding: the juice of the leaves, or they a little bruised and layd to any wound, or place that bleedeth, will stanch the blood;

Wounds & ulcers: and *Matthiolus* saith, that the juice is much commended and used to close the lippes of greene wounds, and so doth the pouder of the dryed herbe strowed thereupon, and likewise helpeth old Ulcers:

Ointment: being boyled with *Axungia* and anointed, it healeth all sorts of hard swellings, or kernells in the throate;

Ear pain: the juice dropped in the eares taketh away the paines of them:

Milk strainer: the herbe serveth well the Country people in stead of a strainer, to cleare their milke from strawes, haires, or any other thing that falleth into it.

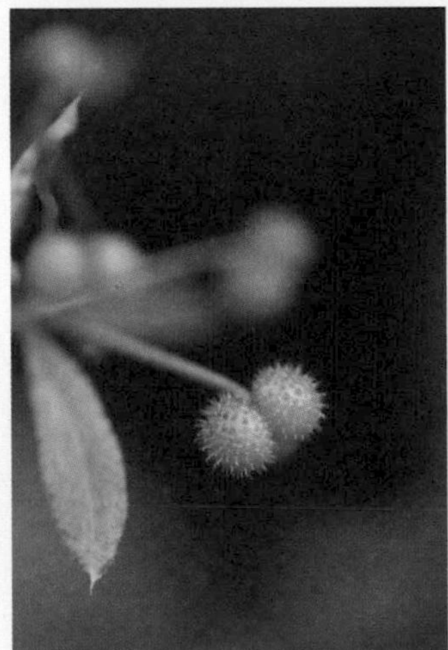

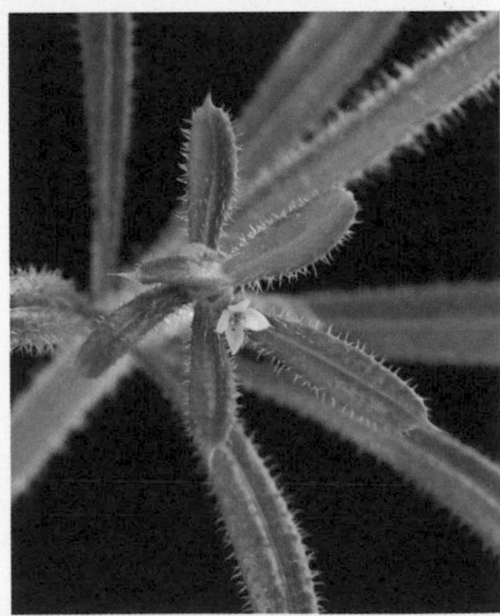

Cleavers *Galium aparine*

Rubiaceae

Cleavers is seen today primarily as a gentle but effective lymphatic cleanser. It is still a remedy for swollen glands in the throat, and has traditionally been used as a cleansing spring tonic. It has a potential role in the treatment of serious diseases such as cancer.

Cleavers is native to Europe, Asia and North America.

Cleavers gets its name from the way that it clings, or cleaves, to anything it touches with tiny little velcro-like hooks. Other common names such as sticky willy also reflect this characteristic.

In the early spring when the plants are small, the tips can be picked and added to salads. Later they become too tough and hairy to be palatable. It is interesting that the juice of the plant still gives a scratchy feeling at the back of the throat, just as if the little hooks were still there.

The furry fruits of cleavers can be dried and roasted to be used as a coffee substitute. Interestingly enough, cleavers is in the same plant family as coffee.

Like the other bedstraws (Galium family), dried cleavers was used to stuff mattresses. It worked well because the little hooks held it together so that it would retain its shape. Cleavers root can be used to make a red dye.

Herbalists today primarily use cleavers as a lymphatic cleanser. This is helpful for toxicity in the body as well as in treatment of infections, especially those that cause the lymph nodes and other lymphatic tissue, such as the tonsils, to become swollen. The fresh or dried herb can be taken as a tea, but for more serious conditions the juice is used. The juice is best preserved by adding vegetable glycerine to it.

By its cleansing action, cleavers would be helpful for old ulcers as well as 'greene wounds', as he says.

Recent research supports Tragus' assertion that cleavers helps the yellow jaundice, showing that the herb has a hepato-protective action.

Because cleavers cleanses the lymph and has beneficial effects on the liver, it is used to treat a range of skin problems, such as seborrhoea, eczema and psoriasis.

It is also considered to be a mild diuretic and is given for cystitis, kidney stones and other urinary problems. As a diuretic, it also helps lower high blood pressure.

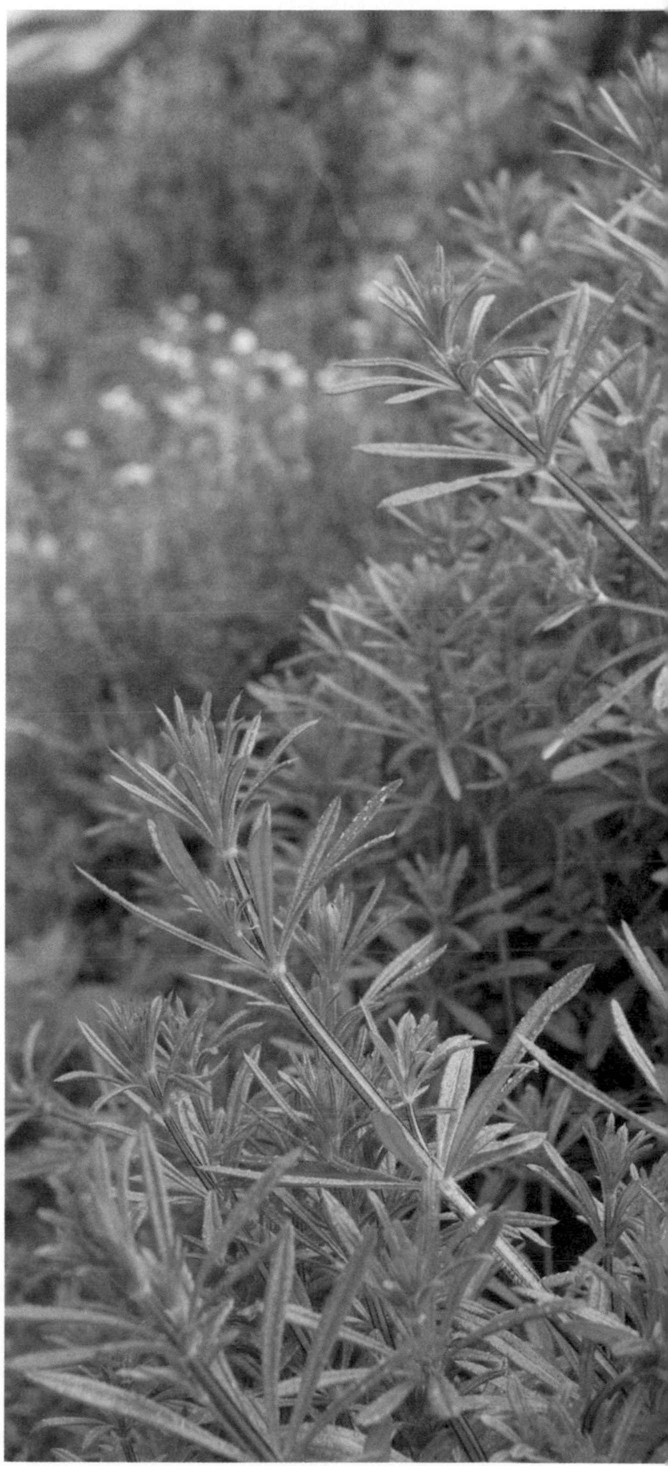

The herbe Coca

Theatrum Botanicum

Tribe 17, Chapter 59, pp1614–15

Coca

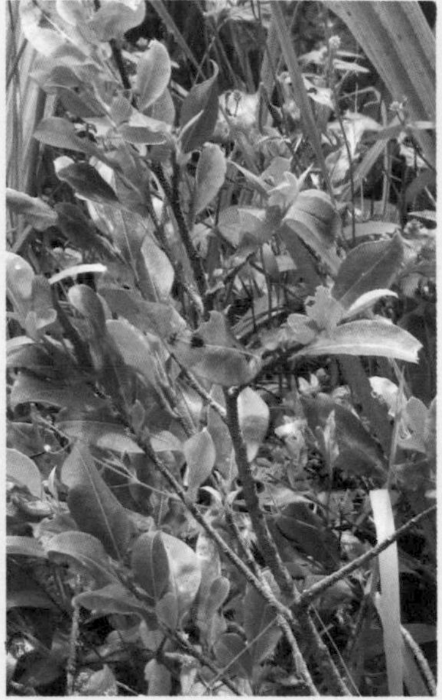

The seed of this Coca is sowne with great care by the West Indians in beds, by rowes, and riseth to be a plant of three or foure foote high, with a stalke as big as a good wand, and somewhat greater leaves then the Myrtle, having as it were another leafe in the middle thereof, being soft, and of a pale greene colour: the berries are red before they be ripe, but blackish afterwards, growing clustring together, and then they gather the leaves, laying them to dry, that they may be kept all the yeare and carryed to and fro into severall Countries, for thereof is the Natives chiefe Merchandise to provide them of all necessaries for life, being instead of money,

which is generally used by the *Americanes* to be chawed, as well in their long journeyes to preserve them from hunger and thirst abroad, as for pleasure at home, which they use after this manner: they burne Oyster shells, and with the powther of them they mix the pouther of the leaves of this *Coca* first chewed in their mouthes, and so made up as it were into a paste or dough (but take lesse of the pouther of the Oyster shells then of the leaves) whereof they make small pellets *trochisses* or *trossis*, laying them to dry, and so use them one by one, holding them in their mouthes, rolling them to and fro, and sucking them untill they be quite spent, and then take another, which maketh them able to travaile many dayes with strength, without either meate or drinke, through uninhabited places, where none is to be had:

If they stay at home, they use the *Coca* alone, chewing them sometimes a whole day without ceasing, untill the substance be sucked forth, and then use another: if they would have them to be stronger, able to intoxicate their braines like unto drunkennesse, or to be as it were senselesse, they put the leaves of Tobacco to it and take great pleasure in those courses.

sowne: planted
West Indians: Parkinson is referring here not to the islands as such but more generically to South America
rowes: rows
wand: long thin stick or stem
clustring: clustering
chawed: chewed
powther, pouther: interchangeable terms for ground-up solid matter
trochisses, trossis: variants of *troches*, small circular tablets or lozenges
travaile: travel
meate: food

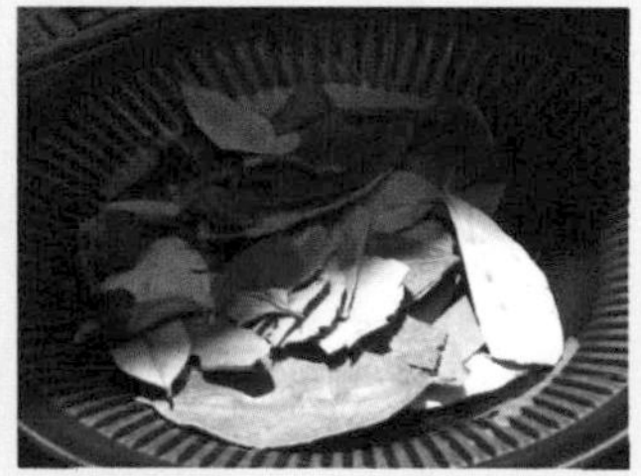

A winning herbal combination Coca-Cola is the most famous brand in the world, and a textbook example of successful global marketing. Less known is how the combination of coca and the West Africa cola or kola nut (*Cola nitida*) was developed as a soft drink because the city of Atlanta brought in alcohol prohibition in 1885. The pharmacist Dr John Pemberton (1831–88) had been experimenting with alcohol-based drinks, his *Pemberton's French Wine Cola* also containing coca and damiana. Once wine was excluded, his marketable insight was to boil coca and cola together and make the syrup palatable by running it through a soda fountain. Until 1902 Coca-Cola actually contained cocaine, but thereafter de-cocainized coca was and remains part of the closely guarded formula.

Coca *Erythroxylum coca* Erythroxylaceae

Parkinson was writing at a time when coca was little known (he includes it his Tribe 17, the *Exoticae*, or strange and outlandish plants), and he may have been reliant on travellers' tales for his account. He would not have been able to grow the plant in England, knows no Latin name, neither illustrates it nor describes its flowers. Yet for all that he is accurate about aspects of its therapeutic and cultural impact in its place of origin, reflecting historic and still-current uses of coca. This was of course a more innocent age, long before the chemical extraction of cocaine from coca (by 1860) or of the development of Coca-Cola (mid-1880s).

Parkinson is vague about where coca comes from, but his comparison of it with myrtle, native to the Mediterranean and known to his readers, is well made. The tidy rows of coca he describes, 3 to 4 feet (1m to 1.25m) high, reflect cultivation practice on the lower slopes of the eastern Andes, in present-day Peru, Colombia and Bolivia, then and now.

He is aware that dried coca leaves were used 'across Countries', as the 'chief merchandise' and indeed currency in what we would call the Inca empire. We now know that the remarkably rapid communication of information and goods through the Incan Andes was by means of runners, *chasquis*, fuelled by coca, taken in porridge, as tea (*maté de coca*) or as chewed leaves. The *chasquis* could carry up to their own body weight of goods in sacks for stints of some 20 miles (32 km) a day in the high mountains. Distance was measured in *cocadas*, the amount of coca needed for a specific journey.

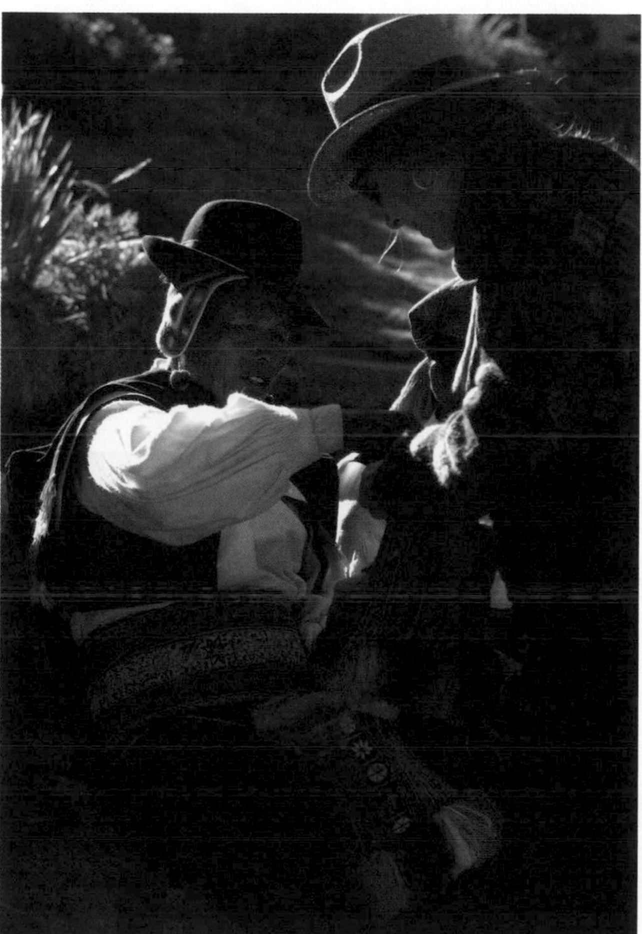

In visiting the rural Andes we saw how local men exchange coca leaves with each other and with visitors, using decorated coca bags as shown in the photograph. The exchange can be called ritualistic in that the giver can use his hands while the receiver takes it in a bag or hat, but the process is cheerfully non-monetary and a good opportunity to talk.

Parkinson also highlights that coca was, and is, chewed as quids or pellets, but not swallowed, and that it is taken along with a source of lime. He mentions oyster shells, but burnt roots of quinoa, or other *Chenopodium* species, are probably more typical. We should explain that the lime helps to extract the tropane alkaloids that provide the stimulant and fatigue-reducing effects of the coca.

Parkinson notes that coca lends great endurance and is a substitute for food and drink, but does not show specific awareness that it is used in the mountains. Nor does he know it is such a good allayer of altitude sickness and as a gastric analgesic. Visitors to Peru and Bolivia are familiar with the free distribution of *maté de coca* in hotels, for altitude acclimatization, and the fact that you can buy coca sweets and other coca goods at the airport, though you are not allowed to carry the tea out of the country, nor import coca into any country, because of drug control laws relating to cocaine.

Coltsfoote

Theatrum Botanicum

Tribe 14, Chapter 14, pp1220–21

Tussilago Herba sine flore.
Colts foote without flowers.

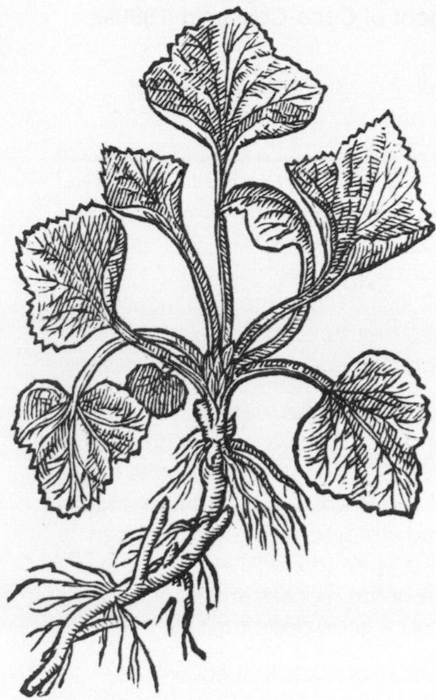

thinne rheums: watery discharge
distillations: trickling mucus
wheesings: chesty, whistling breath
Dioscorides: Greek-speaking Roman physician (fl. mid-first century AD)
Galen: Claudius Galen (AD130–200), Roman physician and writer
nightshade: one of the Solanaceae family
agues: fevers, shivers
clothes: cloths
Saint Antonies fire: erysipelas
wheales and small pushes: pimples and pustules
Matthiolus: Pierandrea Mattiolo (1501–77), physician and author
lye: ashes mixed with water and urine, to form a cleanser
salt niter: saltpetre
stroke: struck

Tussilago

The Vertues

Fresh leaves or syrup: Coltsfoote while it is fresh is cooling and drying, but when it is dry the cooling quality which remained in the moisture, being evaporate it is then somewhat hot and dry, and is best for those that have thinne rheumes and distillations upon the Lungs causing the cough, thereby to thicken and dry it, as the fresh leaves or juyce, or Syrup made thereof, is fittest for an hot dry cough, and for wheesings, and shortnesse of breath:

Smoking: the dryed leaves taken as Tabacco is in the like manner good for the thinne rheumes, distillations and coughes, as also the roote taken in like sort as *Dioscorides* and *Galen* say.

Distilled water: The distilled water hereof simply or with elder flowers and Nightshade is a singular remedy against all hot Agues, to drinke two ounces at a time,

Fomentations: and to have some clothes wet therein and applyed to the head and stomack, the same also applyed to any hot swellings or any other inflammations doth much good, yea, it helpeth that disease called Saint *Anthonies* Fire and burnings also, and is singular good to take away wheales and small pushes that rise through heate, as also against the burning heate of the piles or of the privy parts, to apply wet clothes therein to the places.

Tinder: *Matthiolus* sheweth that in the roote of this Colts foote there growth a certain Cotton or white Wooll, which being clensed from the rootes and bound up in linnen clothes and boyled in lye for a while, and afterwards some salt niter added unto it, and dryed up againe in the Sun is the best tinder to take fire, being stroke from a flint that can be had.

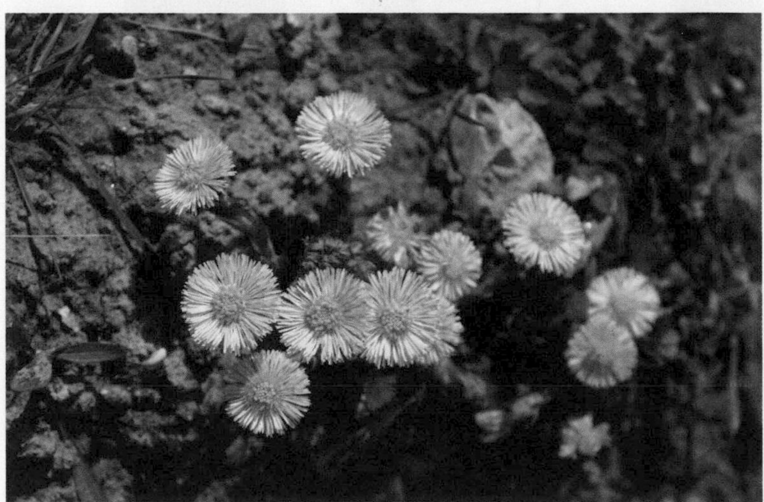

Coltsfoot *Tussilago farfara*

Asteraceae

Coltsfoot has been a favourite cough remedy for at least two thousand years in Europe, and coltsfoot rock candy is still sold for this purpose. The plant is widely naturalized in North America. Its cheery flowers appear in early spring, before the heart-shaped leaves – the old name was 'son before father' – and are followed later by fluffy seed parachutes.

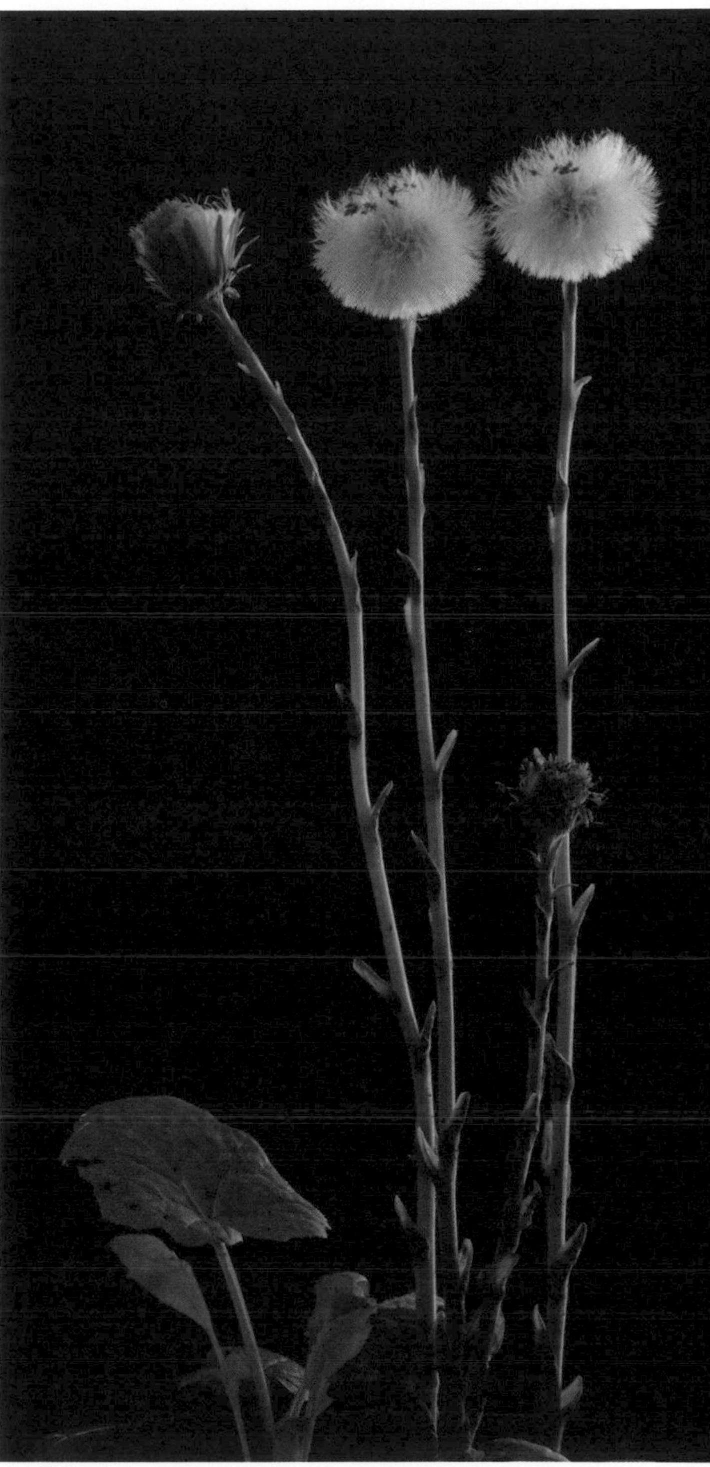

The traditional herbal use of coltsfoot has come into question in recent years with the discovery of pyrrolizidine alkaloids, a group of chemicals that can cause veno-occlusive liver disease in susceptible individuals. Coltsfoot has been banned in some countries as a result, though it contains senkirkine and not senecionine, which is the alkaloid implicated in some case studies. It is possible that adulteration with similar-looking butterbur leaves (which do contain senecionine) was the cause of the reported liver disease.

Fresh leaves or syrup: Parkinson calls attention to the different qualities of fresh and dry coltsfoot, which translate into different aspects of cough treatment, as he describes.

Smoking: Coltsfoot is still popular in herbal tobacco mixes for coughs and asthma.

Distilled water & fomentations: External uses are considered safe, and the tea or distilled water could be used as a fomentation, just as Parkinson suggests, to cool any hot condition.

Many herbalists still consider coltsfoot tea to be a safe and effective remedy for coughs, but it should only be used as needed and not long term (usually understood as more than a month).

More research hopefully will clarify the safety of the different PAs in plants (comfrey and groundsel, among plants in this book, also have high PAs). It would be useful to know whether these alkaloids are present in all parts of the plant at all times of the year, and under various growing conditions, or if they may only be produced when the plant is under stress.

Cautions: coltsfoot should not be taken internally long term, or used at all by pregnant or nursing mothers or by young children.

Comfrey

Theatrum Botanicum

Tribe 5, Chapter 24, pp522–24

3. *Symphitum tuberosum.*
Comfrey with knobbed rootes.

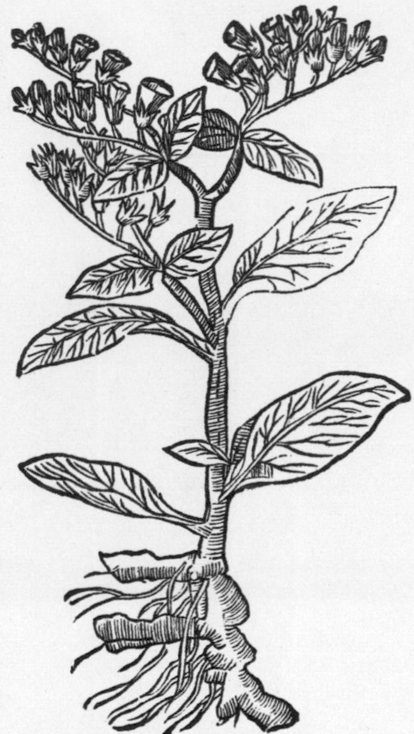

fleagme: phlegm
defluxions of the rheume: trickling down of phlegm
fits of agues: chills of fevers
alay the sharpnesse of humours: moderate the biting quality of the bodily fluids
Camerarius: Joachim Camerarius the Younger (1534–1598), German botanist and physician
Lethargy: extreme tiredness
mortifications: decay, gangrene or necrosis

Symphitum

The Vertues

The great Comfrey is as some say, cold in temperate degree, and others say hot, which is not held true, but drying and binding in a greater measure, for it helpeth those that spit blood, or that bleede at the mouth, or that make a bloody urine:

Healing: as also for all inward hurts, bruises and wounds, and helpeth the ulcers of the lungs, causing the fleagme that oppresseth them, to be easily spit forth, the roote being boyled in water or wine; the same also drunke, stayeth the defluxions of the rheume from the head upon the Lungs, the fluxes of the blood or humours, by the belly, womens immoderate courses, as well the reds as the whites, and the *gonorrhea* or the running of the raines, happening by what cause soever:

Syrup: A syrupe made thereof is very effectuall for all those inward griefes and hurts;

Distilled water: and the distilled water for the same purpose also, and for outward wounds or sores in the fleshy or sinewy parts of the body wheresoever, as also to take away the fits of agues, and to alay the sharpenesse of humours:

Decoction: a decoction of the leaves hereof is availeable to all the purposes, although not so effectuall as of the rootes: *Camerarius* saith, that two ounces of the juice drunke, doth much good in the Lethargy and dead sleepe;

Roots used externally: the rootes being outwardly applyed, helpeth fresh wounds or cuts immediately; being bruised and laid thereto, by glueing together their lips, and is especiall good for ruptures and broken bones; yea it is said to be powerfull to consolidate or knit together, whatsoever needeth knitting, that if they be boyled with dissevered peeces of flesh in a pot, it will joyne them together againe, it is good to be applyed to womens breasts, that grow sore by the aboundance of milke comming into them: as also to represse the overmuch bleeding of the hemorrhoids, to coole the inflammation of the parts thereabouts, and to give ease of paines:

the rootes of Comfrey taken fresh, beaten small, spread upon leather, and laid upon any place troubled with the gout, doe presently give ease of the paines; and applyed in the same manner, giveth ease to pained joynts, and profiteth very much for running and moist ulcers, gangrenes, mortifications, and the like, often experimented and found helpefull.

Comfrey *Symphytum officinale, S.* spp. Boraginaceae

Comfrey, a name that may be a shortening of the Latin *con firma* (making firm), is also known as knitbone, because of its remarkable ability to heal injured tissue, including broken bones. It is also used for sprains, strains and wounds, and in Parkinson's time for running colds and in uneven menstruation.

Parkinson mentions several kinds of comfrey – common great comfrey, great comfrey with purple flowers and tuberous comfrey, *Symphytum tuberosum*. Today, the comfrey most commonly found in gardens is the hybrid Russian comfrey, *Symphytum* x *uplandicum*, or the white flowered *S. orientale*. Any of the comfreys can be used externally.

Decoction of leaves: Comfrey leaf tea is usually made as an infusion today, rather than boiled to make a decoction. Comfrey infusion can be taken to heal broken bones and other injuries but it is recommended that it be taken for six weeks as a maximum, which is as long as is needed for healing a broken bone anyway. *Symphytum officinale* is the best species to use if you are going to drink comfrey tea.

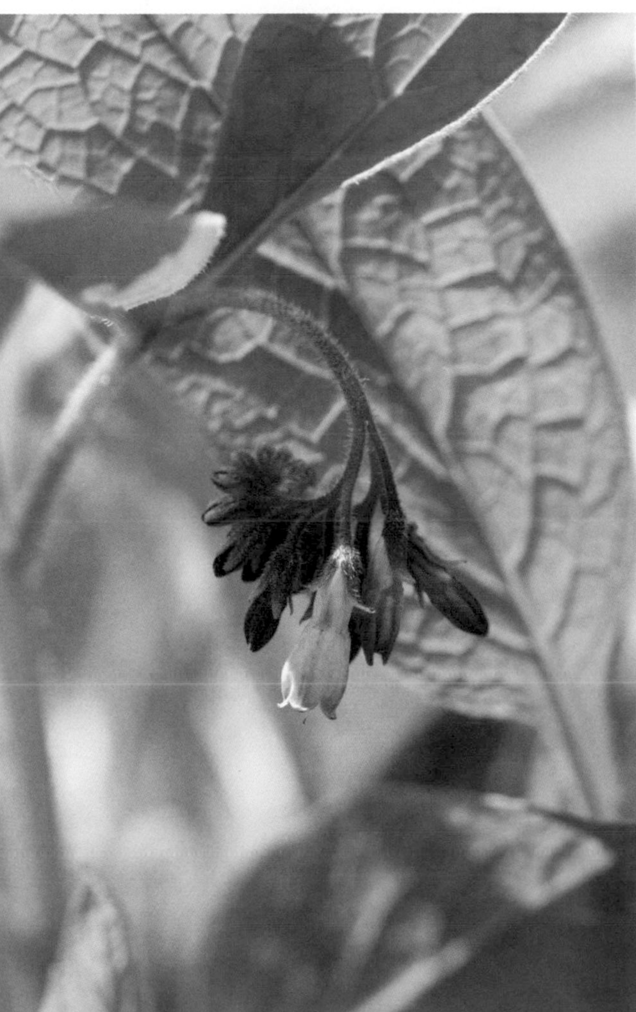

Roots used externally: Like coltsfoot, comfrey contains pyrrolizidine alkaloids, which are found in much higher levels in the root. Comfrey root is no longer recommended for internal use, but it works wonderfully well as a poultice for healing broken bones, sprains and strains. Its allantoin is a cell proliferant that helps repair damaged tissue.

Comfrey should not be used for a break until the bone has been set, as it will knit the bone together in whatever position it is in.

Before using comfrey on a wound, make sure it is clean, as otherwise the rapid healing may trap dirt and pus. Deep wounds are better healed with other herbs first, as comfrey can cause them to heal over at the surface before the underlying tissue has healed.

Comfrey poutices or ointments are great for healing bruises and grazes, and the oil or ointment can be used for skin problems and the treatment of scars.

Leaves used externally: Comfrey leaf also works remarkably well as a poultice for sprains, broken bones and other injuries. The leaf hairs can be irritating to the skin, so it is best to lay a layer of gauze on the skin first before applying the bruised or mashed leaves.

Homeopathic comfrey: Comfrey can also be taken homeopathically for injuries, as the remedy *Symphytum*, removing any danger from pyrrolizidine alkaloids.

Cautions: Comfrey root should not be taken internally at all. The leaf should not be taken internally for more than six weeks, or used internally by pregnant or nursing mothers or by young children, or by anyone with liver disease. Comfrey use is restricted in some countries.

Indian or Turkie Wheat

Theatrum Botanicum

Tribe 12, Chapter 24, pp1138–39

1. *Milium Indicum maximum Maiz dictum sive Frumentum Indicum vel Turcicum.* The usuall *Indian* or *Turkie* Wheate.

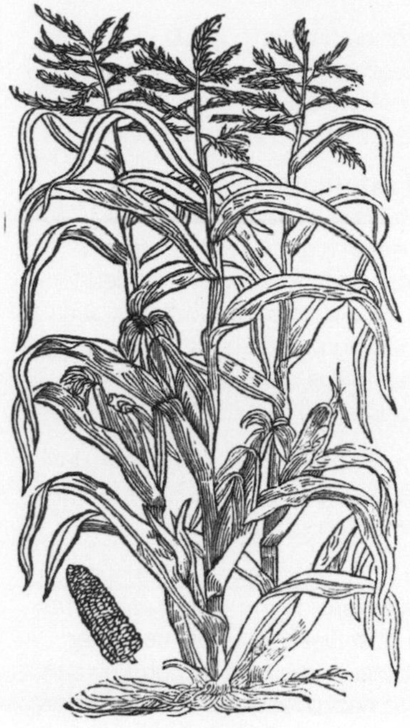

Turkie: in Parkinson's time taken to mean both the Ottoman empire and somewhere vaguely 'Eastern'
Millet: *Milium*, in both Parkinson and currently
Panicke: *Panicum*, foxtail or proso millet
meale: flour
clamminesse: moisture, oiliness
Indians: here, native peoples
suffocate: choke off
cataplasmes: plasters with herbs
Impostumes: deep-seated abscesses
Acosta: Cristóvão da Costa (1515–94), Portuguese doctor, author of 1578 *Tractado* on drugs of the East Indies
grosse blood: sticky, viscous blood
our English plantations: presumably in Virginia
beare: beer
breeding of the stone: growing of gallstones and other stones

Milium Indicum maximum Maiz dictum, sive Frumentum Indicum, vel Turcicum aliquorum

The Vertues

As a food: Many doe condemne this *Maiz* to be dry and of as little nourishment as Millet or Panicke, but they doe not as I thinke rightly consider the thing, for although the graine be dry, yet the meale thereof is nothing so dry as of the *Turkie* Millet, but hath in it some clamminesse, which bindeth the bread close and giveth good nourishment to the body, for wee finde both the Indians and the Christians of all Nations that feede thereon, are nourished thereby in as good manner no doubt, as if they fed on Wheate in the same manner:

External uses: the sweetnesse also of the bread sheweth the greater power of nourishment in it, and as some doe thinke breedeth thicke blood and humours, able to suffocate at the least to breede obstructions, and therefore will not unfitly be put into cataplasmes that are made to ripen Impostumes:

Problems of over-use: *Acosta* saith that by feeding too much thereon it engenders grosse blood, which breedeth itches and scabbes in those that were not used to it.

As a drink: Of it is made drinke also, both in the *Indies* and our *English* plantations, that will intoxicate as quickly as our strong Beare if it bee made accordingly: but is found to be very effectuall to hinder the breeding of the Stone, so that none are troubled therewith that doe drinke thereof,

As animal food: the leaves thereof are used also to fatten their Horses and cattle.

Cornsilk: what Parkinson and others missed

In describing the dried anthers of corn, Parkinson wrote of 'small long bush of threads or haires hanging downe at the ends, which when ripe are to bee cut off'. Like everyone else of his time, he saw corn silk as disposable, when in truth it is the most medicinal part of the plant and its main herbal use.

Cornsilk is now widely known as an effective, gentle urinary demulcent and diuretic, and is still 'official' for these uses in the *British Herbal Pharmacopoeia* (1996). Taken as an infusion or tea, fresh or dried cornsilk assists the body to produce urine and soothes the urinary tract. Conditions treated to good effect include cystitis, urethritis and prostatitis, oedema and kidney dysfunction. Cornsilk is also recognized for treating high blood pressure and stimulating bile production.

Corn *Zea mays*

Poaceae

Parkinson's opening line of the 'vertues' of corn is a hidden attack on John Gerard, whose *Herball* (1597; revised by Thomas Johnson in 1633) describes 'Turky wheat' as 'mean white flour and no bran; hard and dry', which 'hath in it no clamminesse at all'. Gerard says it is hard to digest, offering little or no nourishment.

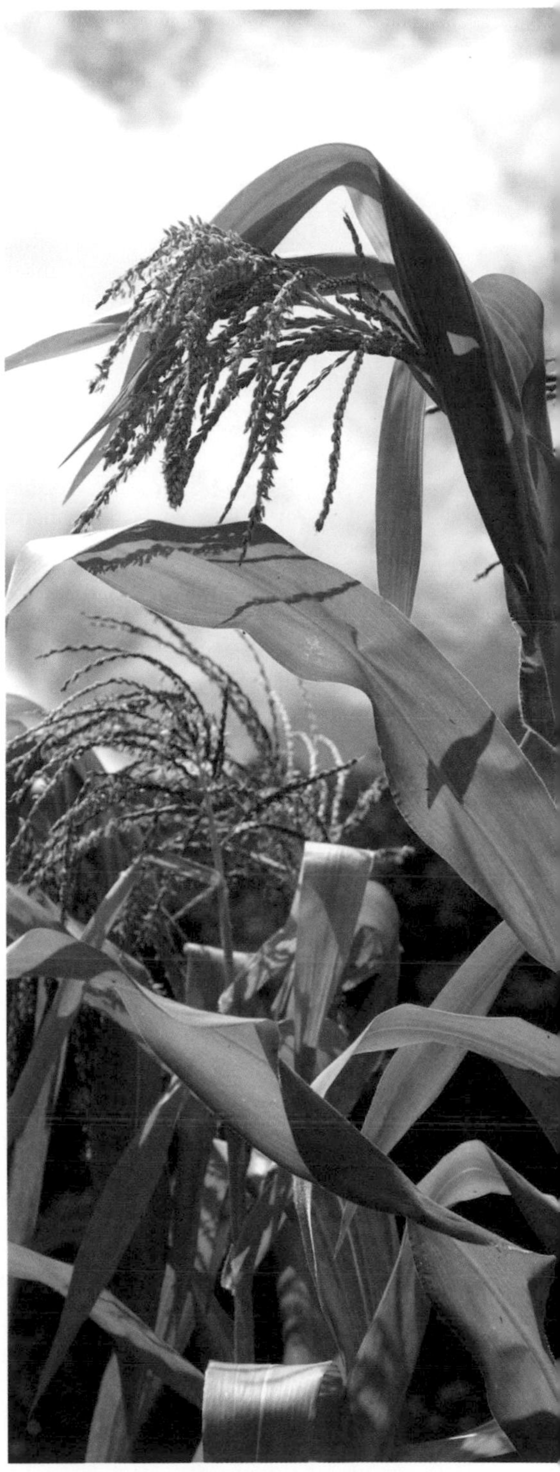

As a food: Gerard's dismissiveness goes on: 'the barbarous Indians, who know no better, are constrained to make a vertue of necessitie, and thinke it a good food'. By contrast, 'we may easily judge that it has little nourishment, and is 'of hard and evill digestion, a more convenient food for swine than for man'.

Parkinson is a much less condescending commentator, and his observations are that both Indians and Christians of all nations make good use of corn, which is as nourishing to them as English wheat. He maintains that it does have 'clamminesse', which suggests corn oil, though he did not know of this.

Gerard was utterly wrong about the pigs, incidentally. Corn is a favoured food for pigs worldwide, but even more for humanity. Its global annual tonnage now exceeds that of wheat or rice, and it is currently expanding as a food source more quickly.

External uses: Parkinson's reasoning about thick blood and humours is not the language of current medicine, but he does recognize the value of corn for use in herb poultices ('cataplasmes') to treat external skin problems, such as itches, boils and abscesses. Cornflour is drying and gentle enough for use on babies' bottoms and for nappy rash.

Problems of over-use: The Portuguese doctor Da Costa recognised the signs of skin inflammations but could not have known that an over-use of maize is implicated in the skin disease, pellagra. This condition was not identified until the 18th century, and was named after the Italian words for 'sour skin', northern Italy being particularly afflicted by the disease.

The original South American cultivators of maize knew that for good health maize needed to be soaked overnight with lime or wood ash before being ground into meal. It took until the 1930s for scientists to explain this process of *nixtamalization*.

Corn contains vitamin B3, niacin, but this is locked in until an alkali like lime of ash releases it. Not doing so can lead to diarrhoea, dermatitis, dementia and death – the '4Ds' of pellagra.

As a drink: Parkinson correctly notes in his introduction that 'The drinke made of *Maiz* is generally in the Indies called *Chica*, but by some *Acua*.' *Chica* or *chicha* remains a favourite corn drink across Central and South America, in both alcoholic and non-fermented versions, and often spiced. He is right too that its use slows the development of kidney and gall stones.

Daisie

Theatrum Botanicum
Tribe 5, Chapter 27, pp528–32

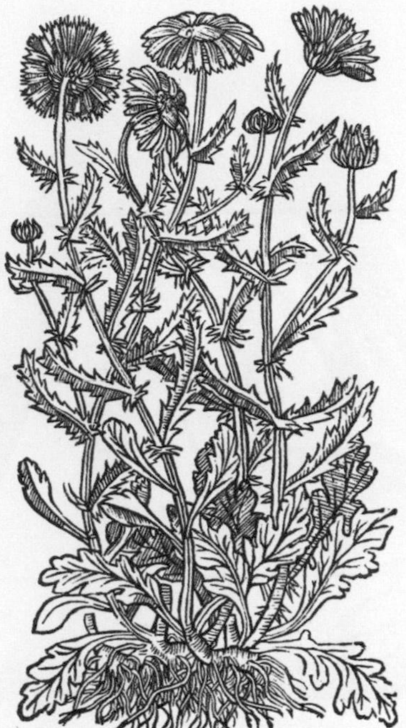
1. Bellis major vulgaris sive sylvestris.
The great white wilde Daisie.

salve: ointment
Dodoneus: Rembert Dodoens (1517–85), physician and author
consolidate: heal
choler: bile, overheating
loosen belly: biliousness
Lobel: Matthias de l'Obel (1538–1616) (Lobelius), botanist and author
sallet: salad
Mallowes: common mallow, *Malva sylvestris*
hollownesse of the breast: concavity of the chest
pustles: pustules
cods: testicles
resolve: heal, settle
Wallwort: *Sambucus ebulus*
Agrimony: *Agrimonia eupatoria*
fomented: cloth soaked in herbs
knots or kernels: hard subcutaneous growths
fals and blowes: falls and blows
moist humours: dampness, mucus

Bellis

The Vertues

Wounds: The greater wild Daisie is a wound herbe of good respect, often used and seldome left out in those drinkes or salves that are for wounds, either inward or outward: both it and the small are held by the most to be cold and dry, yet *Dodoneus* saith they are cold and moist, which none other doth allow of: for the drying qualities doe more properly consolidate,

Cooling: the juice or distilled water of either of them doth much temper the heat of choler, and refresheth the liver and other inward parts.

Salad: It is said that they loosen the belly that is bound (which *Lobel* contradicteth, and true judgement doth the same) being taken in a sallet with oile and vinegar, or the broth of fat flesh wherein the leaves herof and a few Mallowes have beene boyled:

Ulcers: they helpe to cure the wounds of the breast made in the hollownesse thereof, if a decoction be made of them and drunke; the same also doth cure all ulcers, and pustles in the mouth or tongue, or in the secret parts:

Hot swellings: the leaves bruised and applyed to the cods, or to any other parts that are swollen and hot, doth resolve it, and temper the heat;

Palsie, sciatica & gout: they are also much commended that a decoction be made hereof and of Wallwort, and *Agrimony*, and the places fomented, or bathed therewith warme, that are afflicted either with the palsie, the Sciatica, or the gout, to give a great deale of ease of paine:

Growths, bruises & ruptures: the same also dissolveth and disperseth the knots or kernels that grow in the flesh of any part of the body, and bruises and hurts that come of fals and blowes; they are also used for ruptures, or other inward burstings with very good successe:

Ointment: an ointment made thereof doth wonderfully helpe all wounds, that have inflammations about them, or by reason of moist humours having accesse unto them, are kept long from healing, and those are such for the most part that happen in the joynts of the armes; and legges:

Watery eyes: the juice of them dropped into the running eyes of any doth much helpe them:

Small daisy: the small Daisie is held to be more tringent and binding then any other sort.

Daisies *Bellis perennis & Leucanthemum vulgare* Asteraceae

Parkinson describes 13 daisies, including a large white daisy from America and a yellow daisy 'brought me out of Italy, by Mr. Dr. Flud, with many other seedes, that grew in the Garden of Pisa, in the Duke of Florence his dominions, but of whence it is naturall, I have not yet certainly knowne'. Common daisy (*Bellis perennis*) and ox-eye daisy (*Leucanthemum vulgare*) are universal in gardens, and the latter grows wild today.

Wound herbs: Using daisy and ox-eye daisy as wound herbs is unfashionable in our times, but this was their main virtue in Parkinson's day, as an infusion taken inwardly or an ointment externally. Given the ubiquity of the plants, it is good to know you have an effective vulnerary in the lawn or flowerbed.

Cooling: Parkinson reinforces the cooling message by recommending the juice or distilled water for hot conditions and a liver cleanse. In these actions the daisies are similar to chamomile, a distant relative.

Salad: The flowerheads are tasty when fried in a batter, and the buds are like capers. We use the petals as a garnish in summer salads, and taking them with oil and vinegar would be an interesting idea, with or without his mallow buds.

Ulcers: We are not sure why daisy is a specific for breast wounds (though in France it is used for breast enlargement), as Parkinson proposes, but the plants' acridity and slight astringency would make them effective in treating ulcers and pustules.

Hot swellings: Again the cooling qualities of daisy are recommended to temper the heat of swellings. In Australia and the American West, ox-eye daisy, an introduced alien, can cause contact dermatitis in sensitive skins.

Palsy, sciatica & gout: Adding elder and agrimony to a daisy decoction and using this as a warm fomentation will give topical relief in the painful conditions mentioned.

Growths, bruises & ruptures: The old Northern English name of bruisewort for daisy refers to its former reputation; this remains a current homeopathic use, though rarely now a herbal one. John Hill's *Family Herbal* of 1812 (pp107–8) laments that daisy is 'too much neglected for its virtues'.

Ointment: Parkinson returns to the wound theme, adding the detail that daisy is effective as an ointment where there is excess moisture or inflammations.

Watery eyes: In Ireland, ox-eye daisy was popularly used to bathe sore eyes.

Small daisy: The common daisy, as Parkinson says, is slightly more astringent. What he omits to mention is that ox-eye daisy had a reputation as an antispasmodic, being used to soothe whooping cough and asthma; it was also sweat-inducing, and a specific for night sweats.

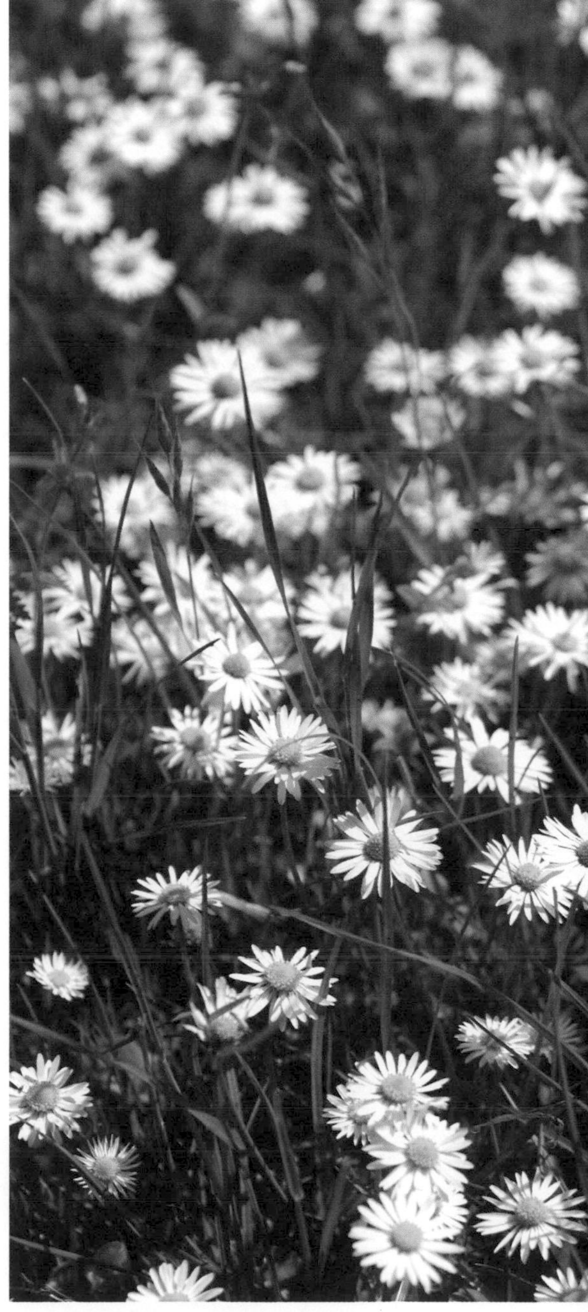

Dandelion

Theatrum Botanicum

Tribe 6, Chapter 26, pp780–82

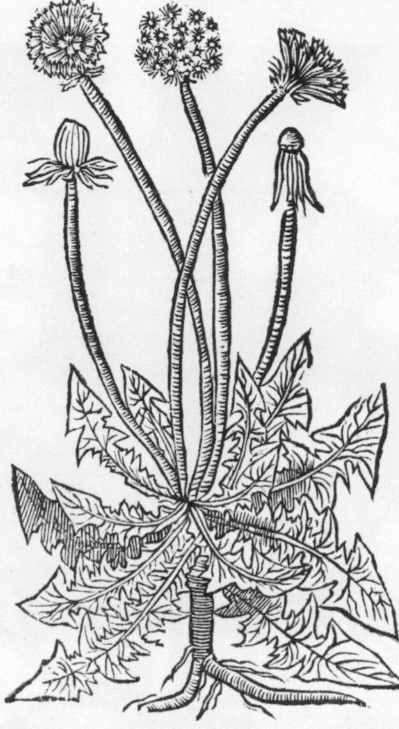

1. *Dens leonis vulgaris.* Common Dandelion.

succory: chicory, *Cichorium intybus*
hypochondriacall passion: hysteria
uritorie parts: urinary system
meseraicall veins: mesenteric veins
apostumes: abscesses
whited: blanched
sallet: salad
allisanders: alexanders, *Smyrnium olusatrum*
macilent: shrivelled or thin
consumption: wasting disease, pulmonary tuberculosis
Cachexia: irreversible loss of bodily mass from chronic illness
ague: fever
pestentiall: pestilential, deadly

Dens leonis

The Vertues

Liver, gall bladder & spleen: Dandelion is neare in propertie unto the wilde Succory, and by the bitternesse doth more open and clense, and is therefore very effectuall for the obstructions of the liver, gall and spleene, and the diseases that arise from them, as the jaundise and the *hypochondriacall* passion,

Diuretic effect: it wonderfully openeth the uritorie parts, causing abundance of urine, not onely in children whose meseraicall veines are not sufficiently strong to containe the quantitie of urine drawne in the night, but that then without restraint or keeping it backe they water their beds, but in those of old age also upon the stopping or yeelding small quantitie of urine;

Urinary ulcers: it also powerfully clenseth apostumes and inward ulcers in the uritorie passages, and by the drying and temperate qualitie doth afterwards heale them, and for those purposes the rootes being buried a while in sand and whited (which taketh away much of the bitternesse, and maketh them the more tender) being eaten as a sallet are more effectuall than the leaves used in the same manner, or who so are not accustomed to such raw sallets may take the decoction of the rootes or leaves in white wine, or the leaves chopped as pot herbes with a few Allisanders boiled in their broth.

Cancer: And who so is macilent drawing towards a consumption, or hath an evill disposition of the whole body, ready to fall into a *Cachexia* by the use hereof for some time together shall finde a wonderfull helpe, not onely in clensing the malignant humors but strengthening the good, and preserving the body sound in all his functions;

Sleep: it helpeth also to procure rest and sleepe to bodies distempered by the heate of ague fits or otherwise:

Distilled water: the destilled water also is effectuall to drinke in pestentiall fevers and to wash the sores.

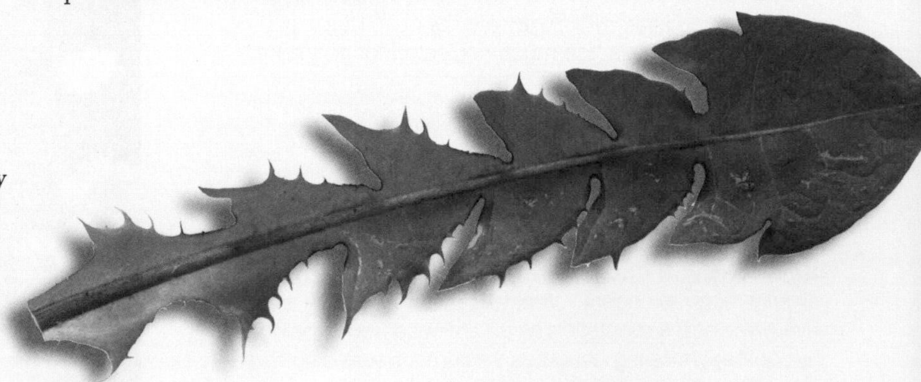

Dandelion *Taraxacum officinale* Asteraceae

Dandelions are still used for liver and gallbladder problems, and as a diuretic, just as in Parkinson's day. They are highly nutritious, being especially rich in potassium and other minerals. They grow all over the world in temperate and subtropical zones and have such a range of medicinal uses that they deserve to be valued, rather than just weeded out!

Dandelions are highly nutritious. Their long tap roots draw up minerals and other nutrients from deep in the soil. All parts of the plant are edible and medicinal. The leaves and roots are bitter, unless blanched as Parkinson describes, but the bitterness is part of their therapeutic value.

The flowers still have a hint of bitterness but are sweeter, especially if picked on a warm sunny day. You can make tasty dandelion fritters by picking and washing the flowers, dipping them wet in flour and sauteeing them for a few minutes. A crunchy mouthful!

All parts of the plant have similar properties, but the roots have the strongest effect on the liver. The leaves have more diuretic qualities, while the flowers have a relaxing effect. Dandelions are often used for skin problems, for their cleansing action through the liver and kidneys. Traditionally they are combined with burdock root for skin conditions as well as in the European root beer known as dandelion and burdock.

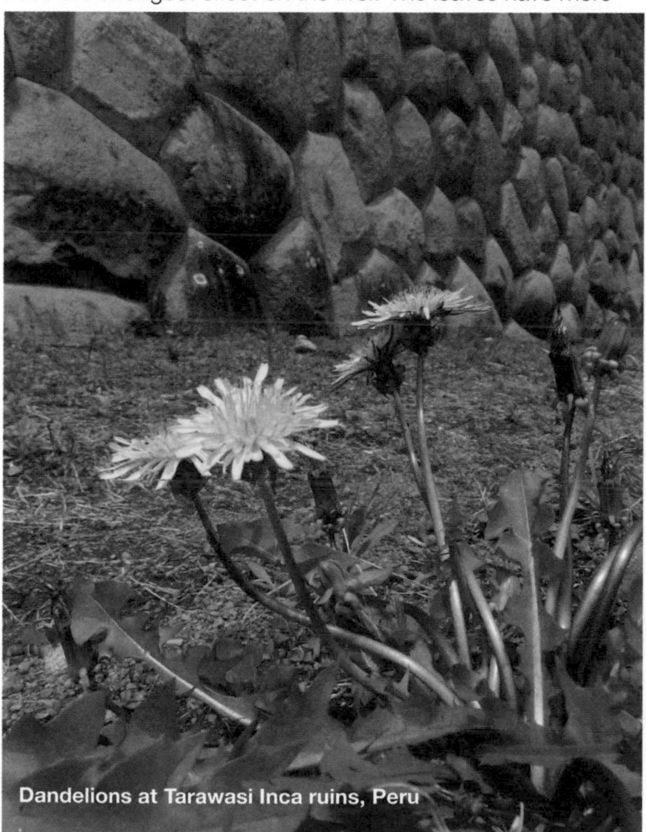

Dandelions at Tarawasi Inca ruins, Peru

Liver, gallbladder & spleen: The bitterness of dandelions stimulates digestion and cools and cleanses the liver, promoting the flow of bile. Parkinson calls their effect 'opening'.

The **diuretic effect** of dandelions is acknowledged in some of its common names such as piss-en-lit and pissabed. Dandelion is the perfect diuretic because it is high in potassium. Potassium is leached from the body when the kidneys are stimulated to excrete more water, and deficiency can result from long-term use of standard diuretic drugs. Being diuretic, dandelion has a role to play in high blood pressure as well as in swellings and dropsy. It is an excellent remedy for older people with scanty urine, as Parkinson notes.

Surprisingly, dandelions are also good to treat bed-wetting, as Parkinson mentions, by strengthening and toning the whole urinary system.

Urinary ulcers: Dandelion is still a remedy for ulcers and for urinary problems, but this use is not so widely known now as in Parkinson's day.

Cancer & cachexia: Dandelions detoxify the whole body, but are also nourishing and building, so the use for cancer and chronic diseases makes perfect sense.

Sleep: Not normally thought of as a sleep remedy, dandelion is cooling and cleansing so would holp give relief in fevers and other hot conditions.

Distilled water: The herbal water is cooling and cleansing, and would still be a valid treatment for measles, chickenpox and similar illnesses.

Docke

Theatrum Botanicum

Tribe 14, Chapter10, pp1224–27

4. *Lapathum sylvestre vulgatius.* The ordinary wilde Docke.

Bloodwort: *Rumex sanguineus* var. *sanguineusia*
Theophrastus: Greek philosopher (c.371–c.287BC)
inter oleracea: pertaining to kitchen gardens
stay laskes: stop diarrhoea
subversions of the stomacke: disorders of the stomach
English rhubarb: *Rheum rhabarbarum*
Munkes Rhubarbe: *Rumex patientia* or *R. alpina*
Dioscorides: Greek-speaking Roman physician (mid-first century AD)
Pliny: Pliny the Elder (AD23–79), Roman naturalist
morphews: skin discolouration
mollifying: soothing

Lapathum

The Vertues

All the sorts of Dockes have a kind of cooling but not all alike drying quality, for the Sorrels are more cold then any of the rest, and the Bloodwort more drying, but the seedes of most of them be drying and binding: some of them besides the Sorrell were used to be eaten.

Leaves: *Theophrastus* therefore put them *inter oleracea,* and for the most part the leaves were stewed or boyled, and so they did the more easily passe through the belly, without giving any great or good nourishment, saving a moisture to the body.

Seed: The seede of most as I said, either of the Garden or the fieldes, doth stay laskes and fluxes of all sorts, and the subversions or loathings of the stomacke through choller, and is helpefull to those that spit blood.

Roots: The rootes likewise of the most of them except the *Rhaes* or Rhubarbs, and the red Dock are drying and binding, conducing to the same effects aforesaid, but all they have an opening quality to them, fit to loosen and make the body soluble, and are therefore of greater use then all the other parts besides, opening the obstructions of the blood, and cooling and clensing the blood, and helping those that have the jaundice, and for that purpose are our *English,* and Munkes Rubarbe, the Garden and the wild red Dockes used with other things to make diet Ale or Beere:

Scorpions: the seede being taken in wine helpeth the bitings of the Scorpion saith *Dioscorides* and *Pliny.*

Skin: The rootes boyled in vinegar, helpeth the itch, scabbes and other breakings out in the skinne, if they be bathed therewith,

Distilled water: the distilled water of the herbe and rootes tendeth to the same effect, and besides clenseth the skinne of freckles, morphews, and all other spots and discolourings therein.

Good King Henry: The *English* Mercury as it is called, or good *Henry* the roote is drying and clensing, the herbe is mollifying and loosening, by reason of the fatnesse or moist slipperinesse therein taken inwardly, but applyed outwardly to woundes and sores, it clenseth the foulenesse and healeth and closeth them up afterwards wonderfully.

Rhubarb & sorrel: The properties of the Rubarbes, and the Sorrels are severally declared before in their proper places.

Good King Henry *Chenopodium bonus-henricus*

This plant is mainly grown as a perennial green vegetable, which can be cooked like spinach. The leaves are too mealy for it to be palatable raw, but it is tasty when cooked, though more popular in times past.

Dock *Rumex* spp.

Polygonaceae

Docks are found around the world, and are used medicinally by people wherever they occur, usually as a cooling and cleansing remedy.

In his treatment Parkinson covers several species of docks and their relatives, and discusses the wild ones or those 'found in the fieldes and wet places where they grow'.

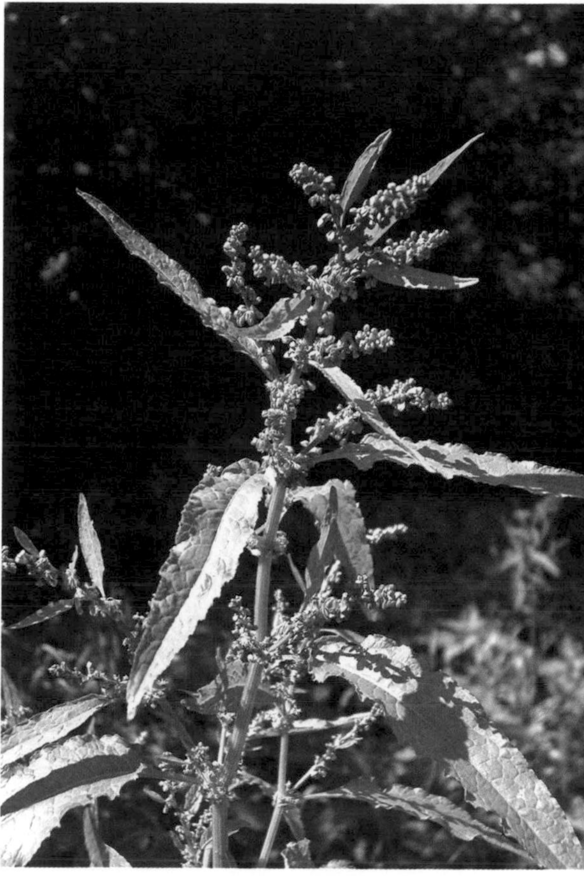

Leaves: The young leaves of curled dock in the spring are very tasty when cooked like spinach. We like to add them to nettle soup, too. They very quickly lose their bright green colour on heating, becoming a shade of olive, but they are delicious – tender, with a lemony tang.

The lemony taste is due to oxalic acid in the leaves, which in theory can cause problems for people prone to kidney stones, which are mostly made up of oxalates or mineral salts of oxalic acid. Boiling reduces the amounts of soluble oxalates present in foods. But to keep it in perspective, spinach and many other green vegetables contain oxalates, as do tea, coffee, chocolate and other foods, and our bodies manufacture their own oxalates from vitamin C.

The young, mucilaginous growing tips of dock are used in Peru to treat tooth abscesses and boils. Young leaves can be applied as a poultice to boils.

Seed: Herbalists today make little use of the seed of dock.

Roots: The roots are the part most often used in western herbalism today. Any of the docks with a yellow root can be used, but the species most often employed and referred to as yellow dock is *Rumex crispus*, the curled dock.

The yellow colour and distinctive smell are from the anthraquinones present in the root. These substances give dock its gentle laxative effect. The related Chinese rhubarb, *Rheum palmatum*, has a much stronger laxative effect.

Dock increases the flow of bile from the liver and gallbladder, which would help clear jaundice, just as Parkinson says. Its cooling action is beneficial to an inflammed liver. Dock is also good for disorders of the spleen and lymph, and therefore helps the immune system generally.

The old name for dock, *Lapathum*, means blood purifier. It has been traditional as such since the ancient Greeks, and is used that way in Chinese medicine and in India today. It is still considered to cleanse the blood in western terms, and is helpful for clearing skin problems such as acne and eczema. Dock root is also used for arthritic and rheumatic conditions.

We consider dock to be a gentle laxative, which fits with the 'opening quality' Parkinson mentions for the roots. The decoction or a tincture work well for mild constipation and lack of appetite, stimulating the digestion.

In an apparent paradox, quite common with herbs, dock is also used to treat diarrhoea and dysentery. It is also used for enteritis, gastritis and rumbling appendicitis.

Dock combines well with dandelion, burdock, nettles and cleavers in a detoxifying formula.

Caution: Do not take while pregnant.

Elder

Theatrum Botanicum

Tribe 2, Chapter 24, pp207–11

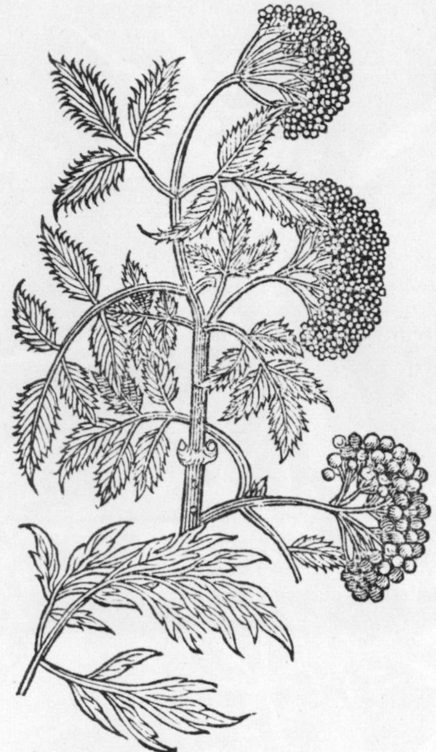
1.&.3. *Sambucus vulgaris & Laciniatis folijs.* The common and the jagged Elder.

Sambucus

The Vertues

Common elder/black elder

Both *Dioscorides* and *Galen* doe attribute to the Wallworte, as well as to the common Elder, (for they account their properties both one) an heating and drying quality, purging watery humors aboundantly, but not without trouble to the stomacke:

Spring shoots: the first shootes of the common Elder boyled like unto *Asparagus,* and the young leaves and stalkes boyled in fat broth, draweth forth mightily choller and tough flegme; the tender leaves also eaten with oyle and salt doe the same:

Bark & berries: the middle or inner barke boyled in water, and given to drinke, worketh much more violently; and the berries also either greene or dry, expell the same humors, and is often given with good successe to helpe the dropsie, by evacuating great plenty of waterish humors:

Root bark: the barke of the roote also boyled in wine, or the juyce thereof drunke, worketh the same effects but more effectually, then either leaves or fruite doe; the juyce of the roote taken provoketh vomit mightily, and purgeth the watery humors of the dropsie; the same decoction of the roote cureth the biting of the viper or adder, as also of a mad dogge, and mollifieth the hardnesse of the mother, if women sit therein, and openeth the veines and bringeth downe their courses:

Berries boiled in wine: the berries boyled in wine performe the same effects; the haire of the head or of other parts washed therewith, is made blacke;

Leaves: the juyce of the greene leaves applyed to the hot inflammations of the eyes, asswageth them: the leaves boyled until they be tender, then beaten and mixed with barly meale, and applyed to hot inflammations asswageth them, and helpeth places that are burnt either by fire or water, cureth fistulous ulcers being layde thereupon, and easeth the paines of the goute, being beaten and boyled with the tallow of a bull or goate, and layd warme thereon: the juyce of the leaves snuffed up the nostrills, purgeth the tunicles of the braine;

Berries: the juyce of the berries boyled with a little honey, and dropped into the eares, easeth the paines of them; the decoction of the berries in wine being drunke, provoketh urine:

Seeds: the powder of the seedes, first prepared in vinegar, and then taken in wine, halfe a dramme at a time, for certaines dayes together, is

Galen: Claudius Galen (AD130–200), Roman physician and author
Wallworte: dwarf elder (*Sambucus ebulus*); also Danewort
watery humors: bodily fluids
fat broth: rich soup
choller: choler: one of humours, bile
tough flegme: tenacious phlegm
oyle: oil
dropsie: oedema
mollifieth: eases
hardnesse of the mother: possibly fibroids in the womb
sit therein: i.e. in a bath
bringeth down courses: causes menstruation to begin
asswageth: relieves
barly meale: barley flour
fistulous ulcers: tubelike ulcers
tallow: rendered suet

Elder *Sambucus* spp. Adoxaceae

Elder has been described as a whole medicine chest in one plant, and Parkinson's account certainly supports this huge variety of uses for the different parts of the plant.

Elders are found in Europe, Asia, North and South America and Australia. Most species have black or red berries, but the Australian species have white or yellow berries.

Black elder *Sambucus nigra*

The black-berried elder is the main species used medicinally and for food. North American (*S. nigra* ssp. *canadensis*) and other black-berried elders and blue-berried elder (*S. nigra* ssp. *cerulea*) are variously considered sub-species or separate but similar species of the European black elder.

Spring shoots: The young shoots are still eaten by some foragers, who usually soak them in salted water overnight before cooking them. We've never tried them so cannot comment on the flavour, but don't doubt that they would have the effects Parkinson describes.

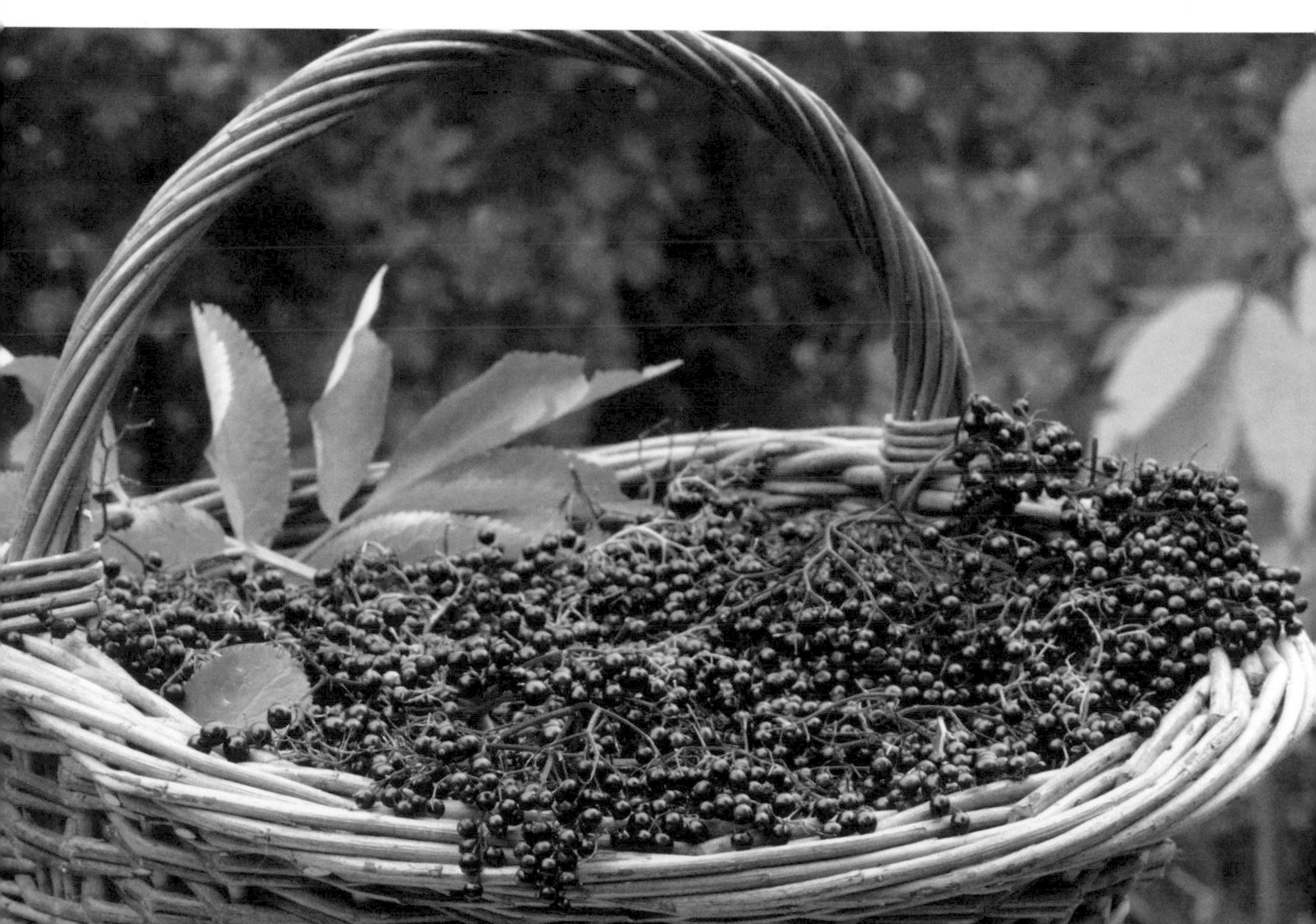

tunicles: membranes
half a dram: 1/16th oz, 1.95 gm
abate and consume: diminish and reduce
white tartar: residue from inside of wine cask
decoction: boiled in water
glisters: enemas
chollick: colic, severe griping pain of stomach
attenuating: thinning, diluting
digesting: dispersing
morphew: discolouration of skin
Matthiolus: Pierandrea Mattioli (1501–77), physician and author
maceration: soaking herb in a solvent
insolation: placing in sun's rays
gratefull: pleasing
quicken: stimulate
Syropus acetosus: medicinal syrup made with vinegar
apostume: large, deep abscess
timpanie: morbid swelling or tumour
taking fasting: refraining from eating
sallet: salad
on the fire: reheat
new wax: beeswax
vernish: varnish
ioyners: joiners, carpenters
Olibanum: frankincense: gum resin of *Boswellia*

a meanes to abate and consume the fat flesh of a corpulent body, and keepe it leane: the berries so prepared, and as much white tartar and a few aniseede put to them, a dramme of this powder given in wine, cureth the dropsie humour, by purging very gently:

Dry flowers: the dry flowers are often used in the decoctions of glisters to expell winde and ease the chollicke, for they lose their purging quality which they have being greene, and retaine an attenuating and digesting propertie being dryed:

Distilled water: the distilled water of the flowers, is of much use to cleare the skinne from sunne burning, freckles, morphew, or the like: and as *Matthiolus* saith both the forepart and hinderpart of the head, being bathed therewith, it taketh away all manner of the headach that commeth of a cold cause.

Elderflower vinegar: The Vinegar made of flowers of the Elder by maceration and insolation, is much more used in *France,* than any where else, and is gratefull to the stomacke, and of great power and effect to quicken the appetite, and helpeth to cut grosse or tough flegme in the chest. A *Syrupus acetosus* made hereof, would worke much better than the ordinary, for these purposes.

Leaves: The leaves boyled and layd hot, upon any hot and painefull apostumes, especially in the more remote and sinewie parts, doth both coole the heate and inflammation of them, and ease the paines.

Distilled water of bark: The distilled water of the inner barke of the tree or of the roote, is very powerfull to purge the watery humors of the dropsie or timpanie, taking it fasting and two houres before supper:

Burns: *Matthiolus* giveth the receipt of a medecine to helpe any burning by fire or water, which is made in this manner; take saith he, one pound of the inner barke of the Elder, bruise it or cut it small and put it into two pound of fine sallet oyle, or oyle Olive, that hath beene first washed oftentimes with the distilled water of Elder flowers, let them boyle gently a good while together, and afterwards straine forth the oyle, pressing it very hard; set this oyle on the fire againe, and put thereto, foure ounces of the juyce of the young branches and leaves of the Elder tree, and as much new wax: let them boyle to the consumption of the juyce, after which being taken from the fire, put presently thereunto, two ounces of liquid Vernish, (such as Ioyners use to vernish their bedsteeds, cupboards tables &c.) and afterwards of *Olibanum* in fine powder foure ounces, and the whites of two egges, being first well beaten by themselves, all these being well stirred and mixed together, put it up into a cleane pot, and keepe it for to use when occasion serveth.

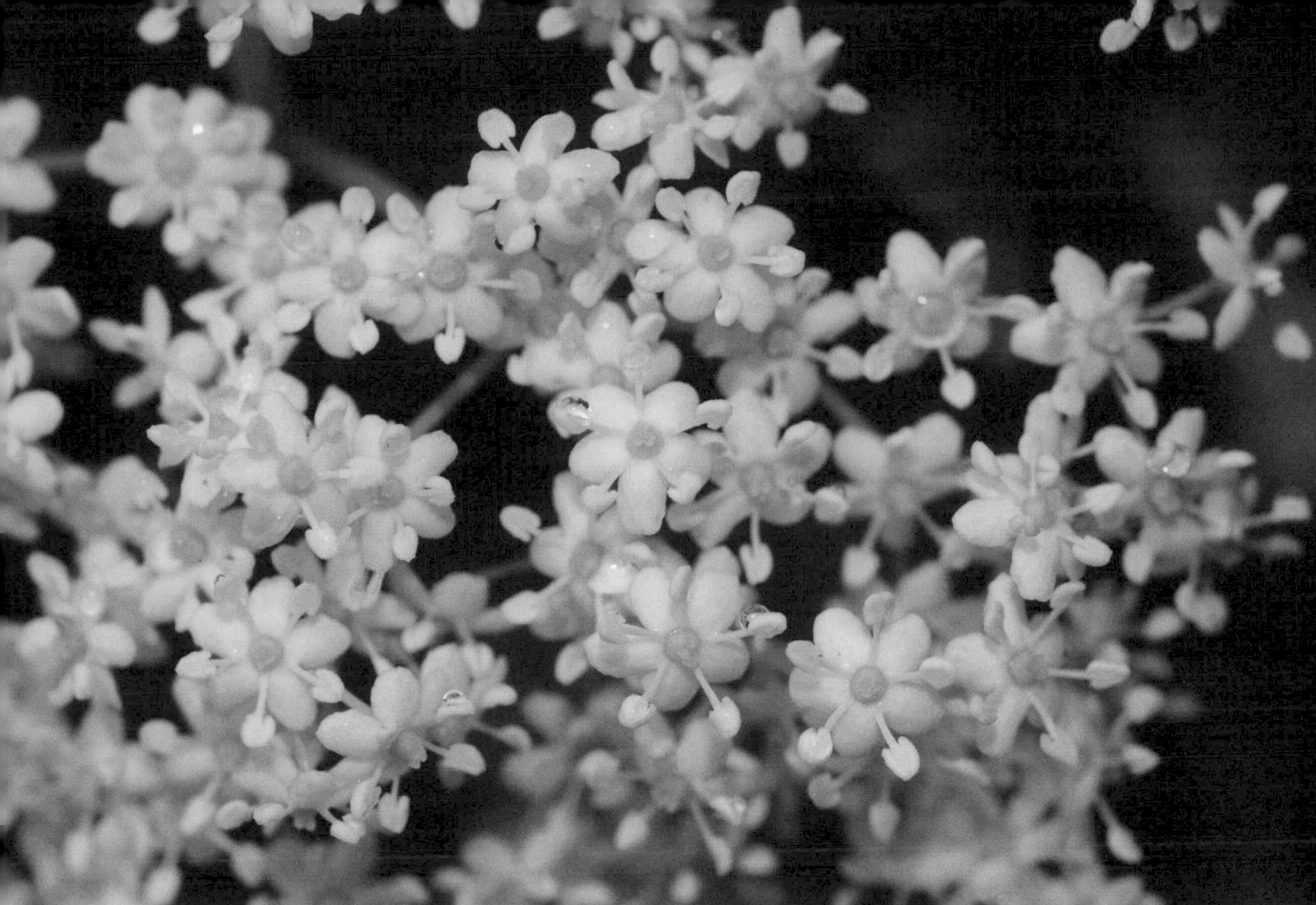

Bark: Elder bark and root bark is little used by modern herbalists, because it produces such a strong purging effect. Vomiting is less popular as a treatment than it was for our ancestors.

Leaves: We use the leaves in an ointment, which is good for bruises, and can also be used for burns after the burned place has been cooled in water for several minutes.

A hot leaf poultice as Parkinson prescribes, with or without barley meal, would be helpful for painful hot inflammations.

Seeds: The seeds aren't used much any more, but they have a purging effect, as you will know if you have ever eaten the raw berries in any quantity. Their qualities change when cooked and probably on drying and powdering, or by soaking in vinegar, as Parkinson suggests.

Flowers: Many people are familiar with elderflower cordial and the fizzy elderflower drinks made by gentle fermentation with the natural yeasts found on the flowers. They are also used to make fritters and to flavour desserts.

It is interesting that Parkinson understood the different effects of the fresh and the dry flowers. We know from our own experience that the fresh flowers made as an infusion and drunk hot produce a stronger fever and sweating than the gentler tea made from dried flowers.

Parkinson suggests using a decoction of the dried flowers as an enema in trying to expel wind and ease colic.

We use the flowers to reduce the symptoms of hay-fever and colds. The cold tea is a diuretic and is used for fluid retention. It also helps reduce night sweats.

Distilled water: We love the distilled water of elderflowers. The fresh lemony tang raises the spirits and reminds us of summer. Julie often adds a little elderflower water to her tincture formulae to lift and activate them, and finds it helpful in cases of depression as it does uplift the spirits.

It has a long tradition of use as a skin remedy to keep the skin clear and free from freckles. Elderflower water can also be used as a soothing eyewash for hot gritty eyes or inflamed and bloodshot eyes,

4. Sambucus racemosa rubra.
Red Berried Elder.

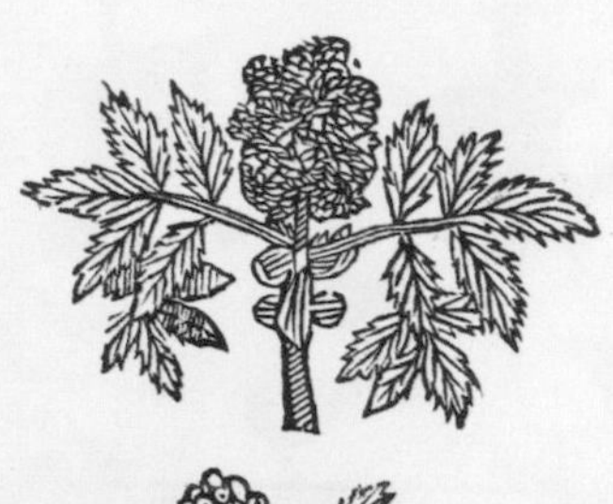

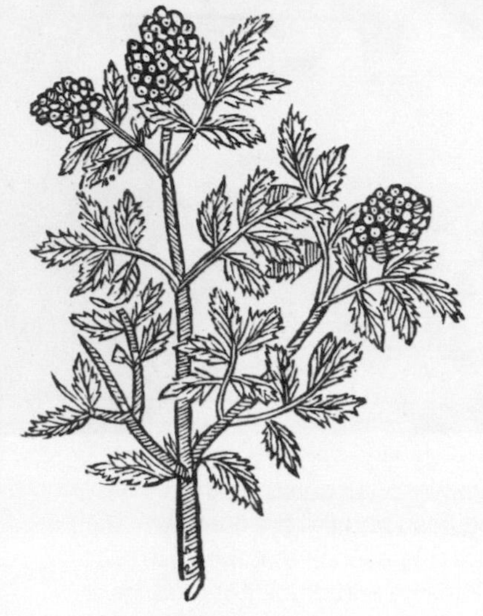

powder: snuff
staieth: stops
tunned up: in casks
Muscadine: sweet wine
fundament: anus or buttocks
piles: haemorrhoids
renued: adding warm water
bloud shotten: bloodshot
palsie: tremors
Fistulous: hollow
stale: stall
Iewes ears: edible brown fungus of Elder, *Auricularia auricula-judae*
Pellitory of Spaine: pellitory, *Anacyclus pyrethrum*

Gout: The young buddes, and leaves of the Elder, and as much of the rootes of Plantaine beaten together, and boyled in old Hogs grease, this being laid warme upon the place, pained with the gout doth give present ease thereto.

Nosebleeds: The leaves also burned and the pouder of them put up into the nostrills, staieth the bleeding being once or twice used.

Flavouring wine & ale: If you shall put some of the fresh flowers of Elders into a bagge, letting it hang in a vessell of wine, when it is new made, and beggineth to boyle (I thinke the like may be tried with a vessell of ale or beere new tunned up, and set to worke together) the bagge being a little pressed every evening, for a seaven night together, giveth to the wine a very good rellish, and smell like Muscadine, (and will do little lesse to ale or beere)

Piles: The leaves of Elders boyled tender and applied warme to the fundament, easeth the paines of the piles, if they be once or twice renued growing cold;

Ulcers: The foule inflamed or old ulcers and sores of the legges, being often washed with the water, of the leaves or of the flowers distilled in the middle of the moneth on May, doth heale them in a short space.

Eyes: The distilled water of the flowers, taketh away the heate and inflammation of the eyes, and helpeth them when they are bloud shotten.

Palsy: The hands being washed morning and evening with the same water of the flowers, doth much helpe and ease them that have the Palsie in them, and cannot keepe them from shaking.

Pith of stalks: The pith in the middle of the Elder stalkes, being dried and put into the cavernous holes of Fistulous ulcers, that are ready to close, openeth and dilateth the orifices, whereby injections may be used, and other remedies applied for the cure of them. It is said that if you gently strike a horse that cannot stale, with a sticke of this Elder, and binde some of the leaves to his belly, it shall make him stale quickly.

Jelly ear fungus

The Mushromes of the Elder called Iewes eares, are of much use being dried to be boyled with Ale or Milke with Columbine leaves for sore throates, and with a little Pepper and Pellitory of *Spaine* in powder, to put up the *uvula* or pallet of the mouth when it is fallen downe. *Matthiolus* saith that the dried Iewes eares steeped in Rosewater, and applied to the temples and forehead, doe ease the paines of the head or headach.

Eldeflower vinegar: We make elderflower vinegar in the summer and use it in salad dressings to add a light lemony flavour. White wine vinegar gives the best flavour, but cider vinegar can be used. It can also be mixed with honey and used as a cordial remedy for colds and sore throats.

Flavouring wine & ale: Fresh elderflowers give a pleasant flavour to wine, and several small British breweries still make an elderflower ale.

Berries: The berries are popular as food in Europe, often being cooked with apple in winter puddings. They keep well in the freezer.

Medicinally, the berries are an effective immune booster and can be used as a syrup, alcohol-based tincture or as a glycerite to prevent and treat colds and flu. We like to make a glycerite that begins with the flowers in summer and then add the berries in the autumn/fall. It is delicious and can be given to children and adults through the winter months.

Elderflowers are used in Sambuca, a strong liquor also flavoured with aniseed and other herbs.

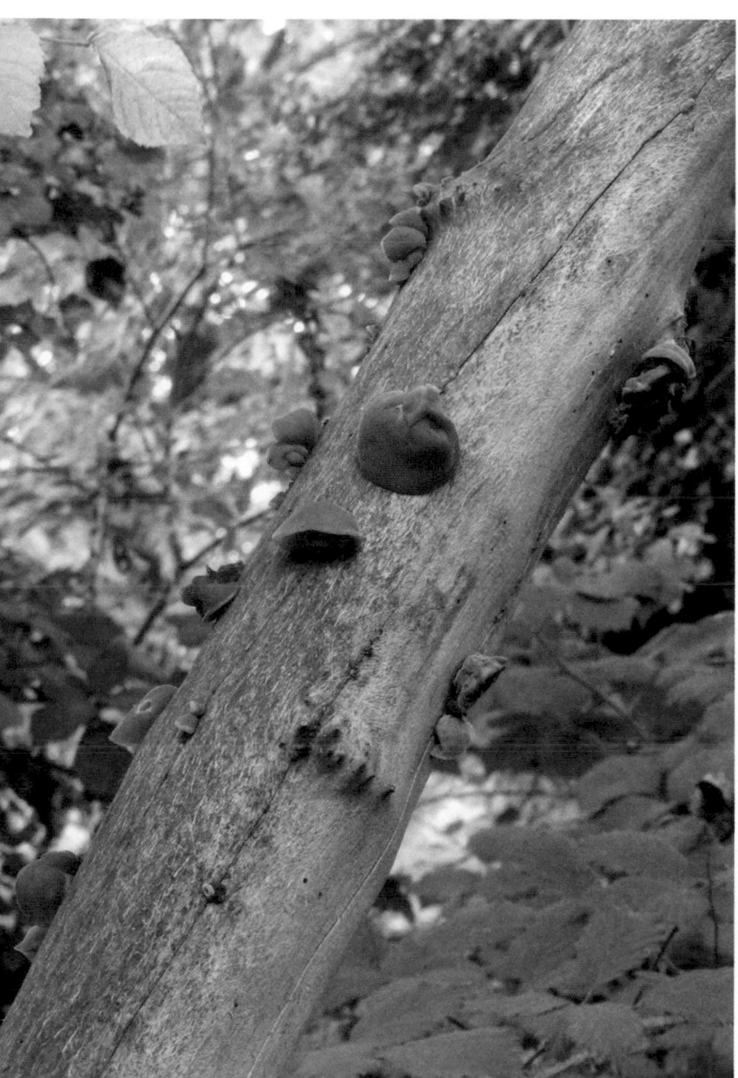

Jelly ear fungus

Auricularia auricula-judae

This fungus is found world-wide, and is used for food and medicine in many cultures. In Europe and North America it mainly grows on elder.

In Chinese food, it is a main ingredient in hot and sour soup, giving its unusual texture to the dish and absorbing other flavours well. It has been used in Chinese medicine for a variety of conditions, including as a strengthening tonic and to treat haemorrhoids.

There have been a number of experiments on jelly ear fungus. It has been found to boost the immune system and have antiviral, antibacterial and antiparasitic effects.

In animal studies it has been shown to reduce blood levels of cholesterol and glucose, making it potentially useful for diabetics and for treating circulatory problems. It has also been shown to reduce blood clotting.

It may have a fertility-lowering effect, so is best avoided by anyone trying to conceive, or by pregnant women.

To eat jelly ear fungus, it can be cooked from fresh or dried and stored, to be rehydrated for use when needed.

7.8. Ebulus vulgaris & laciniatis foliis.
Ordinary Walwort and with fine cut leaves.

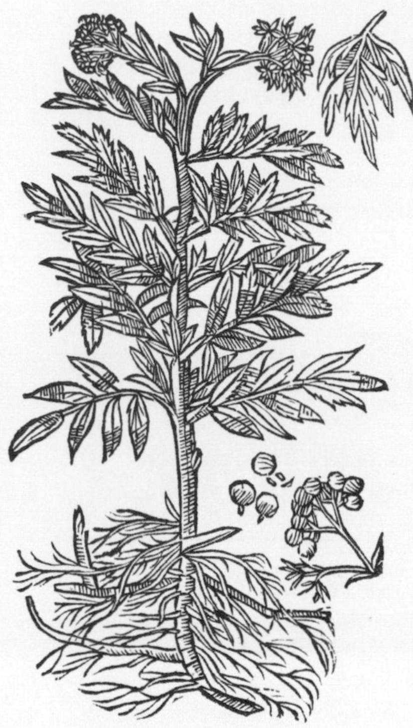

Mountaine elder: red-berried elder, *Sambucus racemosa*
moale: mole
Marsh elder: *Sambucus palustris*
Danewort: dwarf elder, *Sambucus ebulus*
stone: hard, morbid concretion
gravell: sand-like stones
Quinsie: peritonsillar abscess
King's evill: scrofula
Chamaepitys: ground pine, *Ajuga chamaepitys*
French disease: venereal disease
fluent: flow easily
peccant: unhealthy
offensive: causing disease
pouder: dried and powdered
fit of an ague: fevers, shivers
soveraigne remedy: best, most potent

Red-berried elder

The Mountaine or red berried Elder, hath the properties, that the common Elder hath, but weaker to all purposes: the berries hereof are taken to be cold, and to procure sleepe, but the frequent use of it is hurtfull: It is said that if a branch of this Elder be put into the trench that a moale hath made, it will either drive them forth, or kill them in their trench.

Marsh elder

The Marsh Elder is of the like purging qualitie with the common, especially the berries or the juyce of them. Hens and birds doe feede upon them willingly in the Winter.

Dwarf elder

The Wallwort or Danewort, is more forceable or powerfull than the Elder, in all the diseases and for all the purposes whereunto it is applied, but more especially wherein the Elder is little or nothing prevalent; the Wallwort serveth to these uses.

The young and tender branches and leaves thereof taken with wine, helpeth those that are troubled with the stone and gravell, and laid upon the testicles that are swollen and hard, helpeth them quickly:

the juice of the roote of Wallwort applied to the throate, helpeth the Quinsie or Kings evill: the fundament likewise is stayed from falling downe, if the juyce thereof be put therein: the same also put up with a little wooll into the mother, bringeth downe womens courses; the same juyce of the roote is a mighty purger of watery humours, and held most effectuall for the dropsie of all others herbs whatsoever:

the dried berries or the seeds beaten to powder, and taken in wine fasting, worketh the like effect, the powder of the seeds taken in decoction of *Chamaepitys* or ground Pine, and a little Cinamon, to the quantitie of a dramme at a time, is an approved remedy, both for the gout, joynt aches, and sciatica, as also for the French disease, for it easeth the paines by withdrawing the humors from the places affected, and by drawing forth those humors that are fluent, peccant and offensive: the pouder of the roote worketh in the like manner, and to the same effect.

The roote hereof steeped in wine all night, and a draught thereof given before the accesse and comming of the fit of an Ague, prevaileth so effectually there against, that it will either put off the fit, or make it more easie, and at the second taking seldome faileth to rid it quite away.

Red-berried elder *Sambucus racemosa*

Red-berried elder is native to Europe, Asia and North America.

Red-berried elder can be used much the same as black elder, though it is considered more toxic. The berries should not be eaten raw as the seeds contain cyandide-producing alkaloids. Like other elderberries they cause digestive upsets if eaten raw, but removing the seeds or cooking the berries seems to solve the problem.

The flowers of red-berried elder can be used in the same way as other elders, but it is wise to remove the stems before use.

Dwarf elder *Sambucus ebulus*

Dwarf elder or danewort is a herbaceous elder that grows as a small shrub. It is native to Europe, North Africa and the Middle East, and is naturalized in parts of North America. The berries look very like black elderberries, but the flowers are often pink-tipped and have violet anthers. The bush and the flowers have a rather unpleasant smell to most people.

Dwarf elder is little used in medicines today, except locally in areas where it is common.

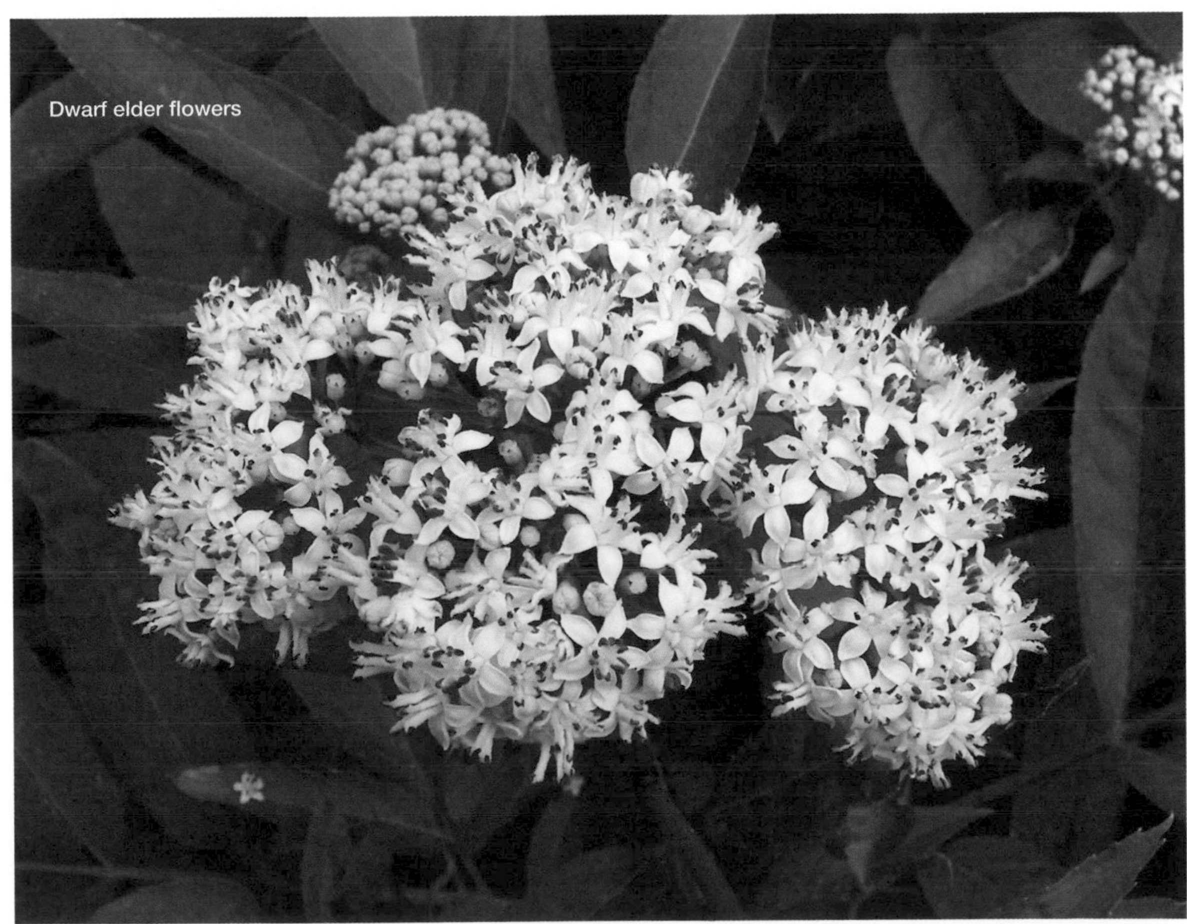
Dwarf elder flowers

moneth: month
starckness: stiffness
casualties: causes
mollifie: soften
grieved parts: affected area
anointed: rubbed with oil
profitable: effective
Tragus: Hieronymus Bock (1498–1554), physician, priest and author
digesting: dissolving
fistulous: hollow
tautologie: needless repetition

An ointment made of the greene leaves, and May butter made in the moneth on May, is accounted with many a soveraigne remedy, for all the outward paines, aches and crampes in the jointes, nerves, or sinewes, for starcknesse and lamenesse by cold and other casualties, and generally to warme comfort and strengthen all the outward parts ill affected: as also to mollifie the hardnesse, and to open the obstructions of the spleene, the grieved parts anointed therewith.

The leaves laid to steepe in water, and sprinkled in any chamber of the house, as it is said, killeth Fleas, Waspes and Flies also, if you credit the report.

Tragus saith, that the tender branches boyled in wine, whereunto some honey is put, and drunke for some dayes together, is profitable for a cold and drie cough, cureth the diseases of the breast, by cutting and digesting the grosse and tough flegme therein.

Briefly whatsoever I have shewed you before in relating the properties of Elder, doth Wallwort more strongly effect in opening and purging choller, flegme and water, in helping the gout, the piles, and womens diseases, coloureth the haire blacke, helpeth the inflammations of the eyes and paines in the eares, the stinging and bites of Serpents or a mad Dogge, the burnings or scaldings by fire and water, the wind-collicke, the collicke and stone, the difficultie of urine, the cure of old sores and fistulous ulcers, and other the griefes before specified, which for brevitie I doe not set downe here, avoiding tautologie as much as I can.

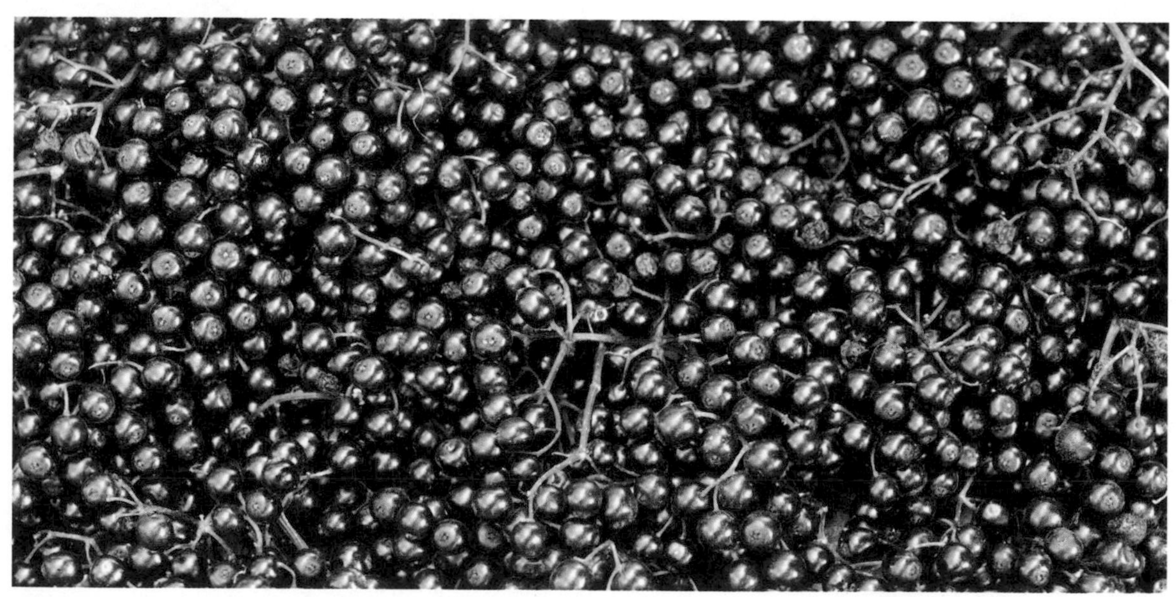

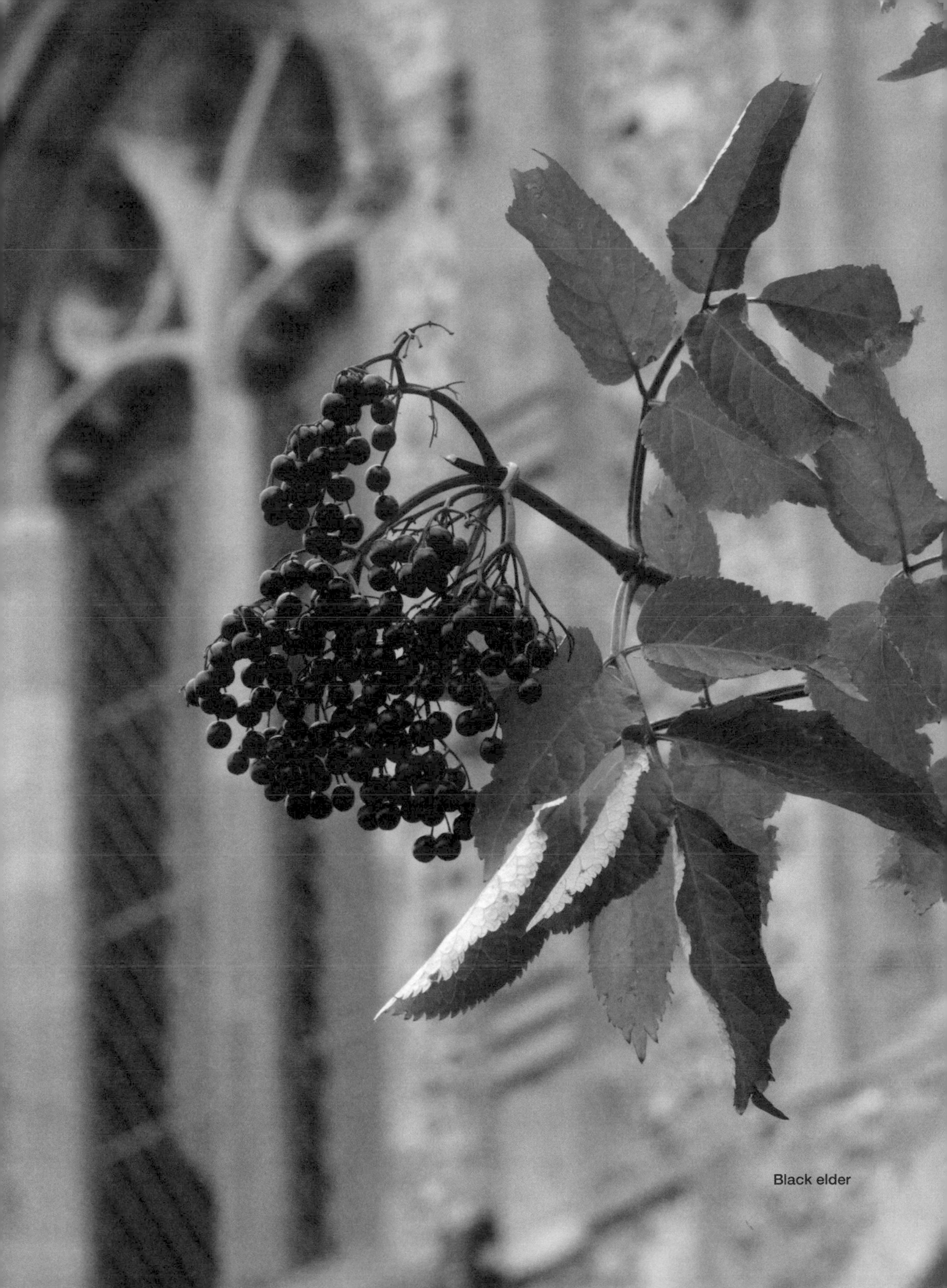

Black elder

Elecampane

Theatrum Botanicum

Tribe 5, Chapter 83, pp654–55

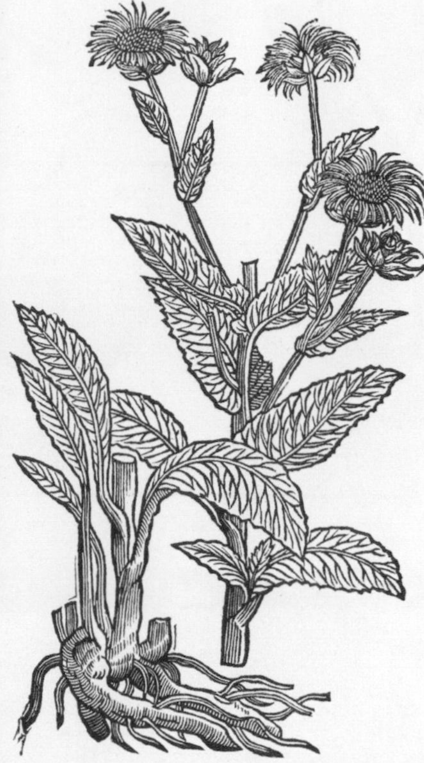

wheesing: chesty, whistling breath
profitable: helpful
menstrues stopped: amenorrhoea
mother: uterus
reines: kidneys
Treakles: theriaca, herbal compounds
Iulia Augusta: Julia Augusta, Livia Drusilla, wife of Roman emperor Augustus
Pliny: Pliny the Elder (AD23–79), Roman naturalist
condited: preserved
beare: beer
quickneth: enlivens
mawe: mouth, gullet or stomach
huckle bone: hip bone
members: limbs
bursten: ruptured
Hogs suet: lard
oyle of trotters: oil from pig's feet

Helenium sive Enula Campana

The Vertues

Fresh roots: The fresh rootes of Elecampane preserved with Sugar, or made into a syrupe or conserve, are very effectuall to warme a cold & windy stomack, and the pricking and stitches therein, or in the sides caused by the Spleene, and to helpe the cough, shortnesse of breath, and wheesing in the Lungs:

Dried roots: the dryed rootes made into powder mixed with Sugar, and taken, serve to the same purposes, and is also profitable for those that have their urine or their menstrues stopped, those that are troubled with the mother, or are pained with the stone in their reines, kidneys or bladder:

Poisons & fevers: it resisteth poyson, and stayeth the spreading of the venome of Serpents, &c. as also of putrid and pestilentiall Fevers, and the Plague it selfe; for which purpose it is put into Treakles, and other medecines for that disease.

Digestion & mirth: *Iulia Augusta* as *Pliny* writeth in his 19. Booke and 5. Chap. let no day passe without eating some of the rootes of *Enula* condited, which it may be shee did to helpe digestion, to expell melancholy and sorrow, and to cause mirth, and to move the belly downewards, for all which they are also effectuall:

Eyesight: the rootes and herbe beaten and put into new Ale or beare instead of wine, as they use in *Germany*, *Italy* and other places, and daily drunke of them that have weake and dim sights, cleareth, strengthneth and quickneth the sight of the eyes wonderfully,

Worms: the decoction of the rootes in wine, or the juice taken therein, killeth and driveth forth all manner of wormes in the belly, stomacke, or mawe,

Loose teeth: and gargled in the mouth, or the roote chewed fastneth loose teeth, and helpeth to keep them from putrefaction:

Cramps, gout & joints: the same also drunke is good for those that spit blood, helpeth to remoove Crampes or Convulsions, and the paines of the Goute, and the huckle bone, or hip-goute called the Sciatica, the loosenesse and paines in the joynts, or those members that are out of joynt, by cold or moisture happening to them,

Ruptures & bruising: applyed outwardly as well as inwardly, and is good also for those that are bursten or have any inward bruise:

Itching: the rootes boyled well in vinegar, beaten afterwards, and made into an oyntment, with Hogs Suet or oyle of trotters, & a little salt and vinegar in powder added thereto, is an excellent remedy for any scabs or itch, in young or old; the places also bathed or washed with the decoction doth the same;

Elecampane *Inula helenium* *Asteraceae*

Elecampane root has been used continuously in European medicine for over two thousand years as a mild bitter to ease phlegmy coughs and sciatica, help digestion, promote urine and menstruation, treat fevers and even plague. Its old uses have been supplemented and to some degree replaced by newer ones, such as treating chronic fatigue, urinary tract infections and some forms of cancer. It was and remains a powerful healing presence.

Elecampane is a perennial in the Aster (daisy) family, classified with the fleabanes, although visually it more resembles a sunflower (one common name is wild sunflower). Parkinson's unusually beautiful woodcut shows this well. It can grow to 7 feet (2 metres), with basal leaves 3 feet (a metre) long, and it needs to be planted allowing for a spread of 10 square feet (say 1 sq. metre).

Its native area is southern Europe and mainland West Asia, from where it spread to the British Isles and thence to eastern North America with the settlers. Its name suggests a wild plant (Parkinson's name *campana* is 'of the fields'), but it is generally a spectacular garden plant these days. We feel lucky to host one in our own garden.

Roots: The roots, where Parkinson begins his account, are the main part used, in both fresh and dried forms. They are at their best from the plant's third year, and dug up in autumn/fall. The rootstock is dense, but the action is powerful and you only need a few fingers' worth – taking some of the side roots is better for the plant.

Wash the reddish-brown root, keeping the bark, and for fresh use cut into chunks of about ¼ inch (say 5 mm). Parkinson suggests a syrup or conserve (jam), or, if drying it, a sugared powder. We like to make a glycerite from the fresh roots.

Why not a tea or decoction? Because, in the words of a herbalist friend, 'it made the most disgusting tea she had tasted in her life'. What happens during the summer is that the plant builds up and stores inulin in the root, until it might make 40% by content. There are also bitters, flavonoids and some essential oils.

Inulin, which gives the genus name, is a type of sugar that humans cannot absorb but which

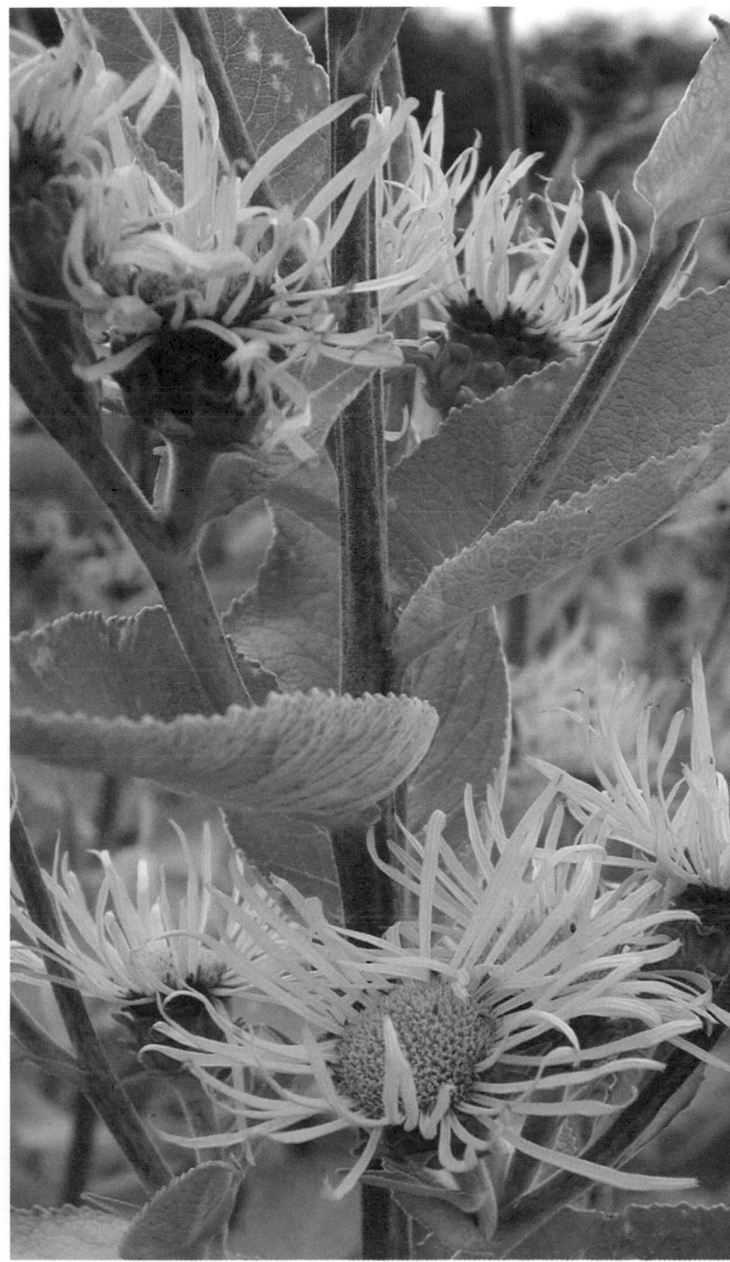

Cankers: ulcers
profitable: effective
morphew: discolouration of skin

Sores and cancers: the same also helpeth all sorts of old putrid, or filthy sores or Cankers wheresoever. In the rootes of this herbe lyeth the chiefe effect for all the remedies aforesayd, yet the leaves are sometimes also used to good purpose:

Distilled water: And the distilled water of them, and the rootes together is used also in the like manner, and besides is very profitable to clense the skinne of the face or other parts from any morphew, spots, or blemishes therein, and causeth it to be cleare.

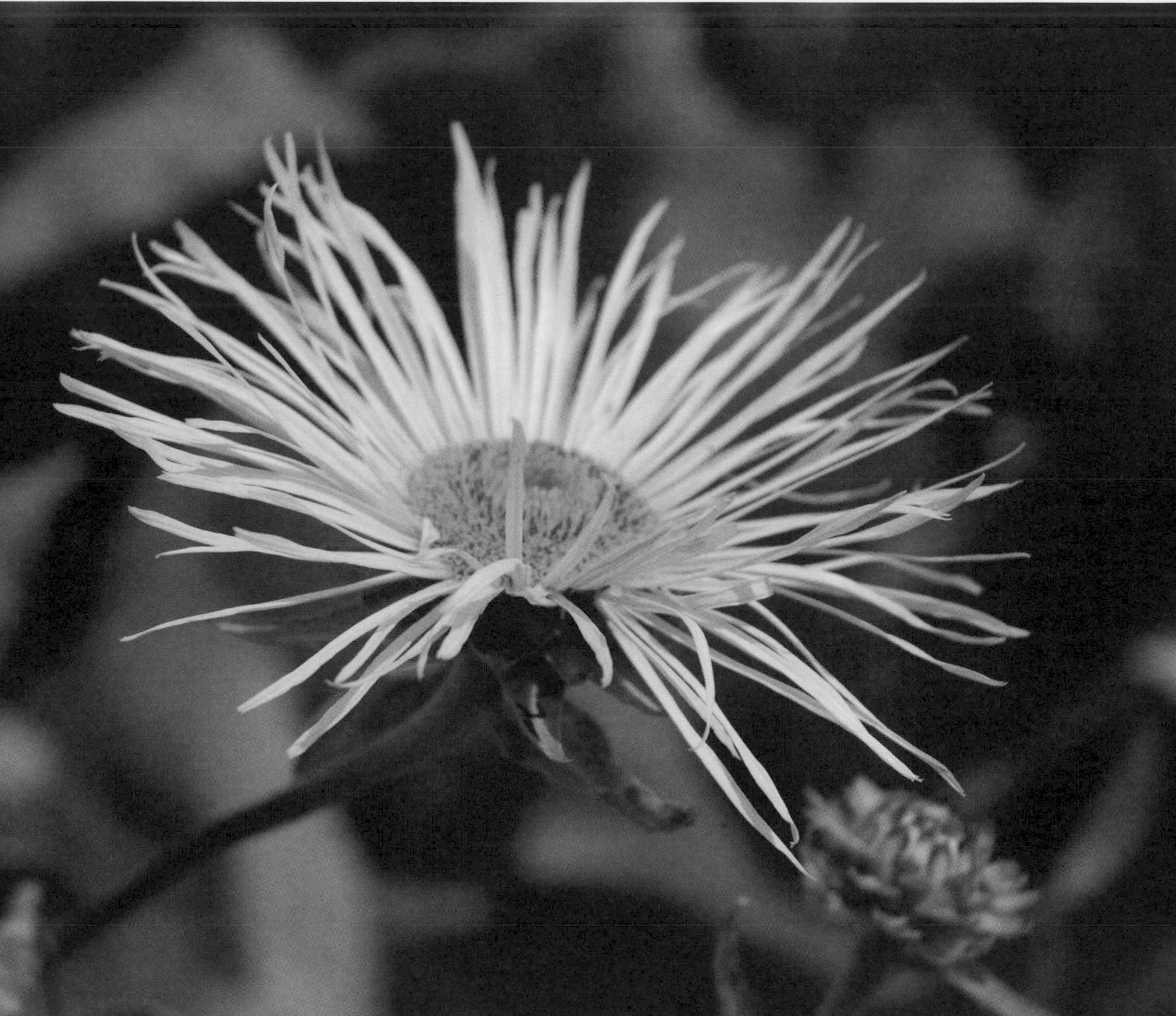

promotes gut-friendly bacteria. An excess can lead to gas and bloating, much as when you take too much Jerusalem artichoke or burdock root. But the other effect of inulin is to lend a certain sweetness in autumn, holding the usually predominant bitters in balance.

In her excellent text *Practical Herbs 2* (Helsinki, 2013), p59, herbalist Henriette Kress explains that the first taste of elecampane root is aromatic and pleasing; after half a minute the bitterness comes in; then after another half a minute for about half an hour there is a tingling sensation in the throat. All are aspects of the plant's medicinal action.

Cough & upper respiratory tract problems: Parkinson begins his 'vertues' by homing in on what has emerged as the leading current use of the plant, as an effective form of treatment for disorders of the upper respiratory tract, both acute and chronic. It is a specific for irritable coughing with wet phlegm, combining antiseptic, bitter and local anaesthetic effects to cut and eject sticky mucus. As Henriette emphasizes, it works best when a cough is related to a digestive problem, which has weakened the immune system.

Parkinson notes the value of elecampane for shortness of breath and wheezing, and it is considered a good treatment for asthma today. He says the fresh root is better for this purpose.

As a diuretic: Parkinson discusses elecampane's diuretic action on promoting urine, menstruation and for the pain of various types of stone.

Poisons & fevers: Parkinson now ups the stakes. Elecampane had a reputation, though probably not overwhelming success, as an antidote to poisons and for treating pestilential fever and the plague, often in the form of a theriac or treacle. The benefit may well have been in the tonic effect of the bitters, the temporary anaesthesia or 'tingling' and the warmth in the chest felt by the patient.

Digestion & mirth: Parkinson relates the story of Pliny prescribing daily sugared elecampane for the emperor's wife, which Pliny took good care to promote in his *Natural History*. This regime was said to help her digestion and to cause 'mirth', which is best understood as contentment, again a likely result of the positive effects of ingesting a source of aromatic/sweetness, bitter tonic and tingling warmth.

Eyesight: We have been unable to find modern experience or research into mixing an ale or beer tincture of elecampane for eyesight. A tincture based on alcohol is the most usual way of taking elecampane today, but this is an intriguing alternative.

Worms: Elecampane is known to have an antiseptic quality, which makes it a good choice in tincture form to treat viral, bacterial and fungal infection, particularly of the upper respiratory tract, and, in Parkinson's context, worms. In North America elecampane is used successfully to treat giardia (*Giardia lamba*) and roundworm (*Ascaris lumbricoides*); other studies have looked at it for treating malarial fever.

Loose teeth: Again this is an under-explored area, but Parkinson is writing about what he knows here.

Cramps, gout & joints: This area of treatment is confirmed by current use of an elecampane wash for treating sciatica and facial neuralgia; it has also been proposed for countering leaky gut syndrome.

An allied possibility is for elecampane to treat the pain and tension that accompany exhaustion, Lyme disease and chronic fatigue syndrome (CFS). The common factor is immune system support.

In a strange repetition of history, this recalls a very old practice in England of using elecampane to treat 'elf-shot'. A man's virility and strength were thought to leak out of his body when arrows fired by elves hit him; elecampane was thus 'elf dock'. Elven arrows could be a useful metaphor in explaining CFS!

Ruptures & bruising, itching: These uses do sound likely to be soothing. Elecampane is known as a skin treatment for sheep scab (with the predictable name scabwort) and for horses (horseheal). As Parkinson goes on to say, the distilled water was used as an effective skin cleanser and treatment for spots and blemishes.

Sores & cancers: Parkinson mentions 'cankers', and research is ongoing into elecampane as a possible treatment in some forms of cancer.

Caution: Elecampane should be avoided in pregnancy or when nursing. In excess, and this usually means the standardized extract rather than the plant, it can lead to contact dermatitis, nausea and diarrhoea. It is best used for moist rather than dry conditions of the upper respiratory tract.

Eyebright

Theatrum Botanicum

Tribe 15, Chapter 3, pp1328–30

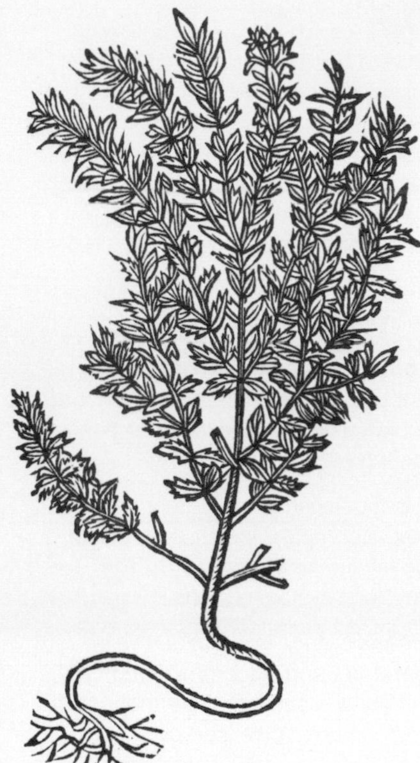

Eufragia

The Vertues

Eyes: The bitter taste that is herein sheweth it to be hot and dry, and is especially used for all the diseases of the eyes, that cause dimnesse of the sight, for either the greene herbe or the dry, the juice or the distilled water is very effectuall for the said purpose, to be taken either inwardly in wine or in broth, or to be dropped into the eyes, and used for divers dayes together: Some also make a conserve of the flower to the same effect.

Memory: Any of these wayes used, it helpeth also a weake braine or memory, and restoreth them being decayed in a short time.

Eyesight: *Arnoldus de Villa Nova,* in his booke of wines, much commendeth the Wine made of Eyebright, put into it when it is new made, and before it worke (which because we cannot make in our land, I could wish that the Eyebright might be tunned up with our strong Beere in the same manner, which no doubt would worke the like effects, their Wine and our Beere having a like working, as we use with Wormewood, Scurvigrasse and the like) to helpe the dimnesse of the sight, and saith that the use thereof restored old mens sight, to read small Letters without spectacles, that could hardly read great ones with their spectacles before: as also did restore their sight that were blinde for a long time before.

Electuary: If this drinke be not to be made or had, the pouther of the dryed herbe either mixed with Sugar, a few maces and Fennell seede, and drunke or eaten in broth, or the said pouthers made into an Electuary with Sugar, doth either way tend to the same effect.

greene: fresh
divers: several
Arnoldus de Villa Nova: Arnaldus de Villanova (1235–1311), Spanish physician and author
worke: ferments
tunned up: put into casks
Wormewood: *Artemesia absinthum*
Scurvigrasse: English scurvygrass, *Cochlearia anglica*
pouther: powder
maces: aril of nutmeg, *Myristica fragrans*
Fennell: *Foeniculum vulgare*
Electuary: medicinal powder mixed with honey or sugar

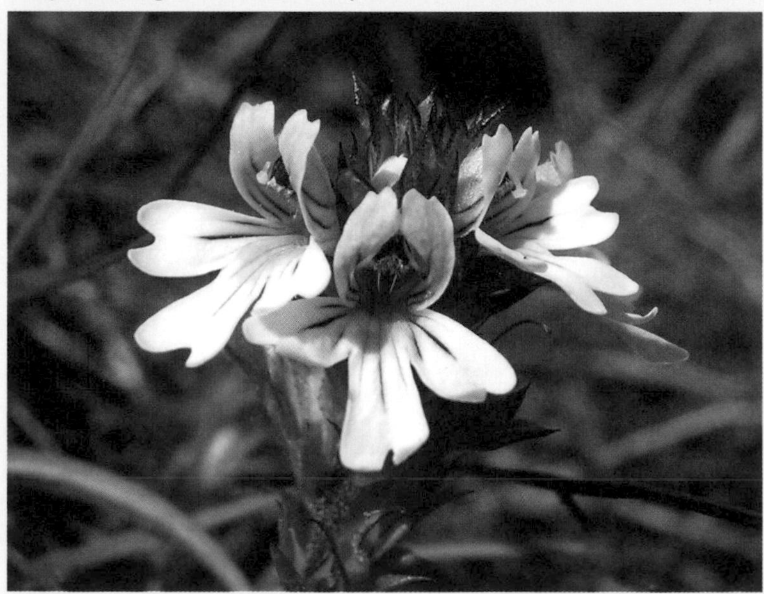

Eyebright *Euphrasia officinalis* Scrophulariaceae

The Latin name looks straightforward: *Euphrasia* is based on Euphrosyne, the 'mirthful' one of the Three Graces of the Greeks, and *officinalis* means used by apothecaries. But in reality it is an aggregate name for the whole genus, with at least 50 subspecies, almost impossible to tell apart – Parkinson describes seven. Eyebright species vary from a few inches to some 2 feet (60 cm) tall, the flowers tending to white with purple veins or tinge, three lobes and a yellow spot in the throat. All are semiparasites, growing on grass, and rather hard to transplant or grow commercially. They are native to Europe and naturalized in North America, mainly in eastern states; most species are medicinal.

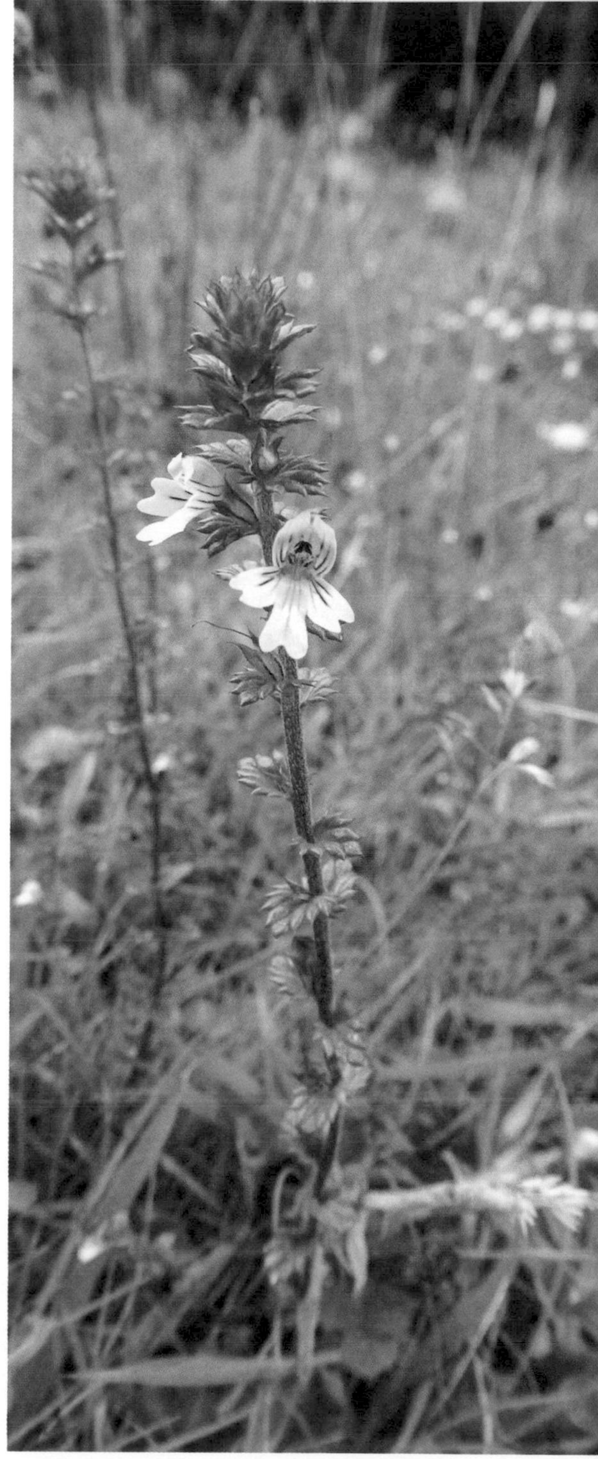

Eyes: In his introduction Parkinson stated that eyebright was not known to the ancient writers, but records two names that were old even in 1640: *ophthalmica* and *occularia,* named 'for the effects'. The German abbess and herbalist Hildegard of Bingen (1098–1179) is often thought to have been the first to write about the virtues of eyebright.

Parkinson is relatively specific in saying the plant was used, in various forms, for 'dimnesse of the sight', including in this term what we now call conjunctivitis and blepharitis. Herbalists today might well combine it with bilberry (*Vaccinium myrtillus*), which is more suited for improving the micro-circulation of the blood in the eye.

Memory: A friend of ours to whom we gave eyebright commented: 'It definitely helps to give me clarity of mind as well as clearing the eyes of the gritty feeling.'

Eyesight: Parkinson cites Arnaldus, whose treatise of 1305, *Luminella* ('little light'), was influential in promoting eyebright. Parkinson laments that the British climate will not allow him to experiment with eyebright wine, and wonders that no one has tried the plant in beer, with its reported 'spectacular' results.

Eyebright's effectiveness is not yet clinically tested (even after all this time), but its action seems to involve soothing, clearing and opening inflamed mucous membranes of the eye, ear, nose and throat. A lotion or eyewash, made from the dried plant, is applied externally for eye infections and poor vision, but usually swallowed as well.

In a related action, it is known to be effective as a cooling astringent for aspects of catarrh, such as blocked sinuses, hayfever, and coughs where mucous membranes are compromised.

Electuary: Parkinson began by noting the bitter taste of eyebright, and his sweetened mixtures would be pleasurable ways of taking it. Adding milk is an option, and eyebright used to be smoked in the prepared formula, British Herbal Mixture.

Featherfew

Theatrum Botanicum

Tribe 1, Chapter 29, pp83–85

1.3. Matricaria vulgaris simplex & bullatis floribus aureis. Ordinary & naked Featherfew. *2. Flore pleno.* Double Featherfew

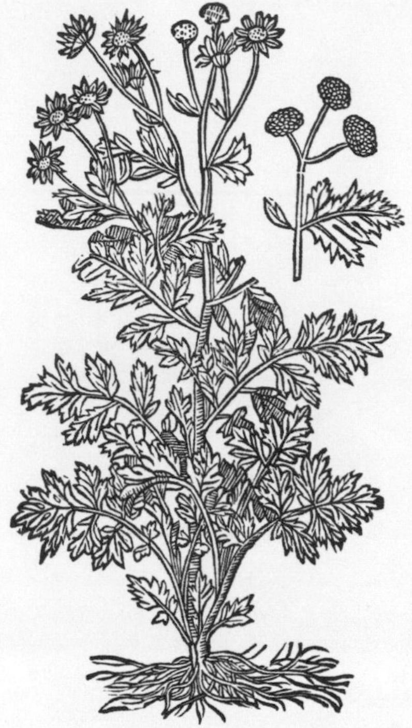

mother: uterus
strangling/rising: displacement
Nutmegge or Mace: *Myristica fragrans*
courses: menstruation
sit over: i.e. a steam bath
stuffing: filling
reines: kidneys
Dioscorides: Greek-speaking Roman physician (mid-first century AD)
Oxymel: spice in honey and vinegar
Epithymum: probably clover dodder, *Cuscuta epithymium*
choler: bile, overheating
availeable: useful
Camerarius: Joachim Camerarius the Younger (1534–98), German botanist
profitable: effective
ague: fever
cornes of Bay-salt: pieces of rock salt
wrestes: wrists
tyle: tile
Opium: opium poppy, *Papaver somniferum*
Tansies: tansy, *Tanacetum vulgare*

Matricaria

The Vertues

Uterus: It is chiefly used for the diseases of the mother, whether it be the strangling or rising of the mother, or the hardnesse or inflammations of the same, applyed outwardly thereunto, or a decoction of the flowers in wine, with a little Nutmegge or Mace put therein, and drunke often in a day, is an approved remedy to bring downe womens courses speedily, and to warme those parts oppressed by obstructions or cold, as also helpeth to expell the dead birth and the afterbirth.

Steam: For a woman to sit over the hot fumes of the decoction of the hearbe, made in water or wine, is effectuall also for the same purposes, and in some cases to apply the boyled hearb warme to the privie parts.

Decoction: The decoction thereof made, with some Sugar or honey put thereto, is used by many with good successe, as well to helpe the cough, and stuffing of the chest by cold, as also to cleanse the reines and bladder, and helpe to expell the stone in them.

Powder: The powder of the hearbe, as *Dioscorides* saith, taken in wine, with some Oxymel, purgeth like to *Epithymum* both choler and flegme, and is availeable for those that are short winded, and are troubled with melancholy and heavinesse, or sadnesse of the spirits:

Head Pain: it is very effectuall for all paines in the head, comming of a cold cause, as *Camerarius* saith, the hearbe being bruised and applied to the crowne of the head;

Vertigo & fevers: It is also profitable for those that hath the Vertigo, that is, a turning and swimming in their head. It is also drunke warme (I meane the decoction) before the accesse or comming of an ague, as also the hearbe bruised with a few cornes of Bay-salt (and some put beaten glasse thereto, but I see no reason wherefore) and applied to the wrestes of the hand, to take away the fits of agues.

Other uses: Some doe use the distilled water of the hearbe and flowers, to take away freckles, and other spots and deformities in the face. And some with good successe doe helpe the winde and collicke, in the lower part of the belly, (and some say it is good also for the winde in the stomack) by bruising the hearbe, and heating it on a tyle, with some wine to moisten it, or fryed with a little wine and oyle in a Frying-panne, and applyed warme outwardly to the places, and renewed as there is need. It is an especiall remedy against *Opium*, that is, taken too liberally.

As food: It is an hearbe among others, as *Camerarius* saith, much used in *Italy*, fryed with egges, as wee doe Tansies, and eaten with great delight; the bitternesse, which else would make it unpleasant, being taken away by the manner of dressing.

Feverfew *Tanacetum parthenium* Asteraceae

Feverfew's changing botanical classification matches its changing herbal reputation. It was a *Matricaria* (mayweed) to Parkinson, later became a *Chrysanthemum* and is now a *Tanacetum*, alongside costmary, tansy and pyrethrum, well known to the gardener and herbalist. Feverfew was chiefly a woman's herb for Parkinson, but has a growing reputation for treating inflammatory conditions like migraine and arthritis.

Women's herb: Feverfew is a cheery native of south-eastern Europe, now naturalized in gardens across the temperate world. It was a herb of Aphrodite/Venus, its name *parthenium* deriving from the Greek for 'virgin', indicating feverfew's value for women's conditions. Parkinson used it for any abnormalities of the 'mother' (uterus), in the form of a compress, decoction in wine (with nutmeg) or steam inhalation, and as a specific for regulating menstruation.

Such uses can be considered today, but be aware it is a uterine stimulant. Research on its possible use for chronic pelvic pain (CPP) is being undertaken.

Decoction & powder: The decoction or powder are very bitter, but with sweetening will be cleansing, if not purgative, for the conditions Parkinson mentions.

Head pain: Modern research confirms the value of feverfew for headache and migraine. Eating a few leaves in a daily sandwich or using a tincture can allay such symptoms as nausea, sensitivity and depression, and reduce the frequency and pain of migraine attacks.

Arthritis: The use of feverfew for arthritis was not prevalent in Parkinson's time, but is an exciting area of research. Its pain-relieving and anti-inflammatory action is found to penetrate deeply into swollen joints.

Vertigo & fevers: Hot, sweetened feverfew tea is still used to forestall or break fevers (the plant's name suggests *febrifuga*, fever-allayer), and for vertigo.

Other uses: This versatile, valuable bitter has more healing potential, and Parkinson relates some forgotten possibilities, including a food idea for a feverfew caudle.

Caution: Avoid in pregnancy; handling leaves may lead to contact dermatitis; eating them may cause mouth ulcers; avoid if on blood-thinning medication.

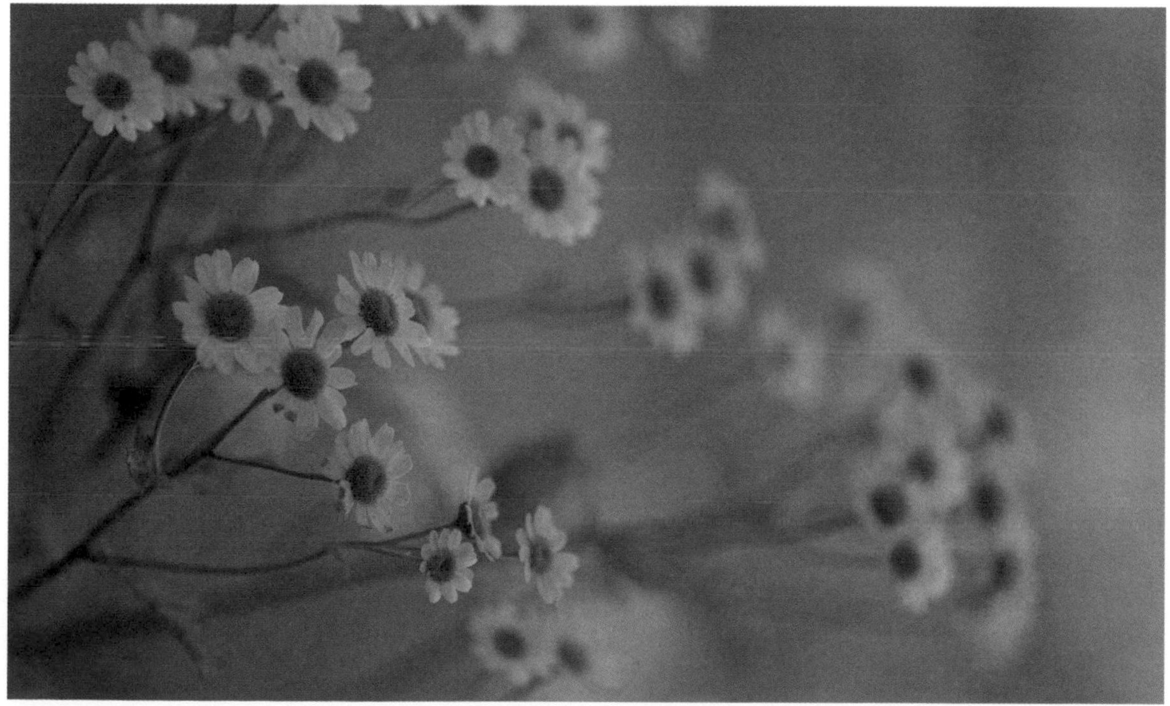

Figwort

Theatrum Botanicum

Tribe 5, Chapter 67, pp609–13

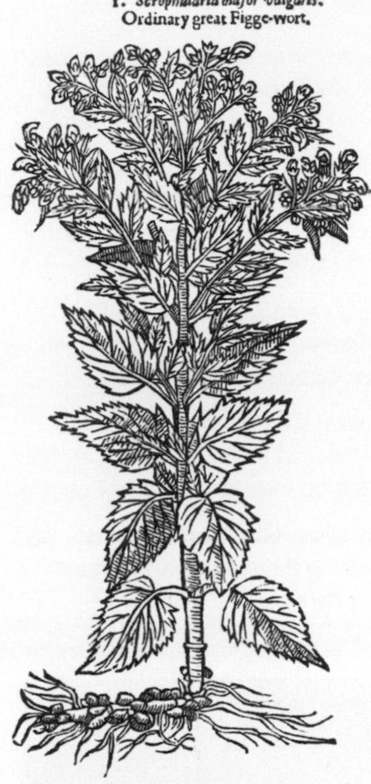

Kings Evill: scrofula
kernels: inflamed glands
bunches: swellings
wennes: boils or cysts
Fundament: anus
moorish: moorland
axungia: soft animal fat, often goose
Lepry: scaly skin condition, leprosy
hollow: fistulous
corroding: chemically damage
stay the malignitie: prevent or stop poison or disease
scurfe: dandruff
inveterate: deep-rooted, old

Scrofularia

The Vertues

Congealed blood: It is very effectuall to dissolve clotted or congealed blood within the body, which happeneth by any wound or by any bruise or fall, both to be taken inwardly by the decoction of the herbe, and by applying the herbe bruised upon the hurt place outwardly:

Cysts & swellings: the same also is no lesse effectuall for the Kings Evill, or any other knots, kernels, bunches or wennes growing in the flesh wheresoever: it is of singular good use to bee applyed for the hemorrhoides or piles, when they grow painefull and fall downe, and for other such knobbes or kernells as sometimes grow in and about the Fundament.

Ointment: An oyntment made hereof in this manner may bee used at all times, when the fresh herbe is not to be had. Wash the rootes cleane, bruise them and put them into a pot with fresh Butter well mixed together, and let them so stand for fifteene dayes close covered in some moyst or moorish place, which afterwards set upon a gentle fire to boyle easily for a little space, which then being strained forth let it be kept in a pot covered to use when occasion requireth: with the roots and leaves likewise bruised and boyled in *axungia* or oyle and wax, is made the like oyntment, exceeding good to heale all sorts of Scabbes and Lepry also.

Distilled water: The distilled water of the whole plant rootes and all, is used for the same purposes, eyther to take inwardly or to apply outwardly by bathings, and serveth well also for fowle Ulcers that are hollow or corroding, to stay the malignitie and dry up the superfluous virulent moysture of them;

Freckles & spots: the same also taketh away all rednesse spots and freckles in the face, as also the scurfe, or any foul deformitie therein that is inveterate, and the Leprosie likewise.

A sign of the times?

Herbalist Michael Moore (*Medicinal Plants of the Mountain West*, Santa Fe, 1979, p78) had his own take on the doctrine of signatures. He agrees that, by chance, figwort worked for skin eruptions as suggested by the nodules, but notes it could have equally been mouth problems (shape of flowers), heart diseases (shape of some leaves), cuts (serrated leaves) or ligament problems (shape of stems). Need led to theory rather than the reverse, for 'So did, and does, Homo sapiens fit the facts to the theory, the theory arising from a need to make a chaotic universe fit neatly into horse stalls.'

Figwort *Scrophularia nodosa* Scrophulariaceae

The Latin and common names suggest the old medicinal uses of figwort, but its main current use is as a lymphatic cleanser. It makes a more palatable tincture and syrup than cleavers, the other leading wild-gathered lymphatic, but is more local in distribution, growing in 'moyst and shadowie woods' in Parkinson's graphic phase. It is a native of Europe and North America, where it is known as woodland figwort, and mainly found in eastern Canada and New England. Other *Scrophulariacae* in the US have similar uses, and the plant occurs in Chinese and Ayurvedic medicine.

'Figs' was a name for haemorrhoids or piles in Parkinson's day, and the knotty roots (*nodosa*) – and perhaps the knobbly purple flowers – gave a visual link between plant and medical condition. Jumping from effect to cause, it followed that the plant would heal the visually similar condition. This was God's design, to give mankind a 'signature' in the plant's appearance to lead the clever physician or herbalist to the secret remedy. Here was the doctrine of signatures in action.

Congealed blood: In this case there was actually a basis of fact, as figwort happens to be a powerful detoxifier, working especially as a stimulant for the body's glandular and lymphatic systems. It softens hard swellings and dissolves congealed blood, at the anus or neck or elsewhere, and as varicose veins, relieving pain as it does so.

Cysts & swellings: Its best known action, as in the name *Scrophularia*, is to treat scrofula, or in modern terms glandular tuberculosis, a painful swelling of the neck. It was devoutly believed that English kings (and queens) could cure scrofula by simply touching the person. The condition was hence called the 'king's evil', and the monarchs of Parkinson's lifetime led organised mass healing sessions. Queen Anne (d. 1714) was the last monarch to apply the regal curing hand.

Parkinson doesn't evaluate this superstition here, or indeed the doctrine of signatures, but calmly goes on to say figwort will also treat other 'knots, kernels, bunches or wennes' anywhere in the body, including piles. The Chinese figwort species, *S. ningpoensis*, *xuan shen*, interestingly, is a specific for 'neck lumps due to phlegm-fire'; the root is dry-fried in salt.

Ointment: Thus far Parkinson has mentioned a decoction of figwort and applying the bruised herb onto a painful area. Now he gives the recipe for an ointment, useful in winter (it is a deciduous perennial). Michael Moore (d. 2009) tried this, changing Parkinson's butter to vegetable oil and suggesting equal herb and oil. Parkinson also uses oil and beeswax, or

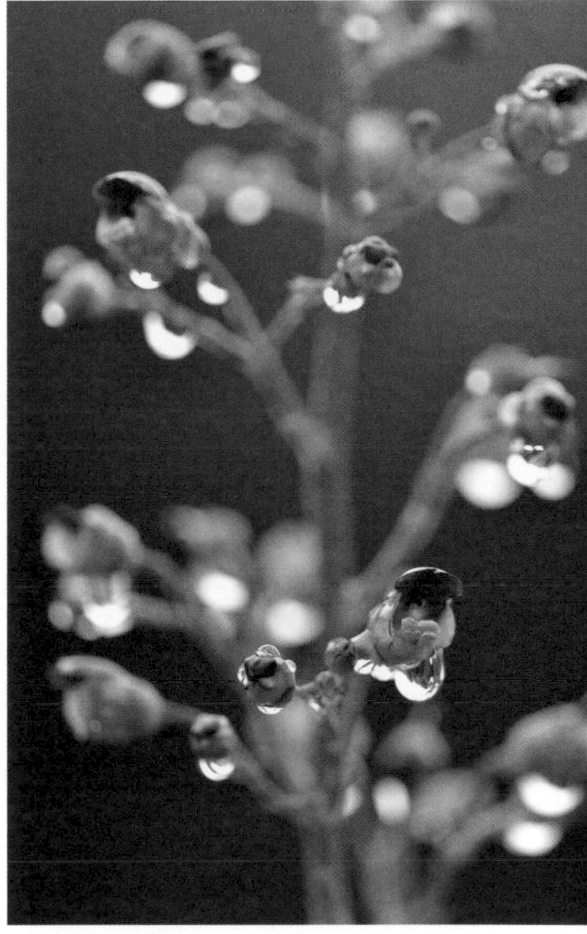

axungia, to make an ointment, as first aid for a raft of skin problems, as in bruises, scratches, fungal infections, burns and small wounds.

Distilled water: This is a more moderate way to take the plant inwardly. The roots taste bitter, so the decoction is a harder swallow, unless honey-sweetened. An alcohol tincture is more usually prescribed today.

Freckles & spots: Parkinson suggests the distilled water – or ointment or compress – for reducing redness of the skin, spots and even a 'foul deformitie' such as leprosy. Given its capacity for fluid detoxification of inflamed tissues, figwort would at least be pain-relieving in such conditions.

Golden Rod

Theatrum Botanicum

Tribe 5, Chapter 33, pp542–43

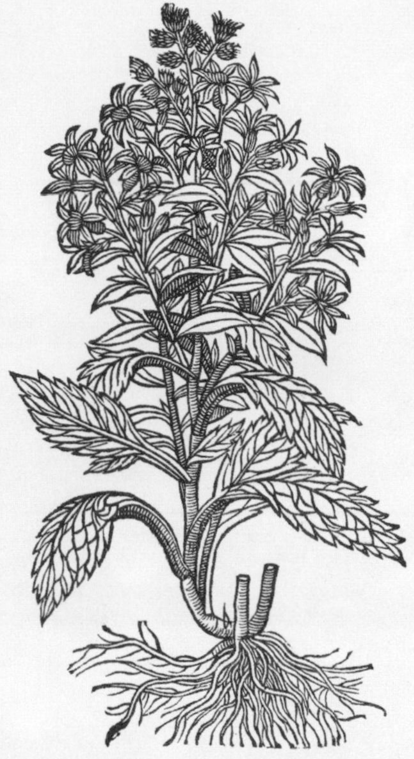

2 *Virga aurea ferratis folijs.*
Golden Rod with dented leaves.

Saracins consound: Saracen's woundwort, broad-leaved ragwort *(Senecio saracenicus* syn. *S. fluviatilis)*
Arnoldus de villa nova: Arnaldus de Villanova, Catalan physician (1235–1311)
gravell: calcareous deposits, calculi
tough flegmaticke humours: sticky, mucus-like secretions
avoided: voided
greene: fresh
stayeth: stops
menstruall courses: periods
blooddy flixe: dysentery
prevalent: powerful
soveraigne: supreme, above others
moist humours: thin liquids
privy parts: genitals

Virga aurea

The Vertues

As Golden Rodde is like unto the Sarasins Consound in forme, but much lesser, so is it also in the properties, not much inferiour, being hot and dry almost in the second degree.

Urinary stone: *Arnoldus de villa nova,* commendeth it much against the stone in the reines and kidneyes, and to provoke urine in abundance, whereby the gravell or stone engendred in the uritory parts, by raw and tough flegmatike humours, may be washed downe into the bladder, from growing into a stone in those parts, and thence may be avoided with the urine:

Bruises & bleeding: the decoction of the herbe greene or dry, or the distilled water thereof is very effectuall for inward bruises, as also to be outwardly applyed: the same also stayeth the bleedings in any part of the body, and of wounds also, and the fluxes of the menstruall courses in women, and the fluxes of the belly and humours, as also the blooddy flixe in man or woman:

Ruptures: it is no lesse prevalent in all ruptures, or burstings, to be both drunke and outwardly applyed:

Wounds: it is the most soveraigne woundherbe of many, and can doe as much therein as any, both inwardly for wounds and hurts in the body, and for either greene wounds, quickly to cure them, or old sores and ulcers, that are hardly to be cured, which often come by the fluxe of moist humours thereunto, and hinder them from healing:

Sores and ulcers: it is likewise of especiall use in all lotions for sores or ulcers in the mouth, and throate, or in the privy parts, of man or woman:

Loose teeth: the decoction thereof likewise helpeth to fasten the teeth that are loose in the gummes.

A flower fit for a king?

In 1816 the radical English journalist William Cobbett (1763–1835), wrote satirically about how the American goldenrod, probably *S. canadensis*, now adorned the king of England's greatest palace: '… an accursed stinking thing, with a *yellow* flower called the "*Plain-weed*," which is the torment of the neighbouring farmer, has been, above all the plants in this world, chosen as the most conspicuous ornament of the front of the King of England's grandest palace, that of Hampton-Court, where, growing in a rich soil to the height of five or six feet, it, under the name of "*Golden Rod*," nods over the whole length of the edge of a walk, three quarters of a mile long, and, perhaps thirty feet wide, the most magnificent perhaps in Europe.' [*The American Gardener*, 1856 edn, p206; online]

Goldenrod *Solidago virgaurea* Asteraceae

The genus name *Solidago* means 'to make whole or sound', an indication of goldenrod's healing reputation; *virgaurea* is literally from the appearance, 'golden rod'. The plant is also called Aaron's rod, as are other tall wild perennials with spiky yellow flowers (such as agrimony and mullein). Goldenrod's origin is in the Middle East, as Parkinson alluded to. While there is one main European species, *S. virgaurea*, growing to 2–3 feet (0.75–1 m), wild and in gardens, there are many taller species in North America, with the Canadian goldenrod *S. canadensis*, with feathery flower plumes up to 6 feet (2 m), most used medicinally.

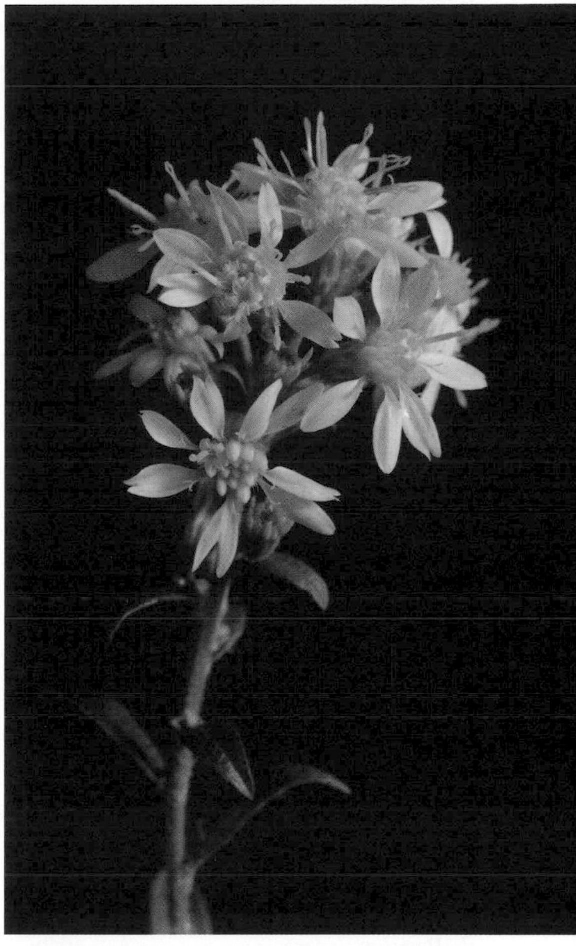

Urinary stone: Parkinson's identification of goldenrod for treating urinary conditions, including kidney stone, remains current today. The plant has strong diuretic qualities, and in Germany goldenrod is a standard kidney treatment, often preferred to pharmaceutical drugs, especially for inflammatory diseases of the lower urinary tract. It is also used in modern irrigation therapy to prevent and break down renal and kidney calculi and gravel. Parkinson is right to say the effect of taking it is to help reduce and move a stone down into the bladder, whence it can be voided in the urine.

Bruises & bleeding: Modern research shows that goldenrod has bioavailable amounts of quercetin, with a reported use for treating haemorrhagic nephritis and other haemorrhagic conditions, described as 'fluxes' in Parkinson's time. The form of treatment in this case, then as now, would be a tea, made of the powdered root or flowers. Modern advice would be to drink plentiful water along with the tea.

Ruptures: A compress soaked in the tea of any astringent herb, including goldenrod, would be soothing when laid on a rupture or hernia, but the usual thing these days would be to go to the doctor.

Wounds: Goldenrod's reputation as a wound-healer (vulnerary) was strong enough in Parkinson's time for him to call it 'the most soveraigne woundherb of many'. He describes it as effective for inner and outer, and old and fresh wounds, adding with the precision of experience that its heat will dry up 'moist humours' that have slowed down healing. This herbal use has all but disappeared today.

Sores & ulcers: Again the plant's heating and drying qualities come into play, with a goldenrod ointment being effective to rub on old and stuck sores and ulcers.

Loose teeth: A herb with astringency from tannins and anti-inflammatory qualities, like goldenrod, will be effective for mouth inflammations and gum disease.

Other: Parkinson doesn't go into detail on goldenrod's value in what we now call upper respiratory infections, including catarrh (for which it is 'official' in the latest *British Herbal Pharmacopoeia* (1996)) and asthma. It also has an old reputation as a carminative, which settles the digestion, and as an effective external treatment for eczema.

Note: Goldenrod is sometimes said to cause summer allergies, but is actually beneficial, as in its use for asthma. In North America the allergic effects of ragweed (*Ambrosia artemisiifolia*) flowers overlap with the innocent goldenrod's flowering season. Ragweed pollen is said to cause over 90% of allergy responses in the US in summer.

Ground Ivie or Alehoofe

Theatrum Botanicum

Tribe 5, Chapter 93, pp676–77

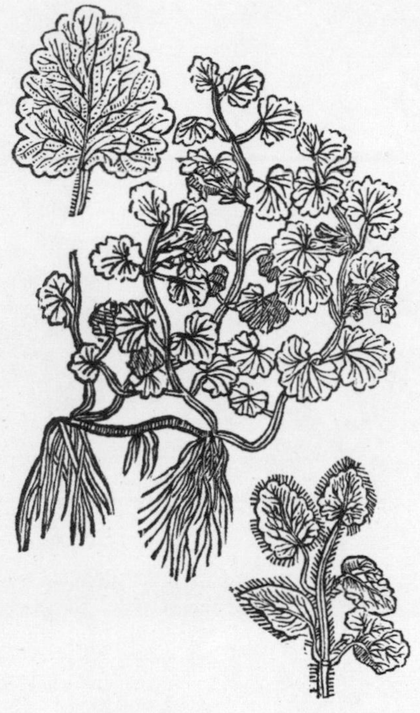

rarefieth: purifies
exulcerated: ulcerated
chollericke: choleric
iaundies: jaundice
women's courses: menstruation
stayeth: stops
peccant humours: disease-causing bodily fluids
allome: alum, a double sulphate salt, often containing aluminium
greene wounds: fresh wounds
vardigresse: verdigris, green pigment from oxidized copper
soveraigne remedy: sovereign or best remedy
pinne, webbe, skinnes or filmes growing over the sight: various eye problems, including pterygium
tunne up: put into casks

Hedera terrestris

The Vertues

Ground Ivie is quicke, sharpe, and bitter in taste, and thereby is found to be hot and dry, it openeth also, clenseth and rarefieth.

Abdominal pain: It is a singular good wound herbe for all inward wounds, as also for exulcerated Lungs or other parts, either by it selfe or with other the like herbes boyled together, and besides being drunke by them that have any griping paines of windie or chollericke humours in the stomacke, spleene or belly, doth ease them in a short space: it likewise helpeth the yellow Iaundies by opening the obstruction of the Gall, Liver and Spleene, it expelleth venome or poison, and the Plague also:

Diuretic effect: it provoketh Urine and womens courses, and stayeth them not as some have thought,

Sciatica & gout: but the decoction of the herbe in wine being drunke for some time together by them that have the Sciatica or Hippe Goute, as also the Goute in the hands, knees, or feete, helpeth to dissolve and disperse the peccant humours, and to procure ease:

Sore Throat: the same decoction is excellent good to gargle any sore throate or mouth, putting thereto some Honey and a little burnt Allome,

Ulcers & cancers: as also to wash the sores and Ulcers of the privy parts in man or woman; it speedily healeth greene wounds being bound thereto: and the juice boyled with a little honey and Vardigresse doth wonderfully clense fistulaes, and hollow Ulcers, and stayeth the malignitie of spreading or eating Cancers and Ulcers: it helpeth also the itch, scabbes, wheales, and other eruptions or exulcerations in the skinne in any part of the body:

Eyes: the juice of *Celandine,* field Daisies and ground Ivie clarified, and a little fine Sugar dissolved therein, dropped into the eyes is a soveraigne remedy for all the paines, rednesse, and watering of the eyes, the pinne, and webbe, skinnes or filmes growing over the sight, or whatsoever might offend them: the same helpeth beasts as well as men:

Ears: the juice dropped into the eares doth wonderfully helpe the noyse and singing of them, and helpeth their hearing that is decayed.

Brewing: The country people doe much use it, and tunne it up with their drinke, not onely for the especiall good vertues therein, but for that it will helpe also to cleare their drinke; and some doe affirme that an handfull put into drinke that is thicke, will cleare it in a night, yea in a few houres say they, and make it more fit to be drunke.

Ground ivy *Glechoma hederacea* Lamiaceae

Ground ivy is found across temperate Europe and Asia, and was taken by early European settlers to North America, where it has become widespread.

It is a low-growing perennial in the mint family, and creeps ivy-like along the ground (hence the name) and has purplish, musty-smelling flowers in early spring.

Medicinally, ground ivy clarifies by removing phlegm. Its current uses are much as Parkinson describes, a significant one being in the treatment of tinnitus or ringing in the ears. It could be tried much more today, as it reported to possess anti-catarrhal, astringent, diaphoretic, anti-inflammatory and tonic qualities, and is also high in Vitamin C.

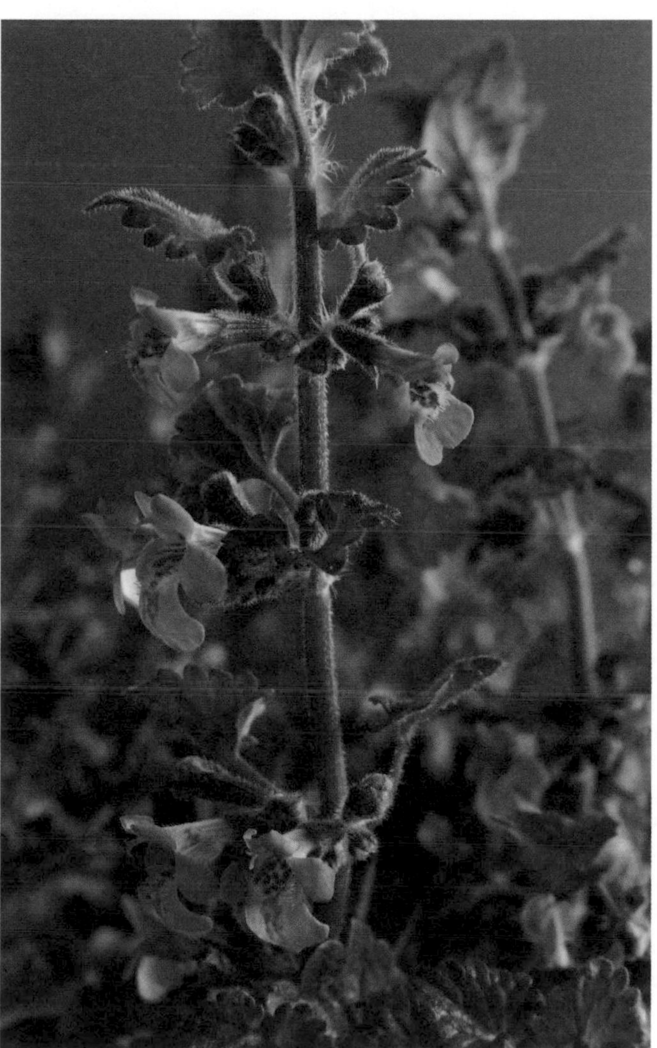

Abdominal pain: Today anyone with internal injuries would go to the hospital for treatment, but ground ivy's ability to clear congestion and its aromatic qualities are still useful for treating griping pains, wind and colic.

Diuretic effect: Parkinson's assertion that ground ivy is diuretic is correct, and it can be used as a tea for cystitis – try it combined with a little goldenseal or some buchu or uva ursi.

Sciatica & gout: Ground ivy would help to 'dissolve and disperse' these 'peccant' conditions, but the wine wouldn't help.

Sore throat: The astringency of ground ivy decoction is good for treating sore throats and mouth problems. Heat wine or water in a small saucepan, then add a few sprigs of fresh ground ivy for each cup of liquid. Put the lid on and simmer gently for about 10 minutes, then strain and cool. Red wine makes the preparation more astringent.

Ulcers & cancers: Ground ivy's cleansing action makes sense of Parkinson's use for treating ulcers and 'eating' cancer.

Skin: It is not used much for skin problems today, but deserves another look.

Eyes: We haven't yet tried Parkinson's recipe, but as ground ivy is so good at clarifying it would be reasonable to predict that it would clear the eyes of humans and animals.

Ears: Ground ivy is still used to treat tinnitus, which causes ringing or buzzing in the ears, and is one of the best herbal remedies for this condition. Today it is more often prescribed by herbalists as an infusion to be drunk or a tincture to take internally.

Brewing: Ground ivy was the main clarifier for brewing ale in Europe until it was largely replaced by hops, in the century before Parkinson, but the home brewers of today still use it occasionally. The old name of alehoofe comes from its use in making ale.

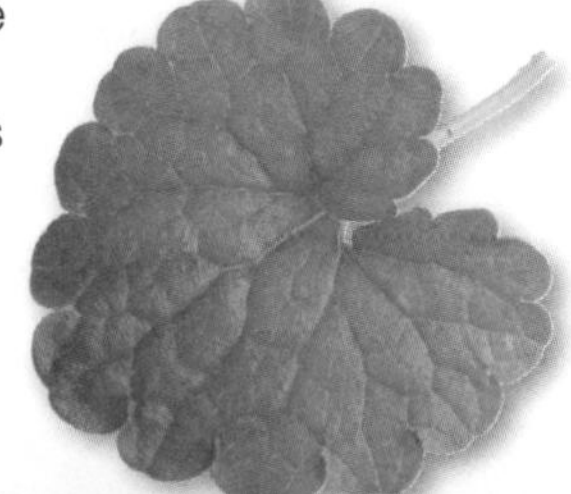

Groundsell

Theatrum Botanicum

Tribe 5, Chapter 90, pp671–73

1. *Senecio vulgaris.* Common Groundsell.

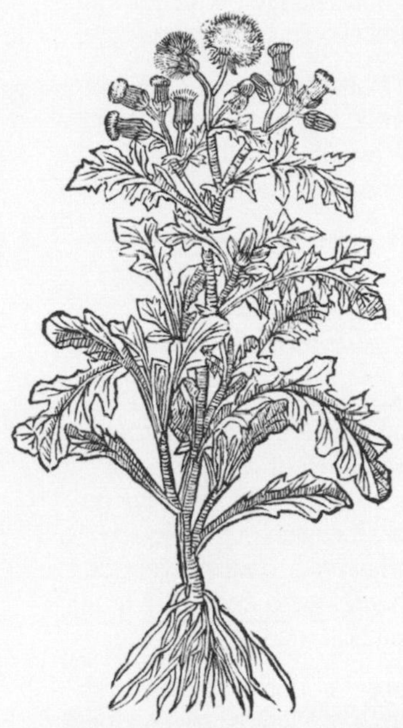

Tragus: Hieronymus Bock (1498–1554), physician, priest and author
Galen: Claudius Galen (AD130–200), Roman physician and author
6. Simp: sixth book of simples (herbs)
digesting: dispersing
Dioscorides: Greek-speaking Roman physician (mid-first century AD)
choller: bile; one of the four humours
Pliny: Pliny the Elder (AD23–79), Roman naturalist
iaundies: jaundice
falling sicknesse: epilepsy
gravell: small kidney stones
oxymel: syrup of vinegar and honey
collicke: colic, griping pains in belly
sallet: salad
courses: menstruation
stayeth the whites: stop leucorrhoea
Matthiolus: Pierandrea Mattioli (1501–77), physician and author
seate and fundament: buttocks, anus
kernells: small lumps, swollen glands
frankincense: resin of *Boswellia* tree
downe: seed parachutes or pappus
defluxion of rheume: watery mucus

Senecio vulgaris

The Vertues

Bile & purging: Groundsell is cold and moist as *Tragus* saith, and therefore seldome used inwardly, *Galen* saith in *6. Simpl.* it hath a mixt quality both cooling and a little digesting: the decoction of the herbe saith *Dioscorides*, made with wine and drunke helpeth the paines in the stomacke proceeding of choller (which it may well doe by a vomit, which our daily experience sheweth, the juice hereof taken in drinke, or the decoction of the herbe in Ale gently performeth)

Kidneys: *Pliny* addeth from others report that it is good against the Iaundies and falling sicknesse, being taken in wine, as also to helpe the paine of the bladder, that is in making water when it is stopped, which it provoketh, as also to expell gravell in the reines or kidneyes, a dram thereof given in *Oxymel*, after some walking or stirring the body:

stomach & liver: it helpeth the Sciatica also and the griping paines in the belly, or the Collicke: some also eate it with Vinegar as a Sallat, accounting it good for the sadnesse of the heart, and to helpe the defects of the Liver:

Female & male herb: it is said also to provoke womens courses, and some say also that it stayeth the whites, which as *Matthiolus* saith cannot be beleeved to be so, in that the one quality is contrary to the other: The fresh herbe boyled and made into a Poultis, and applied to the breasts of women that are swollen with paine and heate, as also to the privy parts of man or woman, the Seate or Fundament, or the Arteries, Ioynts and Sinewes, when they are inflamed and swollen doth much ease them; and used with some salt helpeth to dissolve the knots or kernells that happen in any part of the body:

Wound healer: the juice of the herbe or as *Dioscorides* saith, the leaves and flowers with some fine Frankinsence in powder, used in wounds, whether of the body or of the nerves and sinewes doth singularly helpe to heale them. The downe of the heads saith hee used with Vinegar doth the like, but if the same downe be taken in drinke it will choake any:

Eyes, teeth & fables: the distilled water of the herbe performeth well all the aforesayd properties, but especially for the inflammations of the eyes, and watering of them, by reason of the defluxion of the rheume into them. *Pliny* reporteth a ridiculous fable to helpe the toothach, to digge up the plant without any Iron toole, and then to touch the aking tooth five times therewith, and to spit three times after every such touch, and afterwards to set the herbe againe in the same place, so that it may grow with ease the paines: another as fabulous and ridiculous as that, is this, which some have set downe, that glasse being boyled in the juice of Groundsell, and the blood of a Ramme or Goate, will become as soft as wax, fit to bee made into any forme, which being put into cold water will come to be hard againe.

Groundsel *Senecio vulgaris* Asteraceae

The *Senecio* family (ragworts) are named for the feathery seed heads that resemble the white hair of an older man (Latin *senex*). The common name groundsel, short for 'groundswell', reflects a formidable capacity to colonize bare land throughout the temperate world. Other graphic English names were ground glutton and grundy swallow. A groundsel can complete its life cycle in six weeks and potentially produce five generations a year. The plant was widely used herbally in Parkinson's day, but has been more recently dismissed as toxic to humans and cattle.

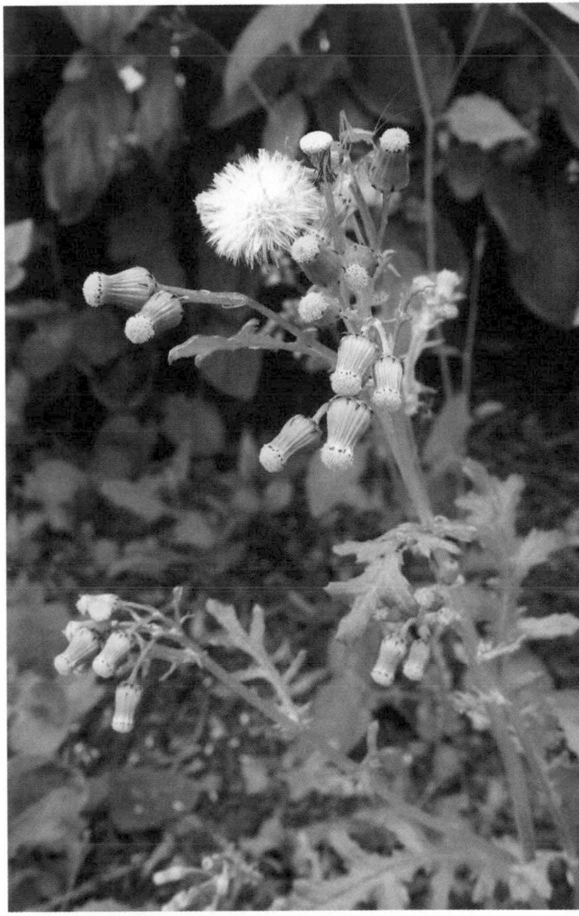

Bile & purging: Groundsel was once seen as a safe remedy without side effects, but in the later twentieth century it was established that it contains toxic pyrrolizidine alkaloids, as do a number of medicinal herbs, including borage, comfrey and coltsfoot (see box on hemp agrimony, page 26).

The science should be heeded: there are certain dangers, yet these occur at the extreme of the range. Dosage influences outcome, from benign to dangerous as amount or frequency increase; there is also the issue of means of preparation. Thus in minute amounts groundsel was given to infants (tempered by being boiled in milk); larger doses made a tea to treat adult constipation; larger amounts still were used, 'as a decoction in Ale', as Parkinson says, for a purge, to clear the bowels or an emetic, to cause vomiting. Continued use over a period or excessive short-term intake was seen as damaging – Parkinson comments that it 'was seldome used inwardly'.

Kidneys: At the same time Parkinson mentions Pliny's report of groundsel taken in wine for treating jaundice, epilepsy and bladder problems, and talks of combining it with vinegar for kidney stone, when accompanied by exercise. These uses arose from the plant's 'cold and moist' nature, which was seen as taking the heat out of painful conditions, but such internal treatments would not usually be recommended today.

Stomach & liver: Parkinson says groundsel will remove biliousness and griping pains in the stomach. In 19th century Ireland, before castor oil was available, groundsel was added to hot milk for constipated babies; boiled with lard it was used for similarly suffering adults. Eating fresh leaves with vinegar as a 'sallat', Parkinson said, could uplift the mood and 'helpe the defects of the Liver', but few herbalists would agree today.

Female & male herb: Like its American cousin, the golden ragwort or squaw weed (*Senecio aureus*), groundsel was once taken for delayed or irregular menstruation and leucorrhoea ('whites'). As a poultice both plants would treat milk retention and hard breasts, and the 'privy parts' of both sexes.

Wound healer: Groundsel poultices for skin problems were known in Gaelic as *am bualan*, the healer. One Scots poultice involved pouring boiling water on groundsel leaves, steeping them and applying the residue warm; the strained water was good for chapped hands. A related *Senecio* species in South Africa, *S. serratuloides,* is a Zulu herb applied on sores and abscesses. Using groundsel with salt for 'knots or kernells', or adding to frankincense for sore wounds, sinews or nerves seem safe external remedies.

Eyes, teeth & fables: Groundsel distilled water for eye inflammations or teeth has probably not been used for many years, nor these 'ridiculous fables' believed for many centuries.

Hawthorne or white Thorne

Theatrum Botanicum

Tribe 9, Chapter 28, pp1025–26

1. *Spina appendix vulgaris.*
The ordinary Hawthorne tree.

dropsie: oedema
divers: various people
Anguilara: Luigi Squalermo or Anguillara (c.1512–70), first director of the botanical garden at Padua
Matthiolus: Pierandrea Mattioli (1501–77), physician and author
Tragus: Hieronymus Bock (1498–1554), physician, priest, author
soveraigne remedy: supreme or highly efficacious remedy
plurisie: pleurisy
flux: excessive flow
laske: diarrhoea
Galen: Claudius Galen (AD130–200), Roman physician and author
sower: sour
bring downe: lower
stay: prevent
monethly courses: menstruation

Spina appendix vulgaris

The Vertues

The Stone: The berries or the seedes in the berries are generally held to be a singular good remedy against the stone, if the powder of them be given to drinke in wine:

Dropsy: the same is also reported to bee good for the Dropsie: but whereas divers have attributed hereunto a binding or astringent qualitie *Anguilara* his judgement was (whom *Matthiolus* confuteth) that *Tragus* who saith that the leaves, flowers & fruit are drying and binding,

Distilled wine: and that if the flowers be steeped three dayes in wine, and afterwards distilled in glasse, the water thereof drunke is a soveraigne remedy for the Plurisie, and for inward tormenting paines:

Distilled water: the distilled water of the flowers by an ordinary way stayeth, saith he, the Flux or Laske of the belly:

Seed: the seed cleared from the downe bruised and boyled in wine and drunke performeth also the same effect:

Splinters & thorns: the said distilled water of the flowers is not onely cooling but drawing also: for it is found by good experience that if clothes or spunges be wet in the sayd water and applyed to any place whereinto thornes, splinters, &c. have entered and bee there abiding it will notably draw them forth:

Galen: the vertues given by *Galen* unto *Oxycantha* doe not pertaine hereunto, for saith he the fruit thereof is not sower or harsh, especially when it is ripe, but sweet and therefore more fit to open then to binde the belly, and fitter to bring downe then to stay womens monethly courses: but the last evinceth this errour.

Sour or sweet?

Once the fruit is ripe, it is not sour or harsh, as Parkinson describes it. Hawthorn berries are slightly sweet when ripe, but are a bit mealy and have little flavour. In our experience, the flowers and leaves are more astringent than the berries, unless unripe berries are used.

Parkinson constructs a learned commentary in his 'Names' section, where he corrects Dioscorides, Galen, Gerard and some contemporaries, saying *Oxycanthus* is not the pyracanthus, pear, myrtle, barberry or a medlar but in truth a hawthorn! He notes it is also called Hedgethorne, White-thorne and May or May-bush, and that Galen's tree is more like a wild pear rather than a hawthorn species.

Hawthorn *Crataegus monogyna, C. laevigata*

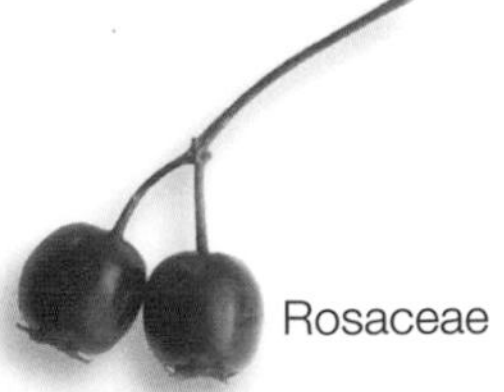

Rosaceae

Hawthorn is a well-known herb with a long history of use – however, current applications are very different from those common in Parkinson's time.

Crataegus oxycantha was the name given by Linnaeus to a species of northern European hawthorn, but there was confusion over species, and this name is no longer used by botanists, though it is still often found in herbal books.

Britain has two native species, *Crataegus monogyna*, the common hawthorn, and *C. laevigata*, the Midland hawthorn, which can be used interchangeably. In eastern and central parts of the USA *C. flabellata* is commonly used medicinally, though other variants and subspecies abound.

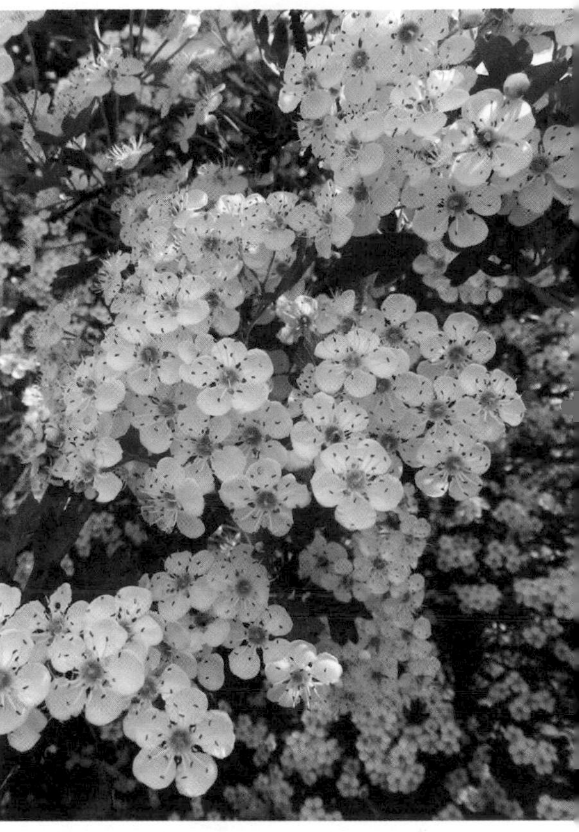

The stone: In the old herbals, the main use of hawthorn is for kidney stones. Drying and powdering the berries and steeping them in wine, as Parkinson does, is a powerful formulation.

Dropsy: The astringent and drying qualities of hawthorn leaf and flower make it useful for treating water retention.

Diarrhoea: A tea made from the leaves and flowers can be drunk to help stop runny tummy and diarrhoea.

Splinters & thorns: The drawing properties of hawthorn are still recognized today. Using a hawthorn thorn to lance a boil will help it heal up rapidly. The drawing power of the distilled water is something we have yet to try, but we imagine it will be soothingly effective.

Hawthorn as a herb for the heart and circulation

Hawthorn today is one of the leading heart herbs, but only began to be recognized and used as such in the 1890s when the secret of the Irish Dr Green's singular success in treating heart disease was revealed to be a tincture of ripe hawthorn berries (see the account in our *Hedgerow Medicine*, Ludlow, 2008, p65).

Hawthorn protects and strengthens the heart muscle and its blood supply, and improves circulation around the body. It also calms the spirit, and is beneficial for anxiety and insomnia.

Our recipe for hawthorn berry tincture

Put the fresh ripe berries in a blender with enough vodka to cover, and blend to a mush. Pour the mixture into wide-mouthed jars – this is important because hawthorn berries have so much pectin that the whole mixture will set solid, and you'll find it impossible to get it out of a narrow-necked bottle. Leave the jars in a cool, dark place for a month, then poke a knife into the jar to chop the contents enough to get them out.

Squeeze the liquid out using a jelly bag – this is good exercise! If you have a juice press, use that as it will be a lot less work. Bottle and label your tincture. It will keep for several years, although it's best to make a fresh batch every year if you can.

Dose: 1 teaspoon once a day as a general tonic; 1 teaspoon three times a day or as advised by your herbalist for circulatory problems.

Hony Suckles

Theatrum Botanicum

Tribe 16, Chapter 48, pp1460–61

Periclymenum sive Caprifolium

1. *Periclymenum sive Caprifolium vulgare.* Woodbinde or Honysuckles.

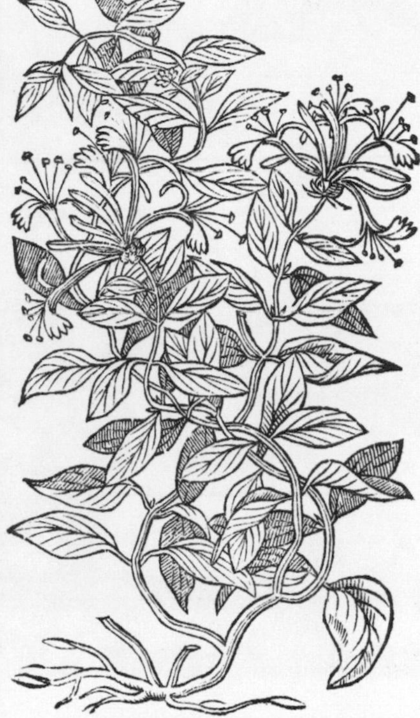

The Vertues

We in our Land have by tradition continued so long in this errour to use the leaves, and flowers, in all gargles, and lotions for inflammations in the mouth, or the sore privy parts of man or woman, that I thinke the custome is growne too strong by time for me with a few words to shew the inconvenience, that it may be reformed, for they are neither cooling nor binding, as they are taken to be:

but are of a clensing, resolving, consuming, and digesting quality, as Hyssope, Origanum, and Winter Savoury are, that with Figges and Licoris, are effectuall to expectorate flegme from the chest and lungs, wherewith they are filled:

Decoction: and that it is not fit to be used in inflammations the very taste of the herbe holding a leafe in ones mouth will declare, by the burning heate will be felt therein, and as *Dioscorides* and *Galen* say, that the decoction thereof being drunke sixe dayes together, will render the urine as blood: although at the first they will but provoke urine onely, the fruite and leaves as well as the flowers, are of one effect:

Seed: but the flowers and leaves are of more use then the seede, which is said to consume the spleene, and to procure a womans speedy delivery, but whereas it is said to bring barrennesse to men that use it, it cannot properly be said of men, but of women to be barren, and of men to be unable to generation, or their seede unprofitable upon sundry causes:

Distilled water: the leaves or flowers in pouther or the distilled water of them, is much commended to clense and dry up foule and moist ulcers, and to clense the face and skinne from morphew, sunburne, freckles, and other discolourings of the skinne.

Infused oil: The oyle wherein the flowers have beene infused and sunned, is good against cramps, convulsions of the sinues, and palsies, and any other benumming cold griefe.

Double honeysuckle: The double Honysuckle may safely be used to all these purposes, when the other is not at hand.

resolving: dissolving
consuming: breaking down
Hyssope: hyssop
Origanum: oregano or marjoram
Winter Savoury: winter savory, *Satureja montana*
Figges: figs
Licoris: liquorice
Dioscorides: Greek-speaking Roman physician (mid-first century AD)
Galen: Claudius Galen (AD130–200), Roman physician and author
consume: shrink
pouther: powder
morphew: discolouration of skin
sunned: set in the sun to infuse
sinues: sinews
palsies: paralysis or tremors
benumming cold griefe: chills or numbness

Hor or cold?

It is the leaf of honeysuckle that Parkinson declares to be hot, and we would have to agree. The taste is slightly peppery in the way that watercress is peppery, but if you nibble a leaf (even a young shoot) the heat builds and becomes quite irritating and burning to the throat.

The effect of the flower, however, we find is cooling for the most part, as mentioned in the text, useful for hot flushes, sunburn and other hot conditions – but they are still used for paralysis and cramps too.

Honeysuckle *Lonicera periclymenum*

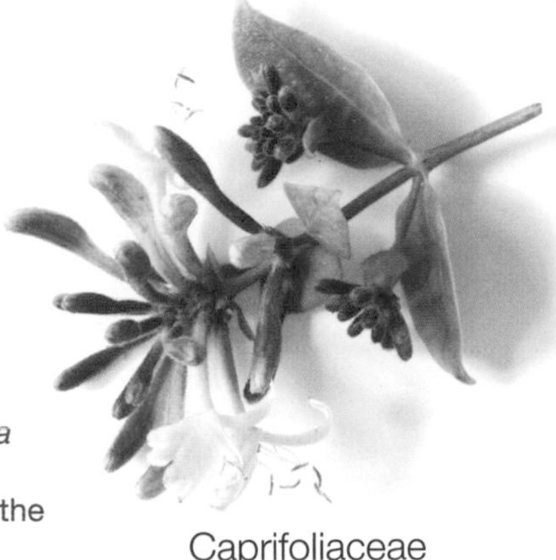

Caprifoliaceae

Honeysuckle is a gardener's delight more than a medicinal in Europe today, but in China the buds of *Lonicera japonica* are a significant herbal treatment. They are used to cool toxic heat and disperse it, as in colds and flu. *L. japonica* is a naturalized weed over much of the US South, and could be a valuable medicinal, as is *L. periclymenum*. Parkinson, as you will see, might argue with the reasoning.

Parkinson declares with some exasperation that the old and prevailing tradition about honeysuckle is wrong, and that its medicinal qualities are to heat, cleanse and consume, as when expelling phlegm. But the modern view sides with the tradition in this case. We now know honeysuckle contains the aspirin-like compound salicylic acid, and that in tea or syrup it acts as an antiviral to cool and soothe a headache, fever, bronchial complaint and some tumours.

Honeysuckle is also used now to cool menopausal hot flushes, sunburn (as in Parkinson's distilled water suggestions) and other heat-sensitive skin issues.

Modern practice corroborates his suggestion of using it for spasm, cramps and paralysis, especially in the respiratory system, for asthma, croup and bronchitis. Parkinson's infused oil put in the sun would taste wonderful. James Duke, the doyen of American herbalists, rates honeysuckle behind only eucalyptus for sore throat relief. It also has strong antiseptic qualities and effectively kills many micro-organisms.

As Parkinson notes, the seed is little used; the berries are bitter, and have a reputation as a poison or to bring on birth; they may well lead to infertility, as he says. Better all round to smell and enjoy the flowers!

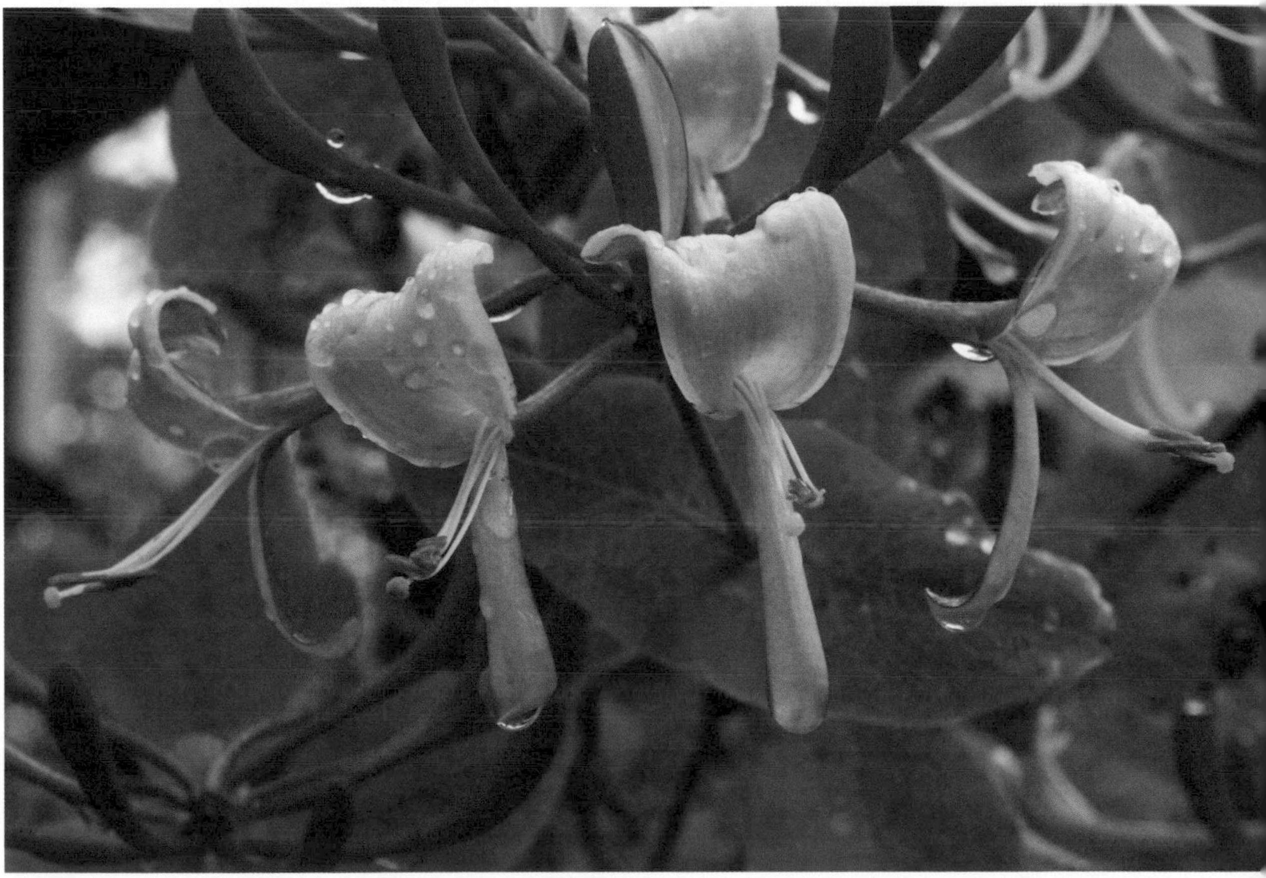

Horsetaile

Theatrum Botanicum

Tribe 13, Chapter 36, pp1200–03

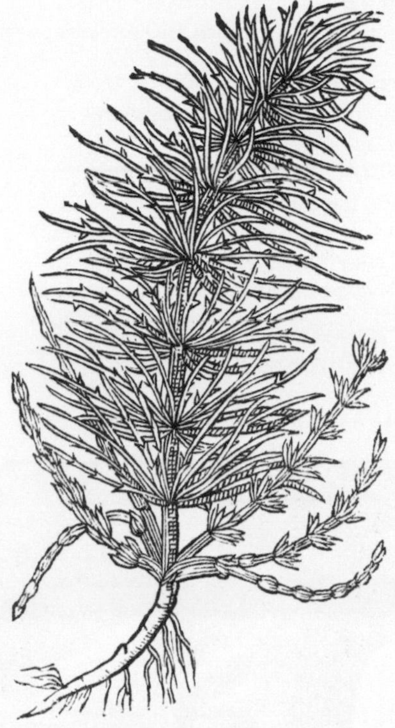

Physicke: medicine
Galen: Claudius Galen (AD130–200), Roman physician and author
sharpenesse: biting quality
stanch, stayeth: stops
Laskes: loose bowels
Fluxes: diarrhoea
excoriations: abrasions, sores
intralls: entrails, intestines
sodereth: fuses
greene: fresh
strangury: slow, painful urination
destillation of rheume: trickling down of watery mucus
wheales: pimples or pustules
fundament: anus or buttocks
peuter: pewter
flower: flour

Equisetum

The Vertues

Horsetaile the smoother rather then the rough, and the leaved then the bare, is both more used and of better effect in Physicke, and is as *Galen* saith with the bitternesse of a binding qualitie, and dryeth without sharpenesse.

Bleeding: It is very powerfull to stanch bleedings wheresoever, eyther inward or outward, the juice or decoction thereof being drunke, or the juice, decoction or distilled water applyed outwardly, it stayeth also all sorts of Laskes and Fluxes in man or woman, and the pissing of blood, and healeth also not onely the inward Ulcers and excoriations of the intralls, bladder, &c. but all other sorts of foule moist and running Ulcers, and soone sodereth together the toppes of greene wounds, not suffering them to grow to maturation:

Ruptures: it cureth also Ruptures in children quickly, in the elder by time, according to the disposition of the partie, and the continuance:

Urinary: the decoction hereof in wine being drunke is said to provoke urine, to helpe the strangury and the stone, and the distilled water thereof drunke two or three times in a day a small quantitie at a time, as also to ease the paines in the intralls or guts,

Cough: and to be effectuall against a cough that commeth by the destillation of rheume from the head:

Swellings & inflammation: the juice or distilled water being warmed, and hot inflammations pustules or red wheales and other such eruptions in the skinne, being bathed therewith doth helpe them, and doth no lesse ease the swellings, heate and inflammations of the fundament and privy parts in man or woman.

Pot scouring: Countrey huswives doe use any of these rough sorts that are next at hand to scoure both their woodden, peuter and brasse vessels,

Eating: the young buds are dressed by some like Asparagus, or being boyled, are after bestrewed with flower and fryed to be eaten.

The silica connection: Horsetail is full of silica, perhaps 30% by weight – in effect it is a silica skeleton – and when burned for ash it has over 80%. It is experimentally established that being water-soluble the silica is readily moved in solution to the body's extremities at a cellular level. Parkinson would not have known this, and omits the use of horsetail to improve the strength and elasticity of nails and hair, and for strengthening connective tissue – all useful modern applications, as is its addition to a hot bath to help restore tissues after sprains and fractures or baths for convalescence more generally.

Horsetail *Equisetum* spp. Equisetaceae

Equisetum, literally horsetail, is an apt descriptive name for this ancient plant, whose ancestors were dominant forest trees up to 400 million years ago. Native and common in moist places in most of the continents, it is also known as lizard tail or mule tail. It is a long-used folk remedy for treating the urinary system, bleeding and inflammation, and as a leading source of plant silica helps supply its deficiency in connective tissue, hair and nails.

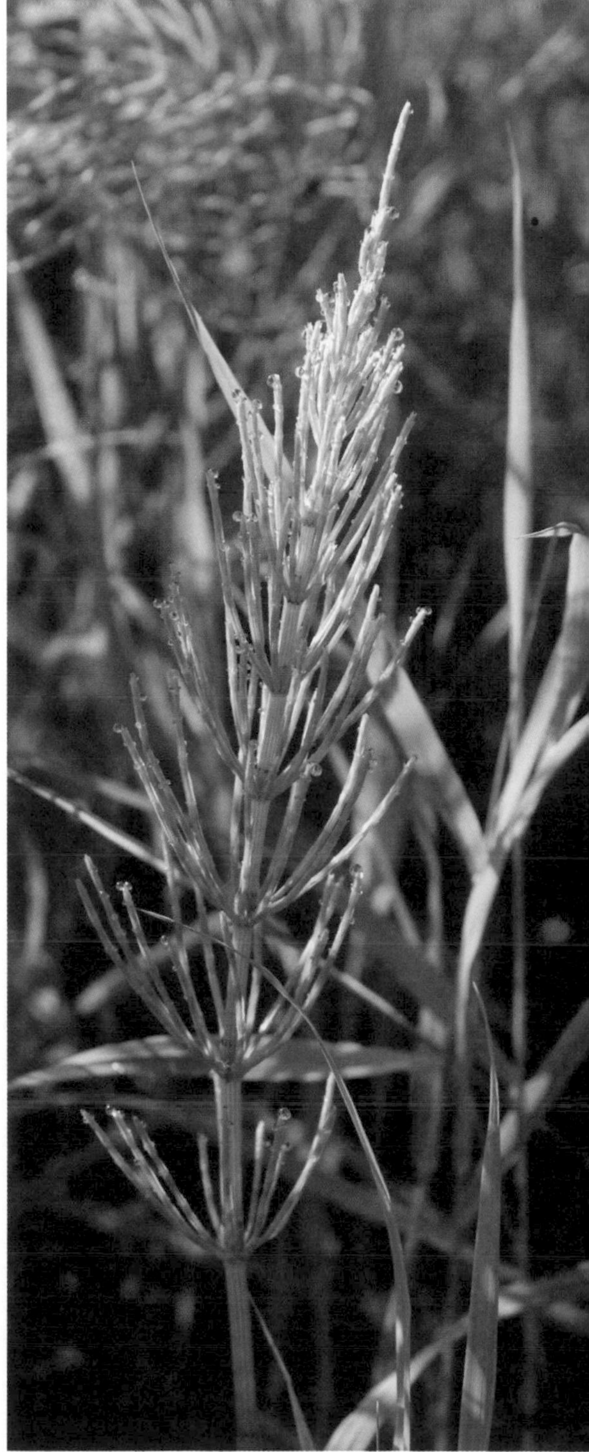

In his introduction to horsetails (which he also calls 'rough joynted Rushes') Parkinson describes 14 species, but is specific about preferring the smooth and leaved. He is right, and modern herbalists use the summer 'grassy', infertile shoots, rather than the earlier cone-like spore-bearing stems, and in particular choose field horsetail, *Equisetum arvense*.

The shoots are harvested by midsummer, dried quickly before they go brown, and shredded for storage. The usual internal preparation is a tea (known as *cola de caballo* in Spanish), but we have also made a tasty syrup. Parkinson suggests the juice, a distilled water or decocting the leaf in wine.

Bleeding: While herbalists would agree with Parkinson on horsetail as a blood coagulant and styptic, it is less used today than, say, yarrow or chili. A traditional wound and burn-healing herb, its parallel capacity to dry 'foule moist and running Ulcers' and close up fresh wounds can also be used.

Ruptures: It is interesting how Parkinson has observed the differential rate of healing for children and the elderly, and takes into account the person's constitution.

Urinary: Horsetail as a wide-ranging treatment for the urinary tract is now probably its major action, and in small, regular doses the tea is considered safe and reliable. It works internally as a diuretic and astringent to promote urine flow, reduce inflammation, clear infection, tone the kidneys and bladder, and equalize moisture levels. Modern usage includes for cystitis, urethritis, prostate enlargement and oedema, and to flush out the lower urinary tract.

Cough: In addition to Parkinson's head cough, herbalists today might turn to horsetail for emphysema and chest pain.

Swellings & inflammation: Horsetail has anti-inflammatory action as a skin lotion, compress, douche or bath. It is also effective on mouth ulcers or puffy eyelids.

Pot scouring: Just as horsetail scours gently within the body, people long ago found out its value for cleaning pots, pewter and silver, in cabinet-making and for polishing glass.

Eating: The 'young buds' made an old Roman tonic salad.

Our common Houseleeke

Theatrum Botanicum

Tribe 6, Chapter 5, pp729–33

Sedum majus vulgare

The Vertues

Cold comfort: Our ordinary Houseleeke is cold in the third degree, moderately drying and binding, and is good for all inward heats as well as outward, and in the eyes or other parts of the body:

Singular good in all hot agues: a Possit made with the juice of Houseleeke is singular good in all hot agues, for it cooleth and temperateth the blood and spirits, and quencheth the thirst, and is also good to stay all hot defluxions of sharpe and salt rheume into the eyes, the juice being dropped into them, or into the eares helpe them, it helpeth also all other fluxes of humors into the bowells, and the immoderate courses of women:

All proceeds of a hot cause: it is sayd also to kill the wormes, and to remedy the biting of the *Phalangium* Spider: it cooleth and restrayneth also all other hot inflammations, Saint *Anthonies* fire, and all other hot eruptions in the flesh, scaldings also and burnings, the shingles, fretting ulcers, cankers, tetters, ringwormes and the like, and easeth much the paine of the goute, proceeding of an hot cause:

Powerful juice: the juice also taketh away warts and cornes in the hands or feete being often bathed therewith, and the skinne of the leaves being layd on them afterwards: it easeth also the headach, and distempered heate of the braine in frensyes or through want of sleepe, being applied to the temples and forehead: the leaves bruised and layd upon the crowne or seame of the head stayeth bleeding at the nose very quickly.

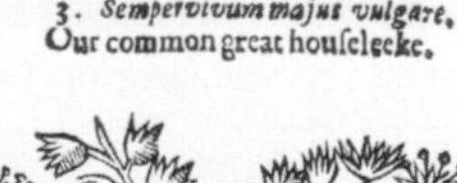
3. *Sempervivum majus vulgare.* Our common great houseleeke.

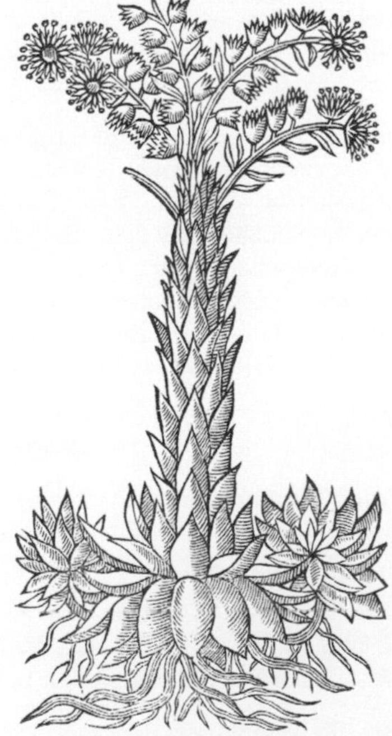

Houseleek water: The distilled water of the herbe is profitable for all the purposes aforesaid: the leaves being very gently rubbed on any place stung by Nettles or Bees, or bitten with any venemous creature doth presently take away the paine.

binding: astringent
possit: posset, a drink of hot milk curdled with an acid, e.g. lemon, often spiced
agues: fevers
temperateth: moderates
stay defluctions: stop flow
rheume: mucus-like secretion
fluxes of humors: flow of liquid
immoderate courses: excessive menstruation
Phalangium spider: a venomous spider, not our modern *Phalangium* or harvestman, which have no venom
Saint Anthonies fire: red facial inflammation; erysipelas
fretting: weeping
cankers: non-healing sore
tetters: pustular skin eruption
distempered: unusual
frensyes: delirium
seame: cranium
stayeth: stops
profitable: effective

Houseleek *Sempervivum tectorum* Crassulaceae

Not many plants spread by imperial edict, but houseleek did. The Holy Roman Emperor Charlemagne in about AD 812 made a list of some 50 plants that by law were to be grown on his imperial estates. Nasturtium, fenugreek, rose and mallow were named, along with houseleek, or Jove's beard, and this was specifically to be grown up on the roof. The modern Latin name reflects this: it literally means plant that lives for ever, and on the roof – the original idea being that by being put there it assuages the god of thunder, Jove or, farther north, Thor, so that he will not send his lightning and burn up the thatch. From the plant's point of view the emperor's intervention was excellent news: it can only spread by 'pups' or offsets, which start a new plant as a clone; human agency and company are what it likes best.

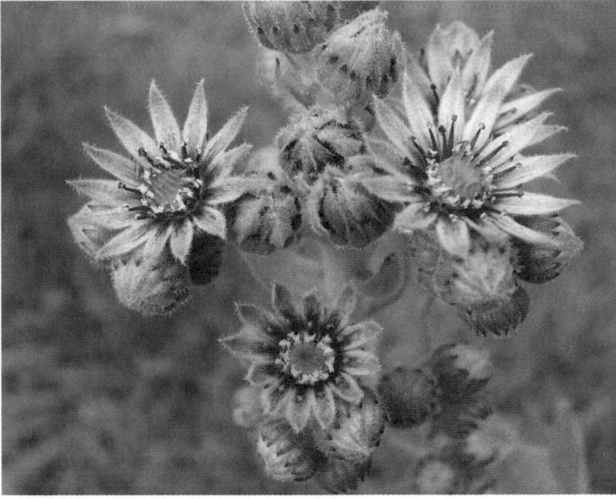

Cold comfort: Parkinson nails the qualities of houseleek that make it beneficial: it is cooling, drying and binding. This combination of virtues is unusual. We have found it is simplicity itself to use: break open one of the gell-filled leaves, and there you have a domestic equivalent of *Aloe vera* ready-made to apply to burns, scalds, headaches and other hot conditions, as Parkinson will go on to mention.

Singular good in all hot agues: Among these conditions are fevers or agues, which can be dealt with inwardly too by a posset or medicinal drink of houseleek boiled in milk. This is cooling and thirst-quenching, and the milk probably prevents it being purgative. Additionally, he says, it will dry up watery mucus of the eyes or ears (the plant was once called 'erewort'), and settle upset bowels or even restart interrupted menstruation.

All proceeds of a hot cause: Parkinson then trumps his previous cards by saying the plant can be used to kill worms, be active in healing skin conditions such as erysipelas, shingles, weeping ulcers and pustular eruptions, and also gout 'proceeding of an hot cause'.

Powerful juice: Applying houseleek onto corns and warts, the juice and cut leaf being kept there by a compress for a few hours, is a reputed country remedy that some older people may still remember. Parkinson would have you apply it to your brows for a hot headache, insomnia or nosebleeds, and there is no reason why it will not be effective.

Houseleek water: A distilled water of houseleek works to the same effect, Parkinson says, and for bites and stings.

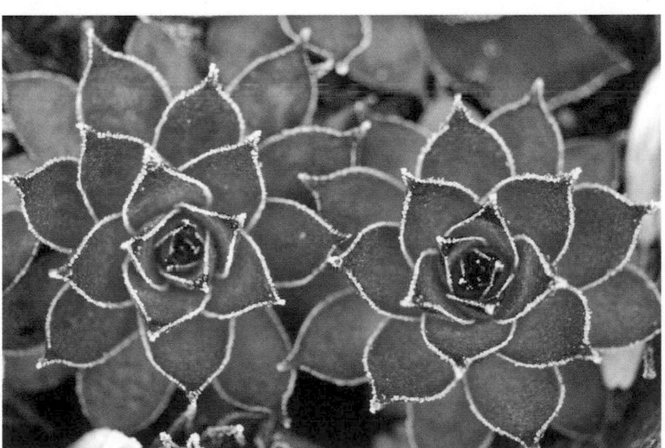

Victorian self-help with houseleek

Some village doctresses would hardly know what to do without it [houseleek], for its cooling leaves are applied to burns and scalds, and freckles and sunburn; and mixed with milk or ale, it is taken for a variety of maladies. Happily it is quite wholesome.
– Anne Pratt, *Haunts of the Wild Flowers* (1866), p197

Hysope

Theatrum Botanicum

Tribe 1, Chapter 1, pp1–4

Hyssopus

Vertues

Dioscorides saith, that Hysope boyled with Rue and Hony, and drunke doth helpe those that are troubled with Coughes, shortnesse of breath, wheesing, and rheumaticke distillations upon the lungs; taken also with Oxymel, it purgeth grosse humours by the stoole, and with hony killeth the wormes in the belly, and taken also with fresh or new figges bruised, helpeth to loosen the belly, but more forcibly, if the roote of the Flowerdeluce and Cresses (yet some copies in stead of *Cardamon* have *Cardamomum*, which I never knew put into any purging medicine in our times, and *Macer* his verse doth intimate Cresses thus; *Cardama si jungas his solves fortius alvum*) be added thereunto:

it amendeth and cherisheth the native colour of the body, spoyled by the yellow-jaundise, helpeth the dropsie and the splene, if it be taken with figges and nitar: being boiled with wine, it is good to wash inflamations, it taketh away the blew and blacke spottes, and markes that come by strokes, bruises, or falles; being applied with warme water;

Throat: it is also an excellent medicine for those, that are troubled with the Quinsie, or swelling in the throate, to wash and gargle it, being boyled with Figges;

Toothache & ears: it helpeth the tooth-ach, being boyled in vinegar and gargled therewith; the hot vapours of the decoction, taken by a funnell in at the eares, easeth the inflamations of them, *Mesues* saith the singing noyse of them;

Pliny: *Pliny* addeth, that it is an enemy to the stomacke, and provoketh casting being taken with figges: being bruised, and salt, hony, and cumminseede put to it, it helpeth those that are stung by serpents.

Galen: *Galen* is very breife herein and onely saith, it is hot and dry in the third degree, and of thin parts.

Matthiolus: *Matthiolus* saith that our Hysope is of thinne parts, and that it cutteth & breaketh tough flegme, it rarifieth or maketh thinne that which is thicke or grosse, it openeth that which is stopped, and clenseth that which is corrupt, the oyle thereof being annoynted killeth lice, and taketh away the itching of the head,

1. *Hyssopus vulgaris.*
Common garden Hysope.

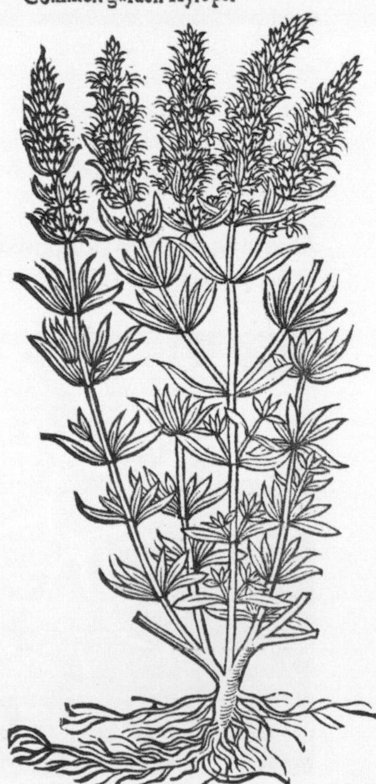

Dioscorides: Greek-speaking Roman physician (mid-first century AD)
rheumaticke distillations: watery mucus
oxymel: honey and vinegar
hony: honey
figges: figs
flowerdeluce: fleur de lys
Cardamon: probably *Cardamine*, bitter cress
Cardamomum: cardamom
Macer: the 1493 book *Macer Floridus de Virtutibus Herbarum*, probably by French physician Odo of Meung
Cardama si jungas his solves fortius alvum: if you mix Cardama with these you will relax the belly more fully
dropsie: dropsy
splene: spleen
nitar: saltpetre
quinsie: a peritonsillar abscess
Mesues: Syriac physician Yuhanna ibn Masawaih (777–857)
the singing noyse: tinnitus
Pliny: Pliny the Elder (AD23–79), Roman naturalist
cumminsede: cumin seed
Galen: Claudius Galen (AD130–200), Roman physician and author
Matthiolus: Pierandrea Mattioli (1501–77), physician and author

Hyssop *Hyssopus officinalis* Lamiaceae

Hyssop is the very first plant in the *Theatrum Botanicum*, and Parkinson places it in the tribe of sweet-smelling herbs. It was popular in his day for strewing on floors to add fragrance to rooms. Its qualities include being warming, gently astringent and anti-inflammatory. Hyssop is still used by herbalists to treat coughs, sore throats and chest infections, for weak digestion and for bruises, sprains and insect bites. It is classified as a calming tonic herb.

Hyssop is often claimed as one of the bitter purging herbs of the Bible, to be used during Passover, but we think that this translation is wrong for the simple reason that hyssop is not bitter. Rather, it has a pleasant aromatic pungency, which was very popular in British cooking in Parkinson's period, and deserves to be tried again in modern cooking. It is quite likely that hyssop is much more strongly flavoured and pungent where it grows in a hot dry climate.

Parkinson says in his introduction to the plant: '*But there is a great controversie among our later writers, what hearbe should be the true Hysope of* Dioscorides, *and other the Greeke authors; for that our common Hysope is not it, but it is the true Hysope of the* Arabians, *as all doe acknowledge except* Matthiolus, *who doth earnestly contend, that our garden Hysope is the same of* Dioscorides, *whose arguments are too weake, to perswade any to be of his opinion...*' and '*Now it is not likely that the Iewes [Jews] had an other Hysope, divers [distinct] both from the Greekes & Arabians ...*' (TB, pp3, 4). The controversy continues!

Modern herbalists cannot even agree on the taste and smell of hyssop – one author describes it as smelling like a skunk, others describe it as lemony and aromatic. So, what can we agree on? Perhaps some of the plant's 'virtues'.

Sore throats: Hyssop tea makes a soothing gargle for sore throat, tonsillitis and quinsy. It can also be boiled with dried figs, as Parkinson suggests, to make a sweeter concoction.

Coughs & congestion: Hyssop is a really good cough remedy. It is particularly good when there is thick phlegm, as it thins it and makes it more liquid, just as Matthiolus said. A hot tea can be drunk several times a day, or try rubbing hyssop infused oil or an ointment on the chest and back twice daily.

Hyssop can be helpful for asthma and bronchitis as well as for colds and flu.

Parkinson's recipe for a decoction of hyssop, figs, muscadine and sugar is really tasty, and very soothing. In fact, it tastes so good that you don't even need a cough as the excuse for taking it!

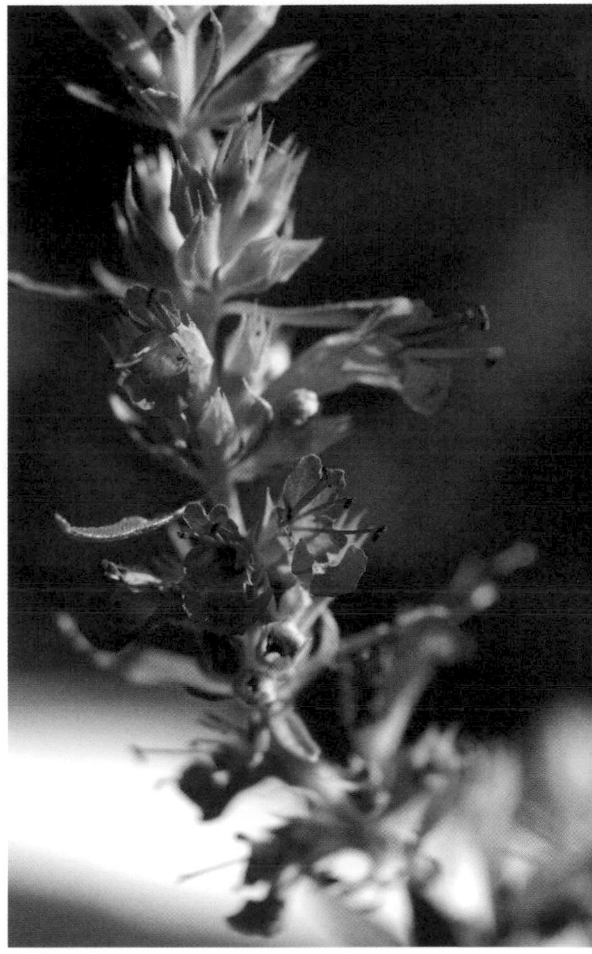

Digestion: Hyssop stimulates digestion and appetite. It also relieves gas, indigestion, bloating and spasm.

Fevers: By promoting sweating, hyssop can help relieve fevers. It also has an antiviral and antibacterial action, and seems to work particularly well during the recovery phase of flus and fevers.

Wounds: Fresh hyssop chewed or chopped for use as a poultice speeds healing of minor cuts and scratches. It will also help bruises and alleviate the pain of aching muscles. The infused oil or an ointment can also be used.

Urine: Hyssop is a diuretic, increasing the flow of urine.

falling sicknesse: epilepsy
Castoreum: exudate from beavers
dragme: dramme, 1/8 oz apothecary weight, 3.89 gm or 3 scruples
pilles: pills
Peonye: peony
Assafaetida: asafoetida (*Ferula assa-foetida)*
scruple: apothecary's weight, 20 grains or 1/25 oz, 1.3g gm
physitians: physicians
cold griefes: chills
stuffeth: blocks
lohoc: a thick syrup
Sugarcandy: sugar crystals
Muscadine: sweet wine
womens monethly courses: menses
sharpe fitts of agues: intense attack of fever
hearbe: herb
greene wound: fresh wound

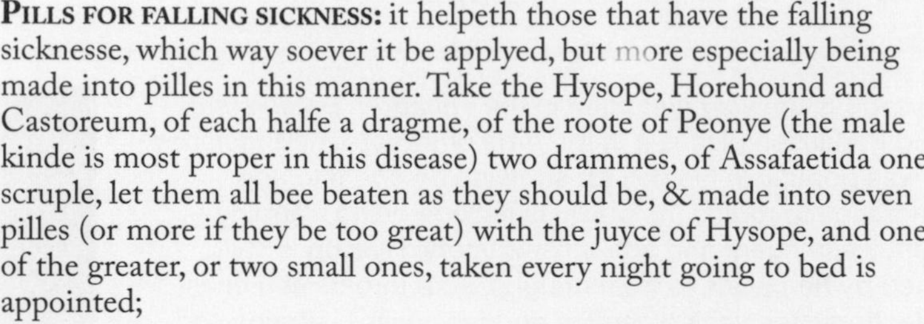

Pills for falling sickness: it helpeth those that have the falling sicknesse, which way soever it be applyed, but more especially being made into pilles in this manner. Take the Hysope, Horehound and Castoreum, of each halfe a dragme, of the roote of Peonye (the male kinde is most proper in this disease) two drammes, of Assafaetida one scruple, let them all bee beaten as they should be, & made into seven pilles (or more if they be too great) with the juyce of Hysope, and one of the greater, or two small ones, taken every night going to bed is appointed;

Lung congestion: the best Physitians of our tymes, assuredly doe account it, to be hot and dry in the third degree, and of thinne parts: for being sharpe and a little bitter withall, they apply it effectually, for all cold griefes or diseases of the chest and lungs, helping to expectorate tough flegme, that stuffeth or oppresseth them, being taken either in a *lohoc* or licking medicine, or in a Syrupe, or any other way,

Cough syrup: and in a decoction thus; Take an handful of Hysope, two ounces of figges, and one ounce of Sugarcandy, boyle them in a quart of Muscadine, untill halfe a pint be consumed, which being strained, & taken morning and evening, availeth much for those that are troubled with an old cough, by causing the tough flegme the more easily to be avoided:

Other uses: it helpeth also to provoke urine being stopped, or that is made by droppes: it helpeth to breake winde, and to cause womens monethly courses, and easeth the sharpe fitts of agues; the greene hearbe being bruised and a little sugar put thereto, doth quickly heale any greene wound or cut in the hand, or else where being applied thereto.

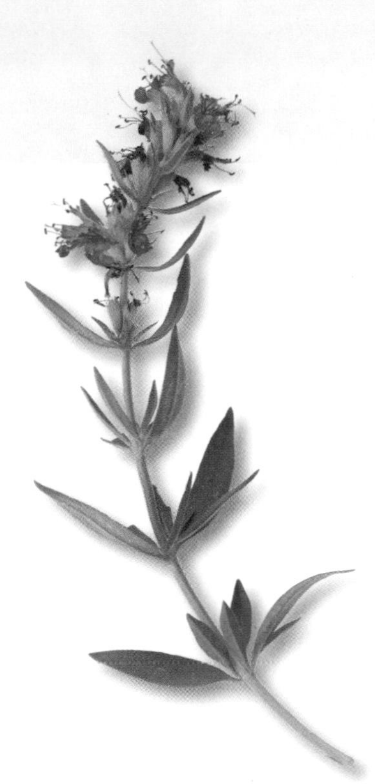

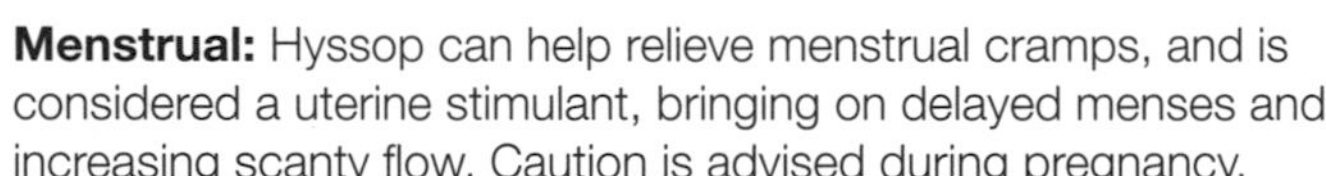

Menstrual: Hyssop can help relieve menstrual cramps, and is considered a uterine stimulant, bringing on delayed menses and increasing scanty flow. Caution is advised during pregnancy.

Other uses: Hyssop relieves jaundice, and through its action on the immune sytem is helpful for the spleen too. It can be given to children as a gentle laxative.

Hyssop essential oil is used as a flavouring in Chartreuse liqueur, and it is also an ingredient in Eau de Cologne.

The fresh or dried leaves are a pleasant addition to soups and stews, and combine well with beans. The flowers are pretty when sprinkled on salads and fruit salads.

Modern research

Hyssop and hyssop essential oil show promise against viral infections including HIV and herpes simplex. Research has also indicated that hyssop has antibacterial and antifungal properties.

Ivie

Theatrum Botanicum

Tribe 5, Chapter 94, pp678–81

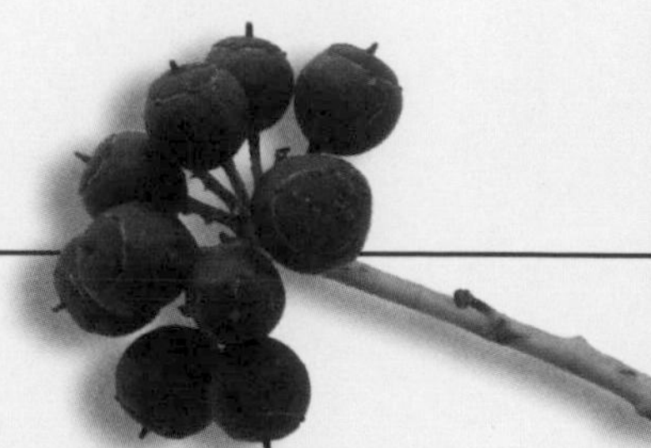

Hedera arborea

The Vertues

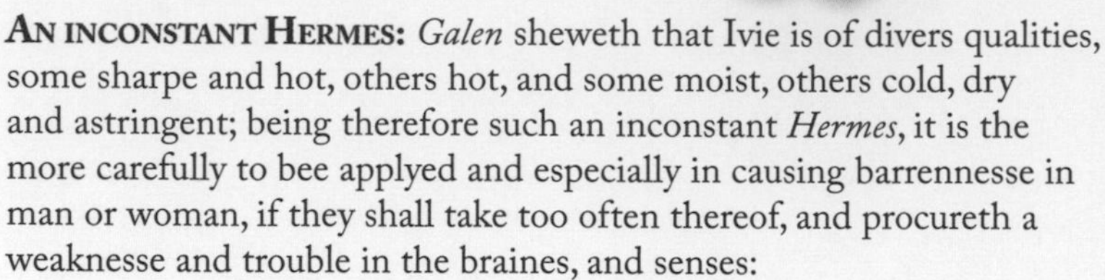

An inconstant Hermes: *Galen* sheweth that Ivie is of divers qualities, some sharpe and hot, others hot, and some moist, others cold, dry and astringent; being therefore such an inconstant *Hermes*, it is the more carefully to bee applyed and especially in causing barrennesse in man or woman, if they shall take too often thereof, and procureth a weaknesse and trouble in the braines, and senses:

Ivy flowers & fluxes: A Pugill of the flowers (that is as much as one may take up with their three fingers together) which may be about a dramme, saith *Dioscorides*, drunke twice a day in red wine, helpeth the Laske and blooddy flix. It is an enemy to the nerves and sinewes being taken too much inwardly, but is very helpefull unto them being applied outwardly:

Ivy berries & bellies: *Pliny* saith that the yellow berries are good against the Iaundies, and taken before one be set to drinke hard will keepe him from drunkennesse, and helpeth those that spit blood, and that the white berries being taken inwardly killeth the wormes of the belly, or applyed outwardly: the juice of the roote is good to be taken against the biting of the *Phalangium*, or deadly Spider: the berries are held by many Empericks Quacksalvers and Chirurgions to be a singular remedy both to prevent the Plague or pestilence, before it be taken, as also to free them from it, that have got it;

Ivy baths & pessaries: by drinking the berries made in powder for two or three dayes together: they being taken in wine do for certaine helpe to breake the stone, provoke urine and womens courses as *Tragus* saith, yea so powerfull they are in those parts, that a bath made of the leaves and berries for women to sit in, or over the fumes, or a pessarie made of them and put up doth mightily prevaile to bring them downe, and to draw forth the dead birth and secondines or afterbirth, but this is to be cautelously used, and not but upon necessitie, or extremetie:

Ivy leaves in vinegar: the leaves of Ivie while they are fresh, boyled in Vinegar, and applied warme to the sides of those that are spleneticke, or troubled with the Spleene, ache or stitch in the sides doth give them much ease: the same also applyed with some Rosewater and oyle of Roses to the forehead and temples, doth ease the headach although it be of long continuance:

Ivy leaves in wine: the fresh leaves boyled in wine, and old filthy sores and Ulcers that are hard to bee cured washed therewith, doth wonderfully helpe to clense and heale them, as also effectuall for greene wounde to heale them quickly and soder up the lippes thereof: the same also is effectuall to heale scaldings of water, and burnings by

1. *Hedera arborea nostras.* Our ordinary Ivie.

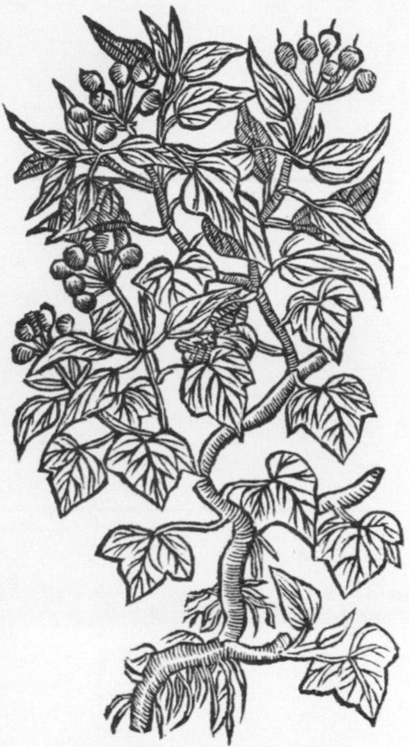

Galen: Claudius Galen (AD130–200), Roman physician and author
Hermes: Mercury, winged messenger of the gods, known to be 'flighty', changeable
pugill: small handful; amount taken up by thumb and first three fingers
dramme: dram, apothecary's weight equal to ⅛ oz or 3.89g
Dioscorides: Greek-speaking Roman physician (mid-first century AD)
laske: diarrhoea
blooddy flix: bloody stools, dysentery
Pliny: Pliny the Elder (AD23–79), Roman naturalist
iaundies: jaundice
Phalangium: venomous spider
empericks: unqualified medical practitioner, but with practical knowledge

Ivy *Hedera helix ssp. helix* Araliaceae

Ivy was widely and respectfully used as a medicine in Parkinson's time, and he gives a full account of its virtues and the associated dangers, often arising from taking it inappropriately internally. The plant has spread almost unfettered in Britain in recent times, as woodlands have been less coppiced, but while its density has increased so its medicinal usefulness has declined. This is a pity as the external application of ivy leaves can be an immediate kitchen medicine for many skin problems.

An inconstant Hermes: Parkinson is right to begin his account of the virtues of ivy by giving a rather scary warning about its potential for causing sterility or brain damage, probably meningitis. The plant was and is so universal – Parkinson says it 'is well knowne to every child almost' – with a complex and powerful chemistry (as we would describe his 'inconstant Hermes') that a note of caution is called for. In the Anglophone world today, ivy leaves are sometimes used for external treatments, such as blisters and corns, while in Germany it remains an authorized remedy for catarrh and chronic bronchial conditions.

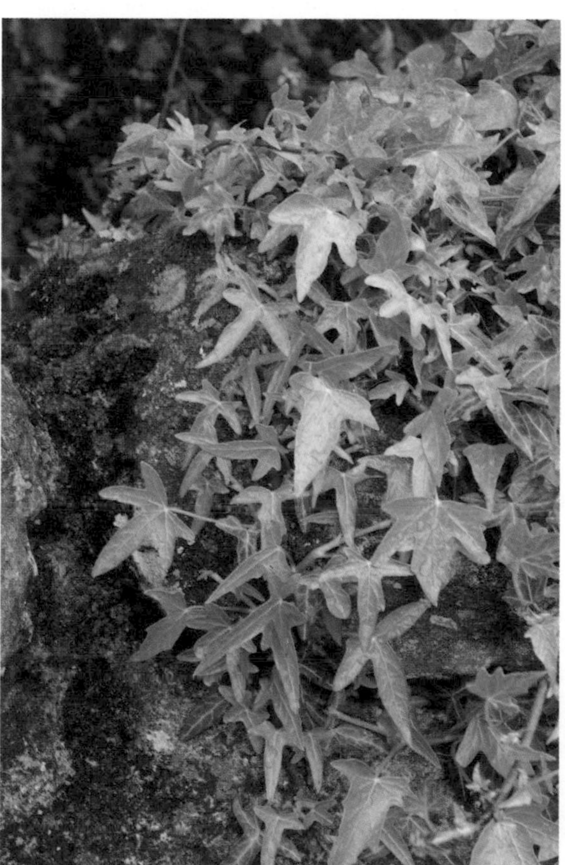

Ivy flowers & fluxes: The flowers are little used currently by herbalists, and Parkinson repeats an ancient Dioscorides recipe combining red wine and ivy flower for treating diarrhoea and dysentery. Again this comes with his caution that too much of such a remedy will damage the nervous system.

Ivy berries & bellies: Parkinson's mention of the berries to treat jaundice was similarly reporting an ancient folk usage. In his day other routine jaundice treatments included bay, betony, dandelion, fumitory, parsley and plantain; modern herbalists might well turn to dandelion, St John's wort or milk thistle. We will return later to ivy and alcohol.

Ivy berries & plague: As an apothecary-freeman Parkinson might be expected to be unsympathetic to unqualified competitors, and especially when it comes to their offering ivy as a useless plague remedy. He shows much restraint in merely reporting their activities. In truth, ivy taken internally in an already compromised immune system could well be a fatal purgative, a pestilence in its own right.

Ivy baths & pessaries: Powdered ivy berries in wine would indeed be a powerful enough treatment to dissolve stones, help urination or stimulate menstruation, at no small risk to the patient. Parkinson goes further, relaying German practices of ivy herbal baths, to immerse in or inhale, or using pessaries, to expel a dead child or the afterbirth of a live child. As he repeats, this is extremely hazardous.

Ivy leaves in vinegar: On the other hand, French herbalist Maurice Mességué describes ivy as a free natural analgesic, and 'the best painkiller you are likely to find a couple of steps away from your house' (*Health Secrets of Plants and Herbs* (1979), pp152–3). Applying the leaves mixed with rosewater and oil of roses is an excellent home remedy for headaches; boiling ivy leaves in vinegar would still 'give much ease' for aching muscles or the spleen area.

quacksalvers: unauthorised pedlar offering chemical cures; from 'quicksilver', mercury
chirurgions: unauthorized surgeons
breake the stone: dissolve bodily concretions
womens courses: menstruation
Tragus: Hieronymus Bock (1498–1554), physician, priest and author
pessarie: pessary
bring them downe: cause to flow
secondines: secundine, afterbirth
cautelously: carefully, cautiously
spleneticke: of the spleen; melancholic, peevish
rosewater, oyle of roses: homemade treatments in Parkinson's day
greene: fresh
soder up the lippes: fuse the edges
exulcerations: ulcerations
sharpnesse: pungent, acidic
salt flegme: sour phlegm
hot humours: warm secretions
thinne rheume: watery mucus
defluxions: flow of mucus, usually with a cold
running sores: suppurating, oozing
pomgranat: pomegranate, *Punica granatum*
issues: discharges
gum: resin
dossolved: probably means: dissolved
aking: aching
holpen: helping
Cato: Marcus Portius Cato Uticensius (95–46BC), Roman politician and Stoic philosopher
Varro: Marcus Terentius Varro (116–27BC), Roman scholar and satirist
gnattes and battes: gnats and bats
noysome: noxious

fire, and the exulcerations that happen thereby, or upon the sharpnesse of salt flegme, and hot humours in other parts of the body:

IVY JUICE: the juice of the leaves or berries being snuffed up into the nose purgeth the head and braine of thinne rheume, which maketh defluxions into the eyes and nose, and cureth the Ulcers and stench therein: the same dropped into the eares, doth helpe the old and running sores of them:

BERRIES & LEAVES AGAIN: five of the yellow berries bruised and heated with oyle of Roses in a Pomgranet rinde and dropped into the eare of such as have the toothache, on the contrary side of the paine easeth them thereof: the berries or the leaves used causeth the haire to grow blacke. The fresh leaves are commonly used to bee layd upon issues wheresoever, in the armes legges, &c. to keepe them open, and to draw forth the humours that fall thither:

IVY RESIN: the Gum of the Ivie, which in the hot countries is gathered from the body and branches, is exceeding sharpe and hot, burning and exulcerating the skinne, yet it is used being dossolved to take away superfluous haire in any place, and to destroy Nits and Lice wheresoever: the same dissolved in Vinegar and put into hollow aking teeth doth ease the same, and being often used will cause them to fall out: Some doe use it as a baite with other things to kill fish:

IVY WOOD: the wood made into a cup, and those that are troubled with the Spleene shall finde ease, and be much holpen thereof, if they continually drinke out of it, so as the drinke may stand some small time therein before it be drunke.

IVY & ALCOHOL: *Cato* writeth an experiment how to finde out the deceit of Vintners and others that put water to their wine, which is this, that if you suspect your wine, you shall put some thereof into such a cup that is made of Ivie wood, and that if there be any water therein it will remaine in the cup, and the wine will soke through; for the nature of Ivie wood saith he and *Varro*, is not to hold any wine, so great an antipathy there is betweene them:

IVY SMOKE: the fume of Ivie branches being burned driveth away Gnattes and Battes, and all other hurtfull and noysome creatures.

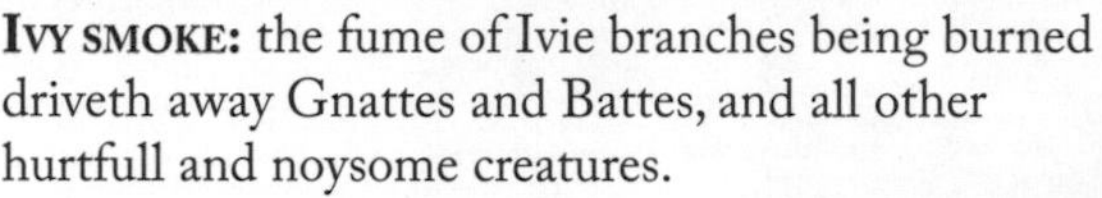

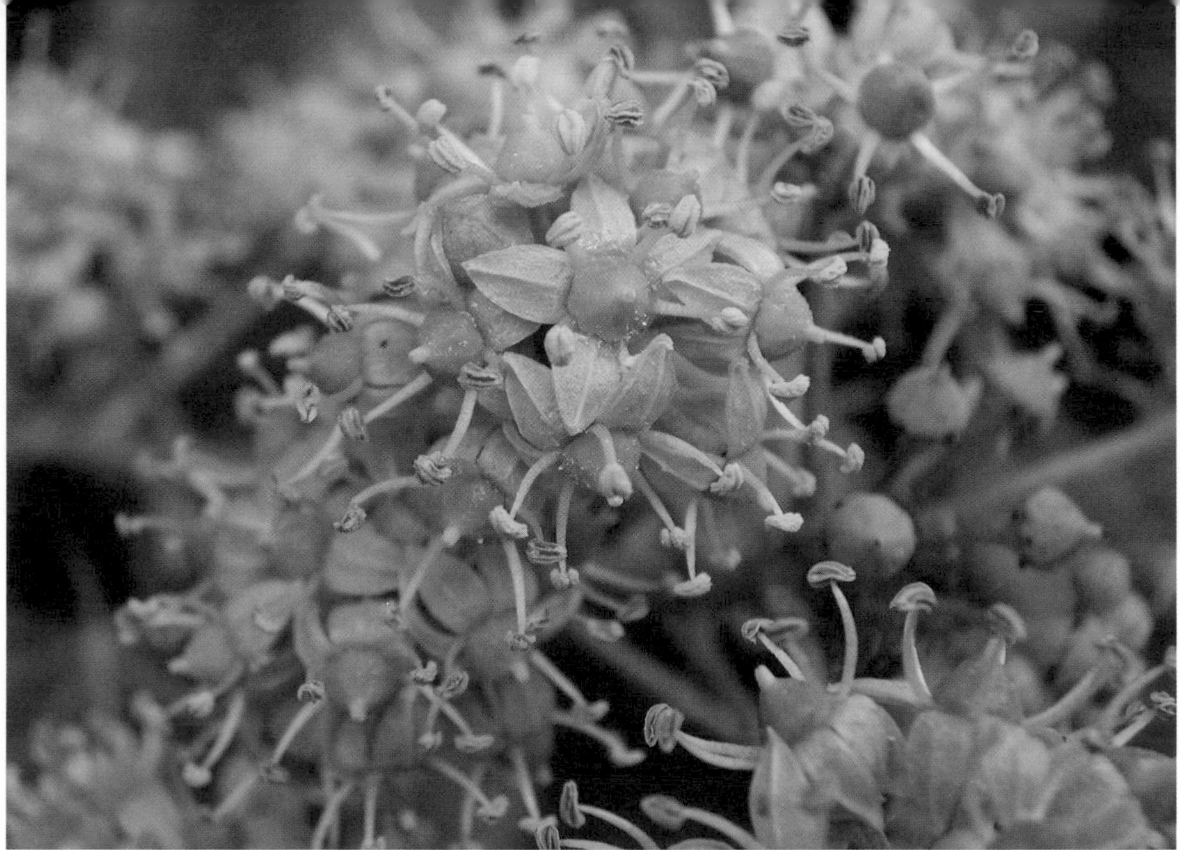

Ivy leaves in wine: Wine is another effective vehicle in which to boil up ivy leaves, and Parkinson talks of this method for treating both old and fresh wounds, for scalds or burns, and to cool 'hot humours' generally. In the Anglo-Saxon Leechbook of Bald, ivy leaves melted into butter were a treatment for sun-burn, and in his book *Grandmother's Secrets* (1972), p161, Jean Palaiseul writes of a French ivy leaf poul-tice. This was made from two handfuls of ivy leaves, chopped up; the leaves are mixed with 4 handfuls of bran and ¼ litre (½ US pint) of water into a thick paste, and warmed on a low heat for 10 minutes. Spread on a suitable cloth, apply to the affected area, and keep on for at least half an hour. Palaiseul says this is soothing for sciatica, phlebitis and neuralgia.

Ivy juice: Snuffing the juice of ivy leaves or berries is indeed expectorant, if not purgative, and clears the head or ears of any mucus – a shock treatment.

Berries & leaves again: Adding pomegranate rind and rose oil to ivy berries is an interesting combination, but we don't know how good it would be for treating toothache; ivy as a restorer of hair colour is well documented (it also refreshes the colour of black silk), and making an ivy leaf compress would be highly drawing for pus and other exudates, and for rheumatic joints.

Ivy resin: Here Parkinson is talking of a species of ivy from 'hot countries', which partakes of the extra heat of its source area. You can well imagine that it would destroy nits and lice, burn the skin, ease the pain of a hollow tooth and then cause it to fall out, or kill fish. Parkinson mentioned earlier that ivy root, even of the common European ivy, was strong enough to coun-ter the bite of the Phalangium spider or harvestman.

Ivy wood: Drinking from a cup made of ivy wood, with the liquid standing for a while, is a specific remedy for spleen problems, Parkinson says. Gabrielle Hatfield reports a child in Cheshire with whooping cough being made to take his potions in a cup of ivy wood (*Hatfield's Herbal*, 2007, p200).

Ivy & alcohol: Ivy has long had a reputation as 'the enemy of the vine', and was thought to prevent drunkenness; this must be why Bacchus, the god of drinking, wears a crown of ivy so that he could drink all the more. Parkinson cites two Roman sources to support the idea that wine soaks into ivy wood while water remains, suggesting this quality can be used 'to finde out the deceit of Vintners'.

Ivy smoke: We can confirm that ivy leaves and wood burn well, producing vigorous smoke that repels any living being, including 'noysome creatures'!

Jasmine or Gelsemine

Theatrum Botanicum

Tribe 16, Chapter 50, pp1464–66

1. *Gelseminum vel Iasminum album vulgare.* The ordinary white Iasmine.

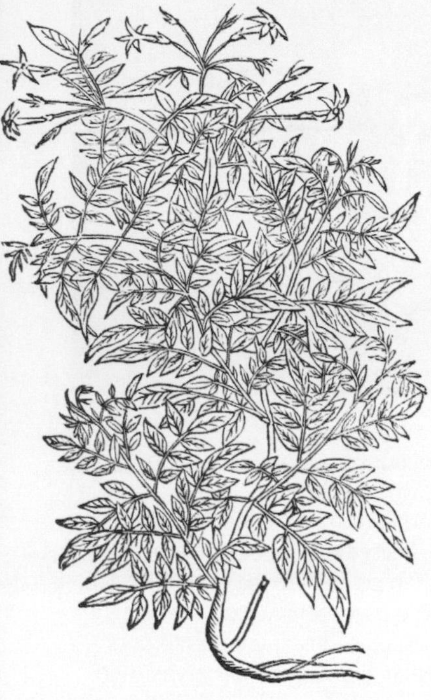

Serapio: probably Serapion the Younger, a 12th century author whose *Book of Simple Medicaments* was translated into Latin in the 16th
delivereth: propounds
discusseth humours: disperses bodily liquids
profitable: effective
tough: sticky
tetters: pustular skin eruption
strow: scatter
sent: scent
insolation: exposure to sunlight
Master Tradescant: John Tradescant the Younger (1608–62), who brought back the plant from Virginia

Gelseminum sive Iasminum

The Vertues

Serapio delivereth it, that the white Iasmine is hot in the beginning of the second degree, that it discusseth humours, is good against salt flegme, profitable to old cold men, and profitable for catarrhs, and the griefes that spring from tough flegme:

Leaves: the leaves either greene or dry, doe clense freckles, spots, and discolouring in the face or elsewhere, and helpeth tetters or ringwormes, and the like: it is not fit that those that are of an hot constitution should use this, for this breedeth the headache.

Flowers: The flowers are very sweete, and therefore they serve to strow in the house for an ornament and good sent, they use also in the warme Countries to lay the flowers among their gloves or fine linnen, to give the better sent.

Infused oil: The oyle that is made of the flowers by insolation is good for any cold part of the body to warme it, and to ease the paines of the crampe, and stitching in the sides.

Parkinson describes five kinds of jasmine: he calls them ordinary white, single Spanish and double Spanish, the Indian most sweete yellow Iasmine, and the sweete climbing Virginian Iasmine. He says the first three were brought from Syria to Spain, and the first (the wild species) is used as a graft for the other two. He is rightly cautious about naming the Sweete climbing Virginian as Jasmine:

'[it] was never mentioned by any before, and but that Master *Tradescant* is confident to call it a Iasmine, and therefore I am content to put it with the rest to give him content, I would be further informed of it my selfe, before I would certainely give my consent' (TB, p1465).

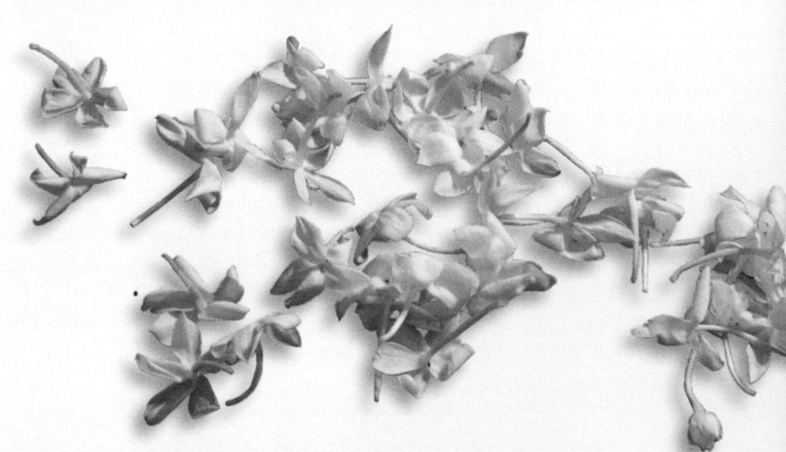

Jasmine *Jasminum* sp.

Oleaceae

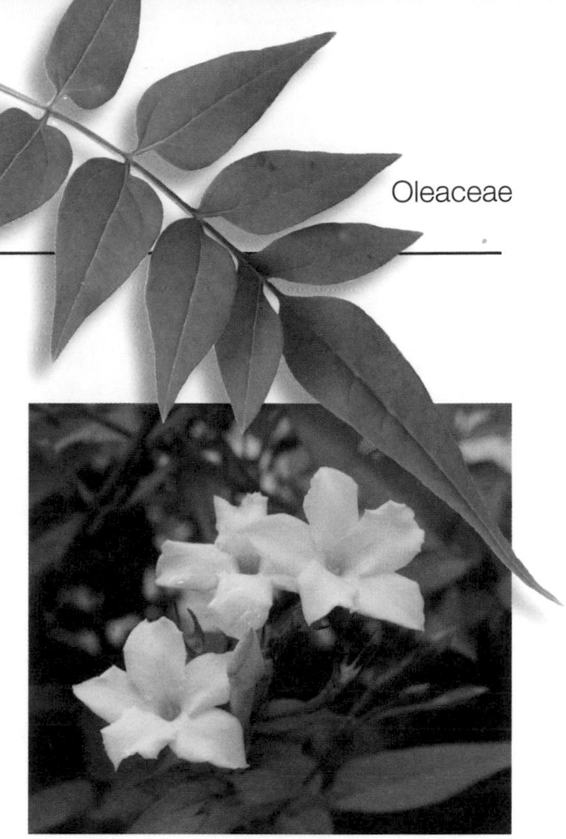

Jasmine is a plant of apparent opposites. It has been considered both male and female, sensuous and spiritual, heating and cooling.

It is thought that Jasmine, *Jasminum officinale,* first arrived in England in the mid-16th century, where it quickly became popular for its sweet scent. Parkinson also talks about the more tender Spanish jasmine, *Jasminum grandiflorum*, which was originally from India but is naturalized in Spain. This is the jasmine most often used in perfumery, and in Ayurvedic and Arabic medicine.

In the Ayurvedic medical system of India jasmine is used to cool, soothe and calm the nervous system, which is helpful in cases of stress, insomnia or depression. It is also used for liver problems, including cirrhosis and hepatitis. Jasmine's bitterness and astringency can help reduce heavy menstrual bleeding, and it is beneficial in soothing inflammations of the skin and mucous membranes.

In Chinese medicine, jasmine is considered more heating, being used to strengthen the yang, stimulate circulation and the flow of energy in the body. It is specific for deficiency cold syndromes.

Infused oil: Jasmine oil is still used for pain relief. Parkinson's method was to infuse the flowers in oil in the sun – sweet almond oil or camellia oil work well for this. Fill a jar with flowers, cover with oil and cover the top with a piece of clean cloth. Leave in a warm, sunny place until the flowers have turned transparent, then strain and bottle.

We have made our own enfleurage of jasmine flowers on coconut oil, purely for the pleasure of it. Pour a thin layer of melted coconut oil onto a baking tray, spreading it evenly by tilting the tray. Allow to cool and set (this only works in a cool climate!), then pick jasmine flowers in the evening or early morning and spread over the set oil. Cover with a clean cloth and leave until the next day, then replace the spent flowers with fresh ones. Keep repeating this for a week or two – until you are satisfied with the fragrance of the oil.

Gelsemium: Parkinson's sweet climbing Virginian jasmine is now known as Carolina Jasmine, *Gelsemium sempervirens.* It is classified as being in the Gelsemiaceae family, even though it still shares the common name of jasmine.

Gelsemium is used in herbal medicine, but in very low doses as its alkaloids are toxic in concentration. It is a safe and important homeopathic remedy.

Our jasmine leaf ointment

Pick a couple of good handfuls of jasmine leaves (about 1 oz or 25 g). Strip them off the larger stems and place in an electric blender with 250 ml extra virgin olive oil. Blend until green.

Leave in a jar overnight or for a couple of days, then strain the oil – a nylon jelly bag works well for this, as it won't absorb the oil.

Let the oil settle in a glass container, so that any watery juice can sink.

Pour the oil into a small saucepan, being careful not to pour in any of the water at the bottom. Add 15 g beeswax and gently heat until the wax is melted. Drop a little onto a cold saucer to see if it is setting hard enough – if not, add a little more beeswax.

Pour the ointment into clean dry jars. Add a few drops of jasmine absolute to each jar if you wish to make it smell gorgeous.

We've found this ointment works well for lightening freckles and liver spots.

Common Knapweede

Theatrum Botanicum

Tribe 5, Chapter 2, pp468–70

1. *Iacea nigra vulgaris.*
The common wild Knapweede.

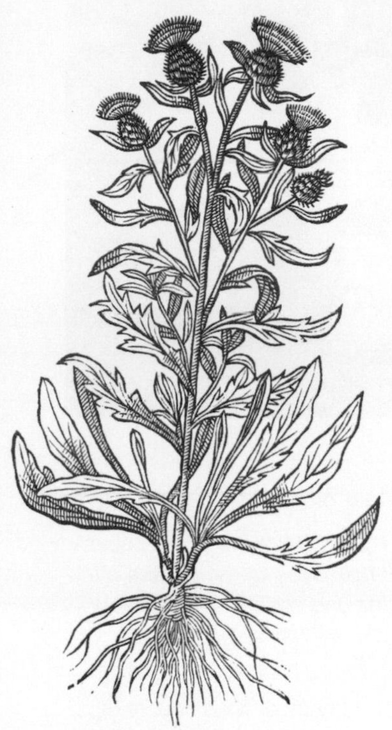

Iacea nigra vulgaris

The Vertues

Similarity to Scabious: This Knapweede being so neare of kindred unto the *Scabions*, are in some part equall to them in their properties:

Astringent & drying: for being of an astringent and drying taste, it thereby helpeth to stay fluxes, both of bloud at the mouth, nose, or other outward parts, and those veines that are inwardly broken, or inward wounds, as also the fluxes of the belly and of the stomacke, provoking castings;

For stopping mucus: it staieth likewise the distillations of thinne and sharpe humours from the head, upon the stomacke and lunges:

For bruising: it is good also for those that are bruised by any falls, beatings and other casualties; it is very profitable for them likewise that are bursten, and have the rupture, by drinking the decoction of the herbe and rootes in wine, and applying the same outwardly to the place:

For non-healing sores: it is singular good in all sorts, of running and cankarous sorts and fistulous also, drying up the moisture, and healing them up gently without any sharpenesse or biting: it doth the like also in the running sores and scabbes of the head or other parts;

For sore throat & fresh wounds: it is of especiall use for the sorenesse of the throat, the swellings of the *Uvula* and jawes, it is also excellent good, for all greene wounds, to stay the bleeding and to close the lippes of the wounds together.

Scabions: scabious
stay fluxes: stop the flow
bloud: blood
castings: vomit
distillations: trickling down
thinne and sharpe humours: clear and acidic mucus
lunges: lungs
profitable: effective
casualties: accidents
bursten: ruptured
decoction in wine: boiling the plant in wine
running and cankerous sores: open and non-healing ulcers
fistulous: tubelike
sharpenesse: acidity
uvula: soft palate above the throat
greene: fresh
close the lippes: fuse the edges

Parkinson's aromatic scabious recipe for respiratory problems

'If you would have it [i.e. a scabious, or by extension knapweed, remedy] more effectuall, take this receipt, *viz.* an handful of dryed *Scabious*, an ounce of Licoris scraped and cut into thinne slices, a dozen figges [figs] washed and cut into peeces, an ounce of Anisseede, and as much Fennelseede bruised, and half an ounce of dried *Orris* [*Iris germanica*, bearded iris] rootes cut into thinne slices: let all these be steeped for a night, in a quart of faire [clean] water, (or rather in so much wine) boyling them the next day, untill a third part be consumed at the least, whereof take a draught every morning and evening, somewhat warme, well sweetned with Sugar or Hony, which worketh wonderfully to helpe all the diseases aforesaid' (TB, p490).

Knapweed *Centaurea nigra* Asteraceae

Knapweed is a common temperate grassland perennial, flowering in the late summer, but its medicinal qualities as a vulnerary, for treating bruising, ruptures and wounds, and particularly for sore throat and inflamed fingernails, are all but forgotten. It is regarded as safe, if rather too astringent for pleasurable use as a tea, but it is one of those lost plants from Parkinson's time that deserve another look.

Similarity to scabious: Parkinson begins the virtues section by likening knapweed to scabious in family and properties. He puts both in his vulnerary tribe, the wound-healing herbs, though modern classification has scabious as a Dipsacaceae, a teasel, while knapweed is an Asteraceae, the former Compositae, or daisy family. Parkinson's delectable scabious respiratory recipe is nonetheless well worth repeating (see opposite) for knapweed, and the two plants can be used interchangeably in herbal medicine.

Astringent & drying: Knapweed has a marked astringent taste in decoction, and it was and remains an effective remedy to stop the outward flow of blood or equally inward veins and wounds, and a bilious stomach. It is a mild purgative.

For stopping mucus: The same astringency serves to stop the flow of mucus downwards from the head into the stomach or lungs.

For bruising: A decoction in wine is Parkinson's preferred style for both inward and outward treatment of bruises and ruptures; herbalists in the 14th century made a knapweed ointment, called *save*, for this purpose.

For non-healing sores: Again the astringency of knapweed serves to dry up the moisture of various open and weeping sores, and it does so without noticeable 'sharpenesse or biting'.

For sore throat & fresh wounds: Knapweed is a specific for sore throat and swellings of the uvula and jaws, taken as an infusion or gargle. It also has a specific historic use for treating whitlows or felons – inflamed fingernails – as remembered in Parkinson's common name of matfelon. Using knapweed for stopping the bleeding of a fresh wound and closing the lips of it was 'excellent good' medicine in Parkinson's day, and could be useful hedgerow medicine today.

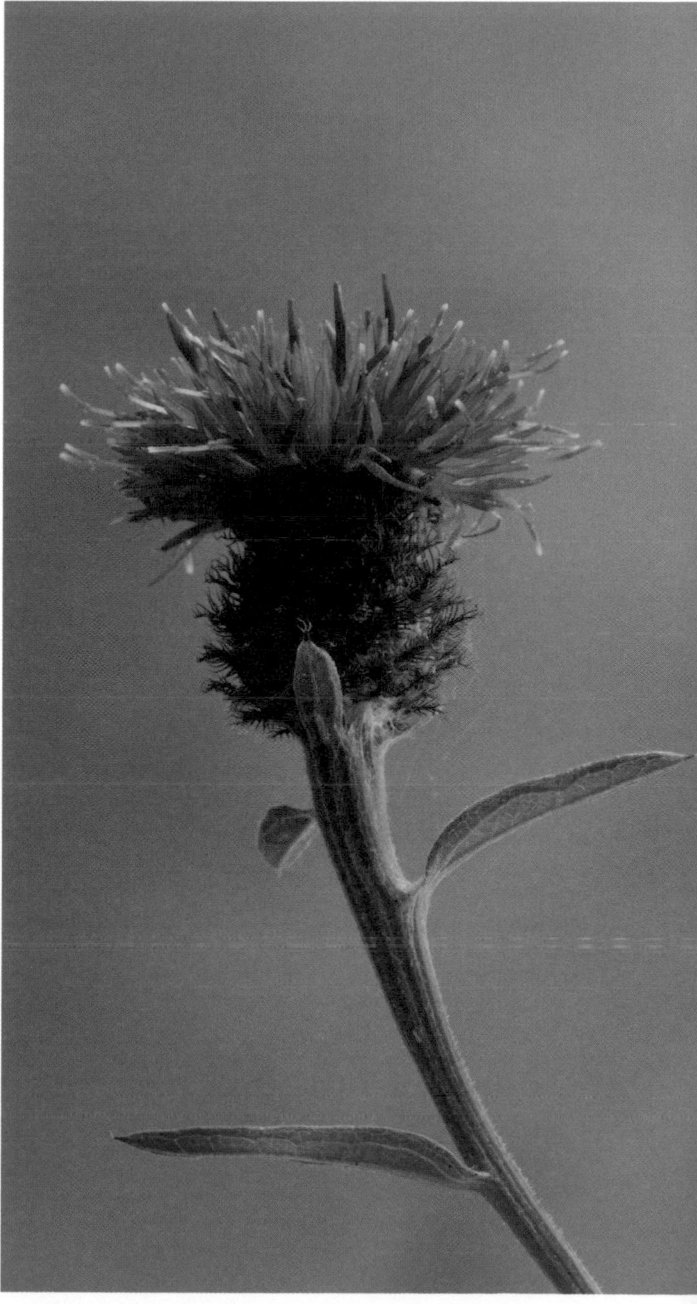

Ladies Bedstraw

Theatrum Botanicum

Tribe 5, Chapter 45, pp564–65

1. *Gallium Luteum.*
Common Ladies Bedstraw.

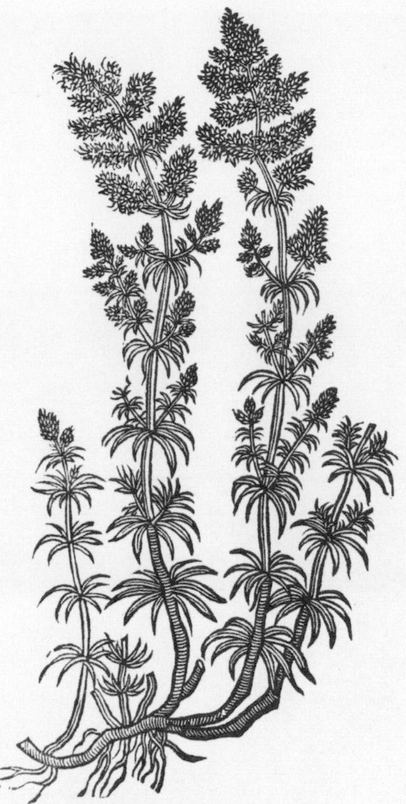

divers: various people
fret: wear away
stay: stop, diminish
nosthrils: nostrils
Dioscorides: Greek-speaking Roman physician (mid-first century AD)
insolated: placed in the sun
Axungia: soft animal fat, often goose
sallet oyle: salad oil, usually olive
traveilers: walkers, travellers
sorbated with travaile: consumed by tiredness
Lackies: servants employed to run
availeable: effective
Clusius: Charles de l'Ecluse (1526–1609), Flemish botanist and author
Gleidkraut: possibly mountain ironwort, *Sideritis montana*

Gallium

Vertues

URINARY: The decoction of the hearbe, I meane the common Ladies Bedstraw, being drunke, is used by divers, to helpe to provoke Urine, and thereby to fret and breake the stone:

BLEEDING: the same also drunke helpeth to stay inward bleedings, as also to heale inward wounds, by the drying and heating qualities therein, the herbe as the flowers being bruised, and put up into the nosthrils, stayeth their bleeding likewise.

APHRODISIAC EFFECT: *Dioscorides* writeth that the roote is good to provoke bodily lust, and some say the flowers doe so also:

BURNS: the flowers and the hearbe likewise made into an oyntment or oyle, in oyle to be insolated or set into the Sunne, and changed after it hath stood some tenne or twelve days, but if it be made into an oyntment, it must be boyled in *Axungia* or sallet oyle, with some waxe melted therein after it is strayned; which will helpe burnings with fire, and scaldings with water:

WEARINESS & STIFFNESS: the same also or the decoction of the herbe and flowers, is good to bath the feete of traveilers, who are sorbated with travaile, and for Lackies or such like, whose running long, causeth not onely wearinesse, but stiffenesse in their sinewes and joynts; for which both the decoction warme is very availeable, and so is the oyntment to use afterwards:

SCABS & ITCHES: the same also as is said before, helpeth the dry scabbe, and the itch in children, whereof the *Germanes* doe make dayly experience:

WHITE-FLOWERED BEDSTRAWS: these sorts with white flowers have beene thought unprofitable, and of no use: but *Clufius* saith, the poore women in *Austria, Hungaria,* and other places in *Germany,* that gather herbes and rootes for their uses that neede them, bringing them to the market to sell, calleth it *Gleidkraut*; and by their experience have found it good, for the sinewes, arteries, and joynts, to bathe them therewith, both to take away their wearinesse, and weakenesse in them, and to comfort and strengthen them also, after travaile, cold, or paines.

Straw and cheese

Harvested lady's bedstraw has a mild scent, which gathers sweetness and a hay smell as it dries (from coumarin build-up). It is soft and giving, but also astringent and deters fleas. So yes, an ideal bedding straw. As for cheese, *galium* is from the Greek for 'milk', and 'cheese rennet' is the plant's old name, referring to its long use in Europe to curdle milk in cheese-making. But modern French cheese-makers say bedstraws just don't work now. Have we lost a secret?

Lady's bedstraw *Galium verum* Rubiaceae

Lady's bedstraw is a bright summer perennial meadow plant, native to Eurasia and naturalized in North America, except for the deep South. Like other herbs named for the Virgin Mary (our Lady), it has a founding myth, which began in medieval Germany and reached Britain in the 16th century. The Virgin's bedding in the stable was bracken and lady's bedstraw, then white-flowered. The bracken refused to acknowledge the infant Jesus, and was prevented from ever flowering again. The bedstraw, which gloried in the newborn, had its flowers turned bright yellow-gold.

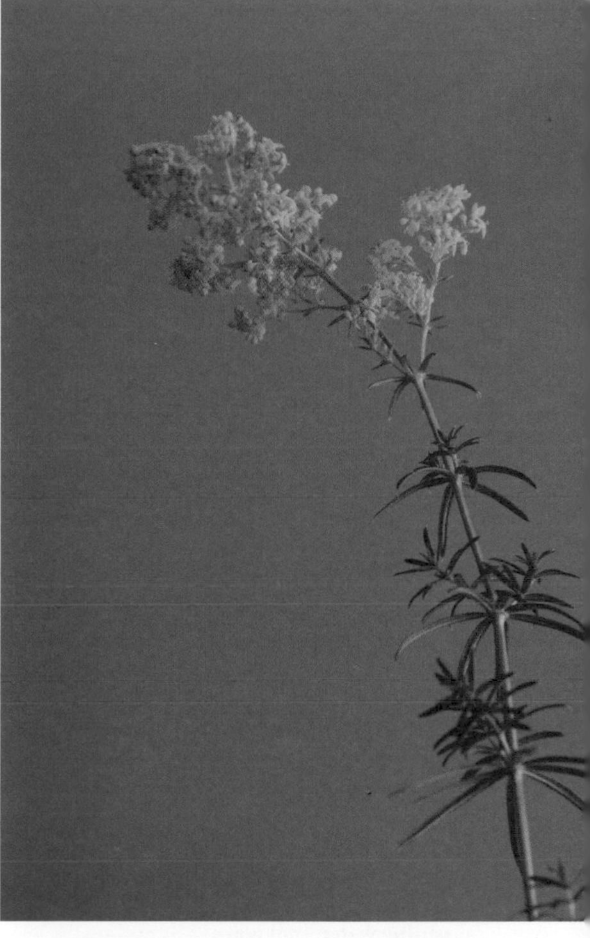

Urinary: Lady's bedstraw in a decoction maintains the reputation Parkinson gives it as a good diuretic, to ease the flow of urine, for cystitis, to break up kidney and bladder stones, and also to treat gout.

Bleeding: Again, it is still used as a heating and drying herb with anti-coagulant and styptic properties to 'stay inward bleedings'; externally, like yarrow, it can be stuffed up the nostrils to stop nose bleeds, as Parkinson says.

Aphrodisiac effect: There doesn't appear to be support for Parkinson's report, among his contemporaries or today.

Burns: Parkinson gives useful preparation hints for an ointment of lady's bedstraw, which will soothe burns or scalds. It can also be used on external wounds.

Weariness & stiffness: Mugwort had a strong reputation as the herb for weary travellers, but lady's bedstraw was not far behind. The warmed decoction was used to bathe feet and other stiff joints, with the ointment added for longer-term relief, as Parkinson says. And weary lackies also had soft bedstraw bedding to look forward to!

Scabs & itches: Like other diuretics, lady's bedstraw is also effective as a skin lotion or wash for a range of skin eruptions, and mild enough for children's use.

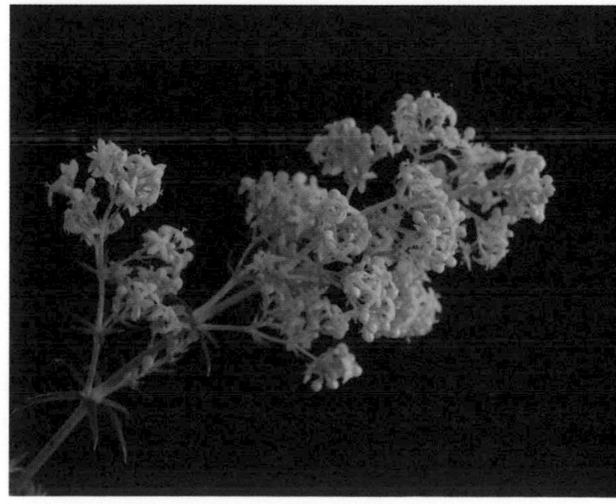

White-flowered bedstraws: Lady's bedstraw is the only yellow-flowered bedstraw, with cleavers, woodruff, and hedge, heath, marsh, fen and slender bedstraws among its white *Galium* cousins. Cleavers and woodruff are described elsewhere in this book, and the other family members can be put to herbal use much as lady's bedstraw.

Other uses: French herbalism had a tradition of using lady's bedstraw for treating epilepsy, but this does not appear to be current. The flowers made a bright yellow dye, much beloved of society women in the time of Henry VIII for colouring their hair, and the roots gave a red dye, but yields of both were too low for sustained commercial use. All the same, for personal purposes it is worth making the experiment.

Ladies Mantile

Theatrum Botanicum

Tribe 5, Chapter 30, pp538–39

1. *Alchymilla major vulgaris.* Common Ladies Mantle.

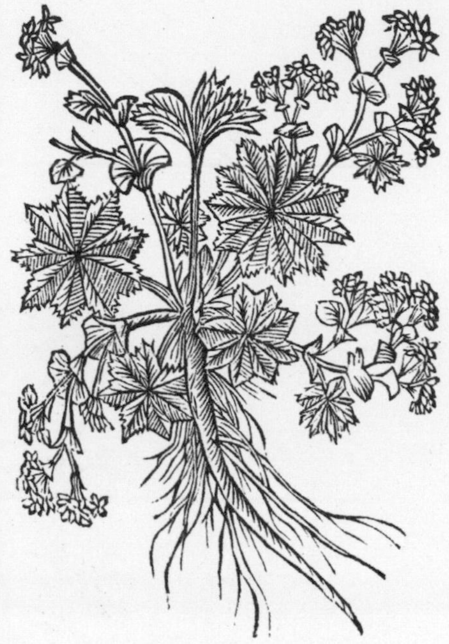

Alchymilla

Unto the Sanicles set downe in the last Chapter, I thinke it fittest to place this next unto it, because both for forme and quality it is so assuredly like it, that it is called of divers the greater Sanicle, and will add thereunto another sort thereof, which hath not beene formerly well knowne. …

It is usually called *Alchymilla* by most writers, because as some thinke the Alchymists gave such commendations of it.

The Vertues

Ladies Mantle is more cooling then Sanicle, and therefore more proper for those wounds that have inflammations, and more astringent binding and drying, and therefore is more effectuall to stay bleedings, vomitings, fluxes in man or woman of all sorts, and bruses by fals or otherwise, and to helpe ruptures,

Sagging breasts & leucorrhoea: it helpeth also such maides or women that have overgreat flagging breasts, causing them to grow lesse and hard, being both drunke, and outwardly applyed, and serveth also to stay the whites in them, wherein it is so powerfull that it is used as a sursuling water also,

Distilled water: the distilled water drunke continually for twenty daies together, by such women as are barren and cannot conceive, or retaine the birth after conception, through the too much humidity of the matrice, and fluxe of moist humours thereunto, causing the seede not to abide but to passe away without fruite, will reduce their bodies to so good and conformable an estate, that they shall thereby be made more fit and able to retaine the conception, and beare out their children, if they doe also sit sometimes as in a bath, in the decoction made of the herbe.

Wounds: It is accounted as one of the most singular wound herbes that is, and therefore the *Germanes* extoll it with exceeding great praise, and never dresse any wound, either inward or outward, but they give of the decoction, hereof to drinke; and either wash the wound with the said decoction, or dippe tents therein, and put them thereinto, which wonderfully dryeth up all humidity of the sores, or of the humours flowing thereunto, yea although they be fistulous and hollow, and abateth also such inflammations, as often happen unto sores:

Fresh wounds: but for fresh or greene wounds or cuts, it so quickely healeth them up, that it suffereth not any quitture to grow therein, but consolidateth the lippes of the wound, yet not suffering any corruption to remaine behinde:

Alchemy: it hath formerly beene much accounted of by Chymists, who have affirmed that the juice hereof will constraine the volubility of Mercury, and make it fixt, from whence as it is thought it tooke the name, but these idle fancies are now quite worne out, as I thinke.

Sanicle: *Sanicula europea* (or any wound herb)
fluxes: diarrhoea
ruptures: hernias
the whites: leucorrhea or thrush
sursuling water: [unknown]
matrice: womb
conformable: harmonious
Germanes: Germans
tents: a cloth tent over a wound
fistulous: hollow
abateth: stops
green wounds: fresh wounds
quitture: discharge
consolidateth: holds together
corruption: infection
Chymists: chemists
volubility: here, flowing quality of mercury; lady's mantle was thought to limit this. The similarity of the dew drop on the leaf (Parkinson calls it a 'pearl') to a drop of mercury also appealed to alchemists

Lady's mantle *Alchemilla xanthochlora, A. alpinus*

Lady's mantle is still considered astringent, cooling and drying. It is used to stop bleeding and strengthen tissue, and like many herbs associated with the Virgin Mary is a revered woman's herb. It moderates heavy menstrual bleeding, regulates the cycle and relieves cramps.

[See pp246–7 for a copy of Parkinson's original pages.]

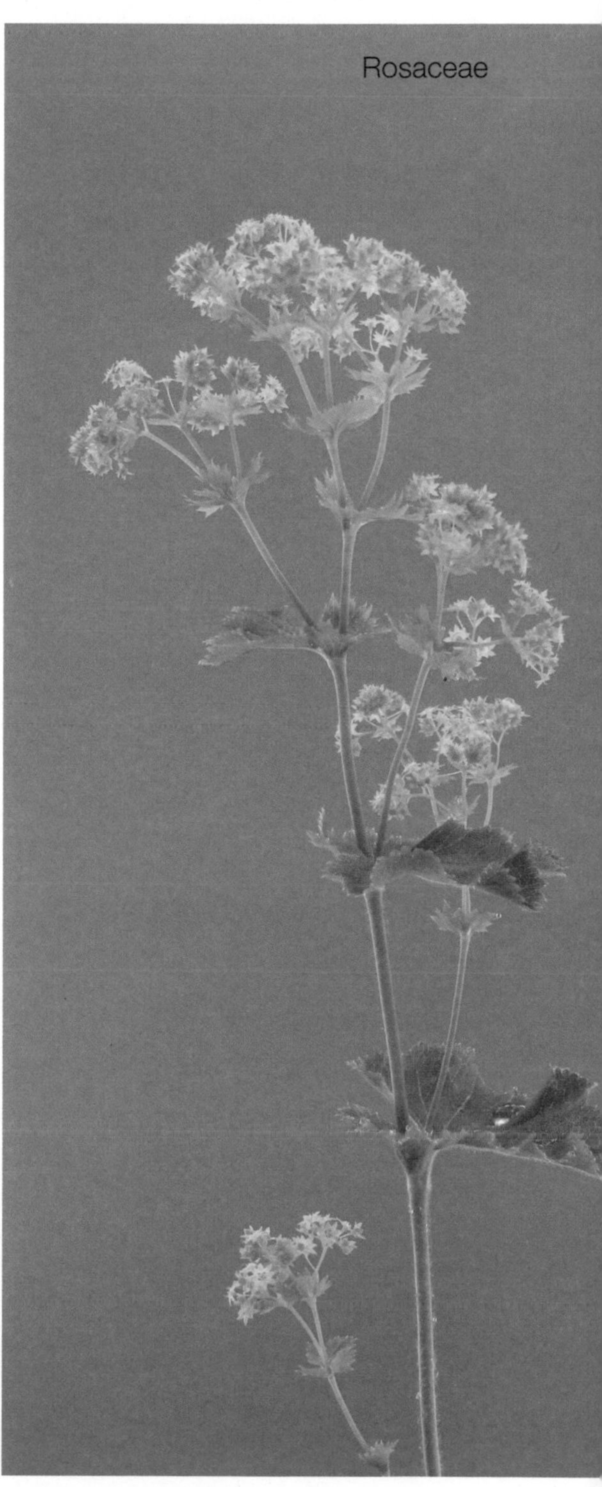

Parkinson describes common Ladies mantle, *Alchemilla vulgaris* (now renamed *A. xanthochlora)*, and cinkefoil Ladies mantle, a smaller variety (possibly alpine Lady's mantle, *A. alpina*). Both species are used medicinally, and in fact give their names to two major groups of *Alchemillas*. There are over 300 *Alchemilla* species found in Europe, Asia and the mountains of Africa and South America. The species most commonly grown in gardens today is *A. mollis*, one of the *vulgaris* group originating from the Balkans.

This genus is fascinating to botanists because many species produce seed without the flowers being fertilized, a process called apomixis. Seedlings are identical to the parent plant.

For women: The astringency of Lady's mantle has the ability to firm up tissue, and its use for sagging breasts was popular in the 16th and 17th centuries, mentioned by many authors. Women in those days did not have bras, so the effects of the herb must have been really appreciated.

Lady's mantle was also used to tone the reproductive organs to help in conception and to prevent miscarriage. It is interesting that Parkinson recommends a sitz bath using the decoction of the herb, as well as drinking the distilled water, for this purpose. The herb was sold for all sorts of women's problems, and even had the reputation of helping those who wished to appear as virgins again.

Today it is used from puberty to menopause, for conditions including leucorrhoea and heavy menstruation, fibroids, prolapses and to tone the womb after childbirth.

Diarrhoea & vomiting: Again, the astringency of this plant comes to our rescue.

Wounds: Lady's mantle is an effective healer for cuts, grazes and other injuries. The tea can be used to speed up healing after surgery, and is effective as a mouthwash after dental extractions.

As Parkinson says, lady's mantle will heal wounds while clearing infection and inflammation at the same time, qualities that make it especially valuable.

For injuries as well as women's problems, lady's mantle is often combined with yarrow.

Licoris Vetch

Theatrum Botanicum

Tribe 11, Chapter 27, pp1098–1100

3. 4. Glycyrrhiza vulgaris siliquosa & echinata.
Codded and rough headed Licoris.

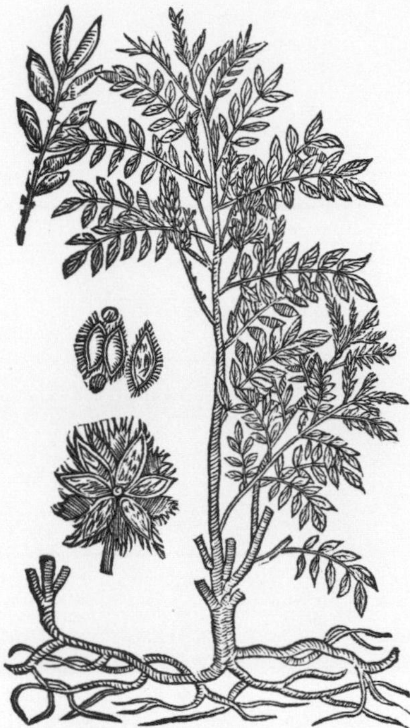

Physicke: medicine
Galen: Claudius Galen (AD130–200), Roman physician and author
familiar: palatable
astriction: drying, astringent
lenifie: moderate
faire water: clear or running water
maidenhaire: maidenhair fern, *Adiantum capillus-veneris*
figges: fig, *Ficus carica*
ptisane: herbal tea
tissicke: dry cough
consumptions: pulmonary tuberculosis
raines/reines: kidneys, adrenals
strangury: 'strangled' urination
Scythians: central Asian nomads
desarts: deserts
staieth hunger: reduces hunger pangs
barme: leaven, alcoholic foam
tunned up: stored in casks
quill: feather used to hold ink

Glaux leguminosa sive Glycyrrhiza sylvestris

The Vertues

Throat & bladder: The two sorts of wilde Licoris are not knowne to be used in Physicke by any, but are wholly neglected: for the other two sorts of true Licoris, their properties being both alike, I shall not neede to entreate distinctly as if the one had some other faculties that the other had not, for they are therein both alike, and as *Galen* saith, is very familiar to our temperature in that it is sweete, and having a little astriction joyned with it, making it temperate in heate and astriction, that it is the nearest unto our temper, and by both these qualities, as he saith, it doth lenifie the hoarsenesse of the throate, and is helpefull for the ulcers in the bladder; it hath also some moisture therein by reason of the sweetnesse, and thereby good to quench the thirst:

Coughs & lungs: Licoris is often boyled in faire water, with some Maidenhaire and Figges, which maketh it a good ptisane drinke, for those that have any dry cough, and to digest the flegme, and to expectorate it, or hoarsenesse, wheesing, and shortnesse of breath, and all other griefes of the breast and lungs, the tissicke or consumptions caused by the distillations of salt humours on them, which doe waste and consume them: it is good also in all the paines of the raines, the strangury, and heate of urine.

Thirst & hunger: The *Scythians* are said by chewing this in their mouthes, that it keepeth them from thirst in their long journies through the desarts for tenne or twelve dayes, and staieth hunger also:

Brewed: Licoris boiled in water, with a little Cinamon added to it, serveth in stead of drinke in many places, especially if it be set to worke with barme as beere is, and then tunned up, and will grow cleere, strong, and heady by time as beare will doe:

Eyes: the fine powder of Licoris blowne through a quill into the eyes that have a pinne and webbe, as they call it, or rheumaticke distillations into them, doth clense them and helpe them:

Juice: the juyce of Licoris is as effectuall in all the diseases of the breast and longs, the reines and bladder as the decoction: the juyce dissolved in Rosewater with some Gumme Tragacanth, is a fine lohoc or licking medicine for hoarsenesse, wheesings, and all other roughnesse in the mouth or throat, and to expectorate tough flegme, as also to condensate thinne rheumes, falling on the lungs; our *English* Licoris is more pleasant to the taste, wanting much of that astriction is in that which commeth to us from beyond sea.

pinne and webbe: two diseases of the eye, caligo and pterygium
rheumaticke distillations: rheumatic symptoms in the eye
Gumme Tragacanth: gum from root of other *Astragulus* species
lohoc: a drinking medicine

Liquorice *Glycyrrhiza glabra*

Fabaceae

Liquorice (or licorice) is an important medicinal member of the *Astragalus* (milk vetch) family, its root having been used in all the leading herbal traditions. It was *gan cao*, or 'sweet herb', in imperial China; *yastimadhu*, or 'sweet stick' in Sanskrit; and *glycyrrhiza*, or 'sweet root' in ancient Rome (Dioscorides used this term in his *De Materia Medica*, written in the first century AD, and the same Latin name remains). Liquorice has become a well-researched herb, and is now termed an adaptogen with a range of effective uses that has increased markedly since Parkinson's time.

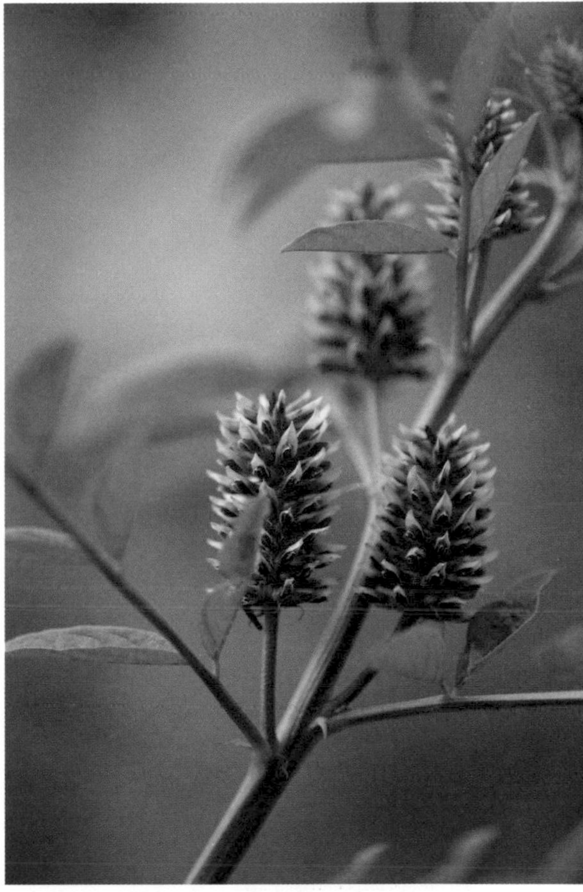

Throat & bladder: It is difficult to be sure which species of liquorice Parkinson begins with, but, as he says, the properties across the species are comparable. There is a corresponding overlap today in the medicinal uses of the main liquorice species – *Glycyrrhiza uralensis* in China, *G. lepidota* in North America, and *G. glabra* in India and Europe.

Parkinson touches on how 'familiar' or palatable liquorice is to 'our temperament', being sweet but with a little 'astriction' or gentle drying quality. This helps a liquorice-based tea to 'lenifie' or moderate a hoarse throat or ease the pain of bladder ulcers. He is hinting at a remarkable feature of liquorice's ability to increase the effectiveness of other herbs while reducing any potential toxicity. It is thus a 'carrier' herb, used in many herbal formulas (it is almost the first plant to go into a Chinese formula). The sweetness of liquorice appeals to the palate but the exceptional modulating quality is key.

Coughs & lungs: Here the old use Parkinson describes accords well with modern practice. Liquorice remains a safe and well-tolerated remedy in a herbal tea for dry and phlegmy coughs, sore throat, shortness of breath, bronchial congestion and 'other griefes of the breast and lungs'. In old herbal parlance, it was specific as a 'pectoral' and 'expectorant'.

Kidneys & urine: He briefly mentions how liquorice eases the pains and reduces the heat of kidney and urinary tract problems. Research has shown that the phytosteroids in liquorice root increase levels of oestrogen and steroids when they are low, in the balancing or harmonizing style of an adaptogen. Addison's disease, brought on by adrenal insufficiency, has been treated with success (and fewer side effects) by liquorice in place of steroidal drugs.

Thirst & hunger, brewing: Parkinson reports how Greek philosopher Theophrastus (c.372–c.286BC) tells of the Scythians chewing liquorice root – which he called *Herba scythia* – to stave off thirst and hunger while travelling. Parkinson's liquorice and cinnamon drink is delicious, and he probably made the beer from liquorice he grew himself.

Eyes: Blowing liquorice powder in the eyes sounds unpleasantto us, but cold liquorice tea can be used as a soothing eyewash.

Juice: He notes the effectiveness of liquorice juice for treating upper respiratory conditions, and prefers the English-grown plant.

Other uses: Research indicates liquorice's value in formulas for treating autoimmune conditions, e.g. lupus and HIV/AIDS, as a restorative sexual tonic, for nourishing chronic fatigue, hepatitis and chronic liver disease.

Caution: Can increase blood pressure, and is best avoided in pregnancy; sodium retention and bloating may occur, but it is safe in small amounts for limited periods. A deglycrrhizinated form, called DCL, is available, but may be less effective.

Ordinary Lovage

Theatrum Botanicum

Tribe 8, Chapter 35, pp936–37

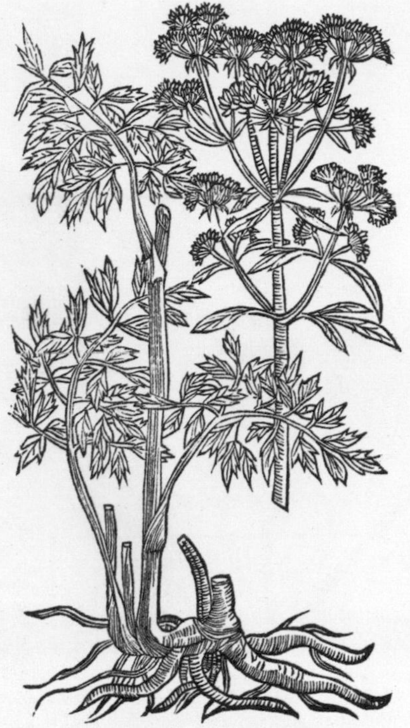

open out and digest humours: clear and disperse bodily fluids
womens courses: menstruation
dramme: ⅛ oz apothecary weight
greene: fresh
moter: mortar
faire water: running or well water
asswageth: relieves
a carouse: a large draught
divers shires: various counties
ague: fever
quotidian, tertian, quartaine: one-, three- or four-day fever
comming: coming
Pepper: i.e. imported black pepper
comfortable: agreeable
quinsie: peritonsillar abscess
dimmenesse: poor vision, glaucoma
hogges lard: pig fat
botch: swelling
bile: boil

Levisticum vulgare

Vertues

Lovage is hot and drie in the beginning of the third degree, and is of thinne parts also, and thereby doth open cut and digest humours, and doth mightily provoketh womens courses and urine, as much as any of the kindes of Parsley:

Dried root: the dried roote in powder taken to the weight of halfe a dramme in wine, doth wonderfully warme a cold stomacke, helping digestion, and consuming all superfluous moisture and raw humours therein, easeth all inward gripings and paines, dissolveth winde, and resisteth poyson and infection effectually:

Fresh root: the greene roote hereof bruised in a stone morter, and steeped for twelve houres in faire water, then strained and drunke first in the morning and last at night two or three spoonefulls at a time, asswageth any drought or great desire to drinke more than a carouse of cold drinke, found true by often experience, although the roote is well knowne to be hot:

it is a knowne remedy, and of much and continuall experience in divers shires of this Land to drinke the decoction of the herbe for any sort of ague, whether it be *quotidian*, *tertian* or *quartaine*, and to helpe the paines and torments in the body and bowells comming of cold:

Seed: the seede is effectuall to all the properties aforesaid, except the last, and worketh more powerfully: the *Germanes* and other Nations in times past, used both the rootes and seede in stead of Pepper to season their meates and brothes, and found them as comfortable and warming to the stomacke:

Distilled water: the distilled water of the herbe helpeth the quinsie in the throate, if the mouth and throate be gargled and washed there-with, and helpeth the pleurisie, if it be drunke three or foure times; the said water also dropped into the eyes taketh away the rednesse or dimmenesse of the eyes, it likewise taketh away spots or freckles in the face:

the leaves of Lovage bruised and fried with a little hogges larde, and laid hot on any botch or bile will quickely breake it:

Fresh root preserved: the greene rootes may be kept in pickle made with salt and vinegar for a long time, but preserved with Sugar is more pleasant.

Lovage *Levisticum officinale* Apiaceae

Lovage is a tall garden perennial in the carrot and parsley family, which Parkinson says 'grows eight foote high in my Garden'. It is still an easily cultivated and architectural border plant, and one with useful but mostly forgotten medicinal qualities. American herbalist Peter Holmes calls it 'an inappropriately neglected plant, both as a draining diuretic and digestive remedy' (*Energetics of Western Herbs*, Berkeley, 1993, I, 176).

Parkinson immediately identifies lovage as effective at stimulating menstruation and urine, because it is hot and drying while also dispersing bodily fluids or humours. He notes that this action is similar to related kinds of parsley (indeed, the 'age' of lov-age is from the medieval name 'ache' for parsley; similarly, celery was once 'small-age').

Dried root: Parkinson's description of powdered lovage root in wine as a warming drink for a cold stomach is echoed today by the revival of the cordial drink 'Lovage' (made from brandy and sugar, and the seed rather than the root), which was an English pub favourite of the earlier 20th century. Again lovage dries up 'all superfluous moisture and raw humours', which extends to easing stomach pains, improving the appetite and helping the body resist poison and infection.

Fresh root: Parkinson specifies freshly dug lovage root, crushed gently in a stone bowl and soaked in pure water, then strained and drunk. This is a remedy for undue thirst, he claims, and is 'found true by often experience'.

Again he refers to practical experience of treating fevers of shorter or longer duration by boiling up lovage root (other parts of the plant would be equally good, one can add) in water as a decoction. The premise is that the warming and tonic effect will ease the pain 'comming of cold'.

Seed: Parkinson mentions the use of lovage seed instead of expensive black pepper to season savoury food, and lovage is currently making a comeback in the kitchen. One contemporary cook calls it a 'punchy substitute' for parsley and celery, and stronger than both; he suggests baking the seeds in biscuits or bread, steaming the stems or braising the roots. The taste is something of an acquired one, though.

Distilled water: Using this gentlest form of lovage is recommended by Parkinson as a gargle for infected tonsils, a drink for pleurisy, an eyewash and to treat freckles and spots of the face. Frying the leaves in cooking oil can be used as a mini-compress for boils, he adds. It is good first-aid advice.

Fresh root preserved: Preserving the stems or young roots in sugar makes a tasty candy, but angelica, a close relative, enjoys a more enduring reputation in this respect.

Caution: Parkinson does not say this directly, but modern herbalism calls lovage a uterine tonic, and as such it should be avoided in pregnancy.

Scots lovage (*Ligusticum scoticum*) or Scots parsley is a closely related species, probably not known to Parkinson. It grows wild on rocky coastlines of Scotland and northern England, but is much smaller than English garden lovage (at about 2 feet, 65 cm). The livid green leaves were and are foraged, eaten raw or boiled as a vegetable (*shums* in Gaelic). Medicinally, it was taken as a breakfast appetizer, and to counter scurvy and infection.

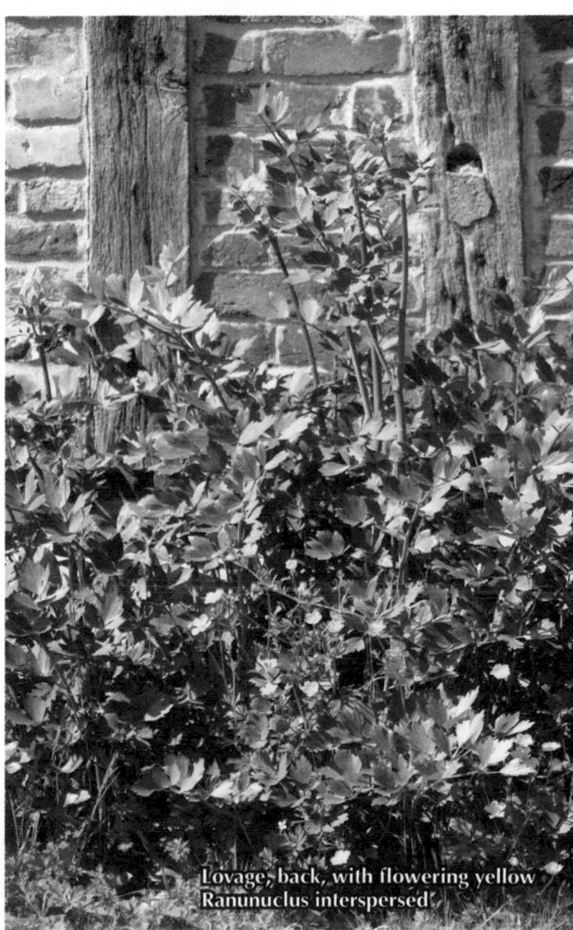

Lovage, back, with flowering yellow Ranunuclus interspersed.

Marjerome

Theatrum Botanicum

Tribe 1, Chapter 5, pp11–14

1. *Majorana vulgaris.* Swεete Marjerome.

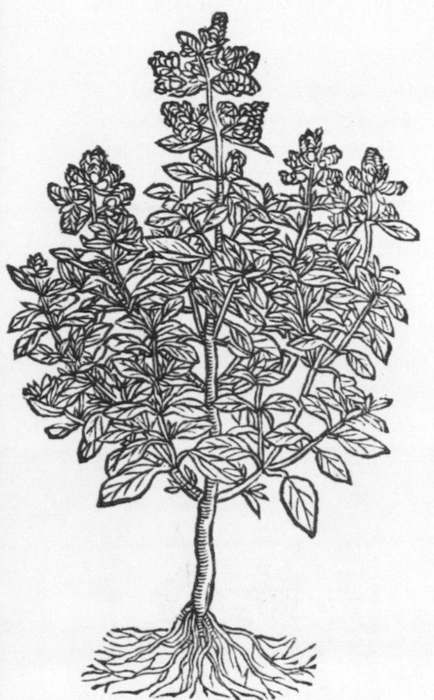

Majorana

Vertues

Our common sweet Marjerome is hot and dry in the second degree, and is warming and comfortable in cold diseases of the head, stomack, sinewes, and other parts, taken inwardly, or applyed outwardly: it digesteth saith *Matthiolus*, attenuateth, openeth, and strengthneth:

Lungs: the decoction thereof, being drunke helpeth all the diseases of the chest, which hinder the freenesse of breathing:

Liver & spleen: it is likewise profitable for the obstructions of the liver and spleene, for it not onely cleareth them of those humours did stuffe them, but strengthneth also and confirmeth the inward parts:

Womb: it helpeth the cold griefes of the wombe, and the windines thereof, or in any other inward part:

Speech: it helpeth the losse of speech by the resolution of the tongue: the decoction thereof made with some *Pelletory* of *Spaine*, and long pepper, or with a little *Acorus* or *Origanum*: *Dioscorides* and *Galens Sampsuchum* is hot and dry in the third degree of thin parts, and of a digesting quality:

Decoction: the decoction thereof drunke is good for those that are beginning to fall into a dropsie; for those that cannot make their water, and against paines and torments in the belly,

Pessary: it provoketh also womens courses, if it be put up, being made into a pessary,

Other uses: and applyed with salt and vinegar, it taketh away the venome of the Scorpions sting: being made into powder and mixed with hony, it taketh away the black markes of blowes or bruises applied thereto: it is good for the inflammations and watering of the eyes, being mixed with fine flower, and laid unto them:

Ears: the juyce thereof dropped into the eares easeth the paines in them, and helpeth the singing noyse of them:

Ointments: it is profitably put into those oyntments and salves, that are made to warme and comfort the outward parts or members, the joynts also and sinewes, for swellings also and places out of joynt:

Powder: the powder thereof snuffed up into the nose, provoketh neesing, and thereby purgeth the braine, and chewed in the mouth draweth forth much flegme.

Oil: The oyle made thereof is very warming and comfortable to the joynts that are stiffe, and the sinewes that are hard, to molifie, supple, and stretch them forth.

For pleasure: Our Marjerome is much used in all odoriferous waters, powders, &c. that are for ornament and delight.

sinewes: sinews
Matthiolus: Pierandrea Mattioli (1501–77), physician and author
windines: windiness
pelletory of Spaine: Spanish chamomile, *Anacyclus pyrethrum*
long pepper: *Piper longum*
Acorus: sweet flag, *Acorus calamus*
Dioscorides: Greek-speaking Roman physician (mid-first century AD)
Galen: Claudius Galen (AD130–200), Roman physician and author
Sampsuchum: an *Origanum* species
dropsie: dropsy, fluid retention
womens courses: periods
hony: honey
flower: flour
singing noyse: tinnitus
neesing: sneezing
flegme: plegm
oyle: oil
molifie: soften

Marjoram *Origanum majorana, O. vulgare* Lamiaceae

Marjoram, a popular culinary herb, is also a powerful medicinal plant. Sweet marjoram is native to the Mediterranean, while wild marjoram will grow happily in colder climes.

Sweet marjoram is a relaxing tonic to the nervous system, while both plants are used by herbalists for digestive problems and chest infections.

Marjoram and oregano are two herbs that cause a lot of confusion, even today, with common names often being interchanged and the Latin genera having evolved. But it is clear which species Parkinson is talking about (he describes nine species of marjoram). His sweet marjoram is now *Origanum majorana*, with white flowers, and his wild or field marjoram is modern *Origanum vulgare*, which has purplish flowers, and is called oregano in some countries. Pot marjoram is *Origanum onites*. The genus has numerous species, subspecies and hybrids, with similar but subtly different actions.

Marjoram was a symbol of love for the Greeks and Romans, and was considered protective against evil influences.

Marjoram is one of the many aromatic herbs that was popular in Tudor times for strewing in rooms, and Parkinson says it is used in perfuming waters and powders 'for ornament and delight' – both uses that are lost to us.

Sweet marjoram both relaxes and tones the nervous system. It relieves stress and anxiety without making one sleepy, and has an antispasmodic action.

Lungs: Marjoram is warming and clearing, with a marked expectorant quality. Its tonic properties will strengthen weak lungs over time if used regularly, and its antispasmodic action makes it helpful for a tight chest, coughs and asthma. Today's herbalists tend to use it as an infusion rather than a decoction.

Liver & spleen: Parkinson builds on Matthiolus' statement of the actions of marjoram by saying it will open obstructions of the liver and spleen, clear the blocking liquids while also strengthening the healed organs.

Uterus & pessaries: Sweet marjoram has long been recognized as having stimulating action in the pelvic area. Parkinson uses its warming, supportive quality for 'cold griefes' in the uterus and recommends a pessary to bring on menstruation, an example of the wide range of herbal preparations available at his time. Pessaries are still used by herbalists as an effective way of administering healing plants for the female reproductive system.

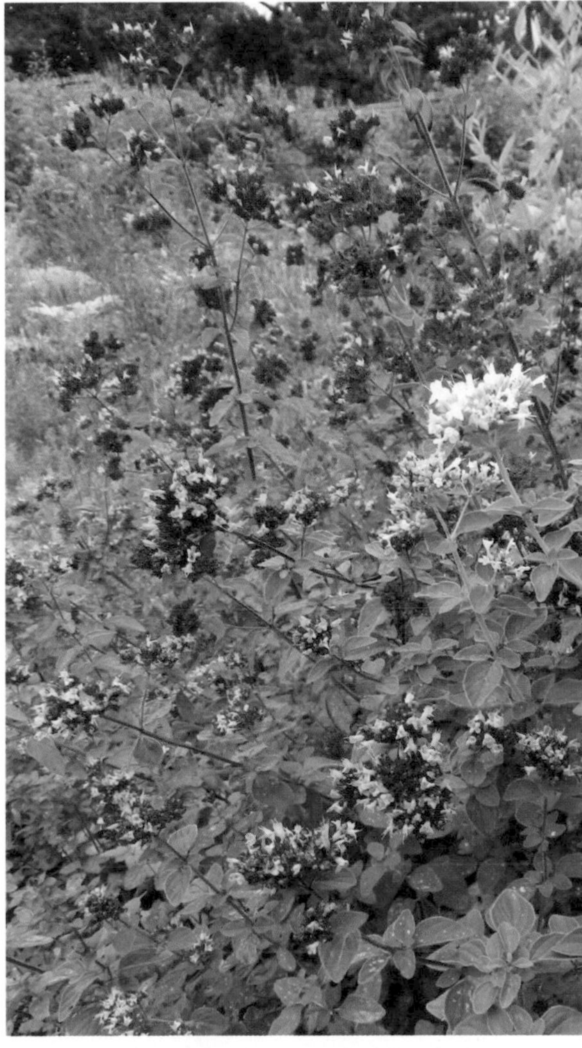

Wild marjoram and sweet marjoram growing together

Speech: Parkinson's recipe for freeing up the tongue uses a combination of warming herbs to relax and soothe.

Ears & eyes: Parkinson suggests a poultice of sweet marjoram mixed with flour to soothe inflamed or watery eyes, and the juice for earache and tinnitus.

Oil & ointment: Marjoram makes a lovely warming, relaxing oil when infused in the sun in olive oil. If distilled, an orangey yellow essential oil is obtained. Sweet marjoram

pot Marjerome: *Origanum onites*
wilde Marjerome: *Origanum vulgare*
Hearb Mastick: Parkinson gives the Latin as *Marum vulgare*; today it is known as *Thymus mastichina*, Mastic thyme or Spanish marjoram
Marum: possibly *Teucrium marum*
Trochisci Hedychroi: herbal lozenges – see box below
Andromachus: Andromachus the Elder, physician to Roman emperor Nero and inventor of the compound *Theriaca Andromachi*
treacle: theriac or poison antidote formula
effectuall: effective
still: distill

Pot marjoram: The great or pot Marjerome because it is more mild and lesse bitter than the former, is lesse used in Physicke, but more in meates and brothes to give a rellish unto them, and to helpe to warme a cold stomack, and to expell winde:

Wild marjoram: the wilde Marjerome is more hot than it, and therefore more effectuall to heat, warme, comfort, and strengthen both inwardly and outwardly in all things whereunto it is applyed:

Mastic thyme: Hearb Mastick is more temperate in heat than Marjerome, and is used by our Apothecaries, in stead of the true *Marum* (which may well bee admitted untill a truer may be knowne) in the composition of the *Trochisci Hedychroi* which *Andromachus* thought fit to make a principal part of his Treacle, accounting it effectuall against all poisons, especially of vipers, and other Serpents.

Our daintiest women doe put it to still among their other sweet hearbs, to make sweet washing water.

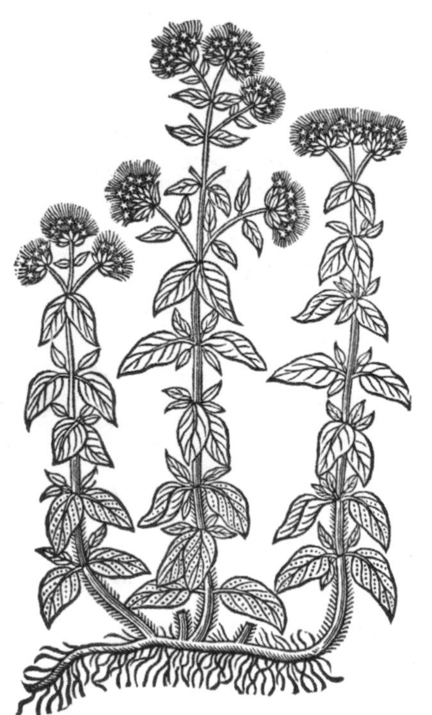

essential oil is calming and relaxing, good for releasing tension and reducing high blood pressure. As with most plants, those grown in a hot dry climate have stronger volatile oil content than those from a cooler, wetter climate.

Distilled water: The distilled water of marjoram is a wonderful mouthwash, and helps promote digestion. It is relaxing to abdominal spasms, such as irritable bowel syndrome (IBS), and makes an aromatic water for the complexion of 'our daintiest women'.

Culpeper writes on *Trochisci Hedychroi*

Nicholas Culpeper's *Pharmacopoeia Londinensis*, or, *The London Dispensatory* (1649, rev. 1653) was his attempt to set right the wrong he called 'Ignorance in Physick'. Culpeper did this by translating into plain English the exclusive-to-apothecaries and Latin-based *London Pharmacopoiea*, and publishing the resulting book cheaply for the common man.

Among the apothecaries' recipes he reveals are a number for troches or pastilles, including *Trochisci Hedychroi* (his p148). As a sample of the compound treacles it is interesting to see how complex, expensive and hard to source this actually was.

The ingredients Culpeper lists are: Aspalathus, or yellow sandalwood; Mastich leaves; Asarabacca; Rhupontick; Castus; Calamus Aromaticus; Aloes; Cinnamon; Squinancth; Opobalsamum or Oyl of Nutmegs; Cassia Lignea, Indian Leaf or Mace; Indian Spicknard; Mirrh; Saffron; Amomus or Cardamoms the less; Mastich; and Canary wine.

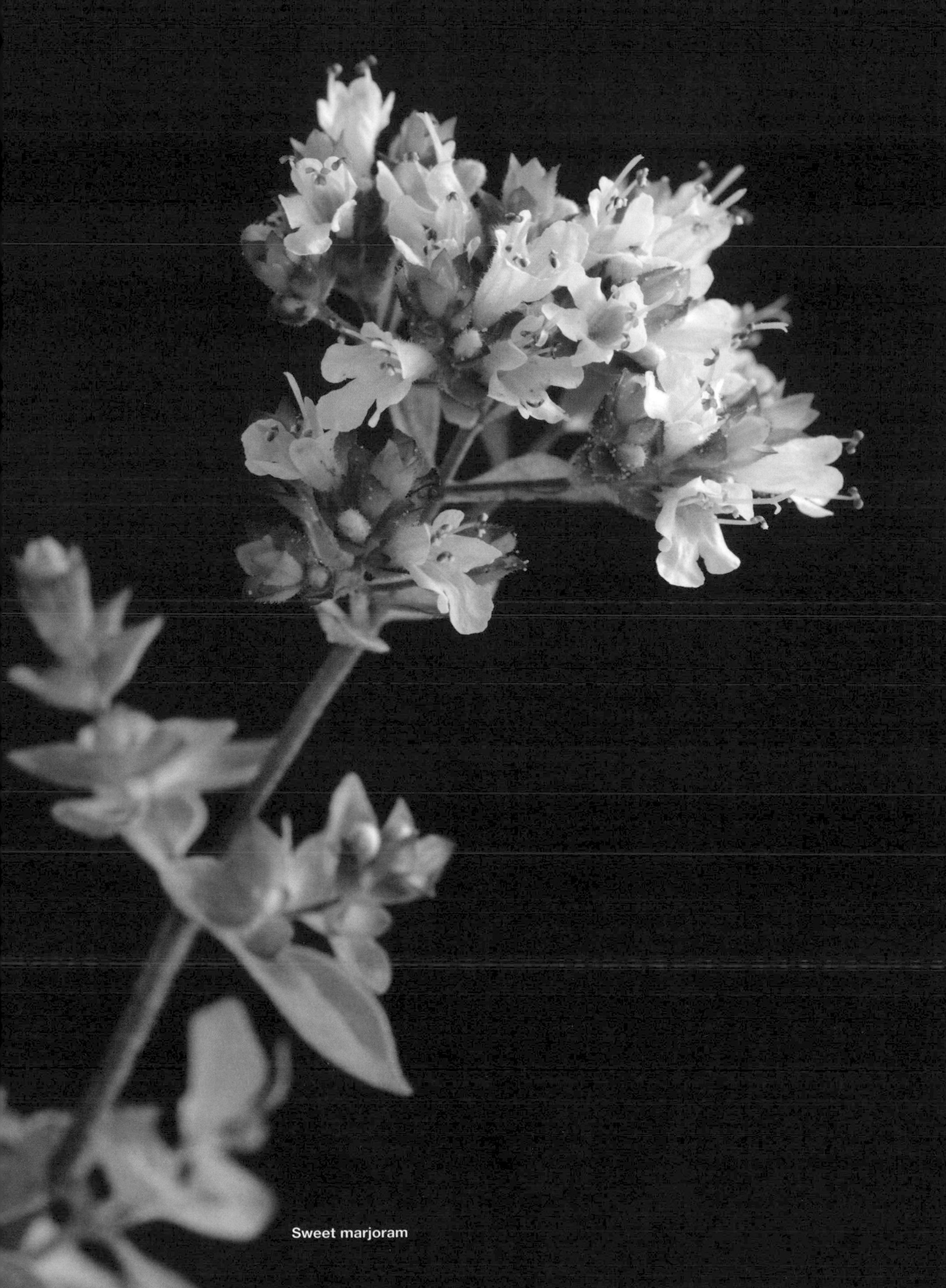

Sweet marjoram

Medowsweete

Theatrum Botanicum

Tribe 5, Chapter 58, pp591–93

1. *Vlmaria vulgaris.* Common Medeſweete.

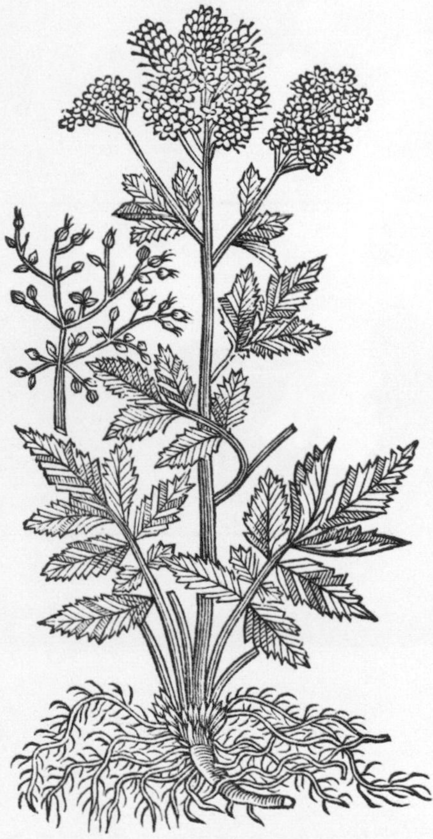

Burnet: *Sanuisorba officinalis*
Tragus: Hieronymus Bock (1498–1554), physician, priest, author
stay: stop
fluxes: irregular flows
womens courses: menstruation
whites: leucorrhea or thrush
quartaine Agues: four-day fevers
collicke: colic
Bottes: infestation by bot fly larvae
cancrous: non-healing
fistulous: tubular
secret parts: sexual organs
Camerarius: Joachim Camerarius the Younger (1534–98), German botanist
parlars: parlours
quick: lively
rellish: tang

Ulmaria

The Vertues

Astringency: Being neare a little in taste and smell with Burnet, they are most likely to bee neare of the same facultie, yet *Tragus* accounteth them more hot and dry, they are also used in the same manner and for the same purposes, to stay all manner of fluxes, bleedings, and vomitings, and womens courses, as also their whites:

Fevers & depression: it is sayd to alter and take away the fits of quartaine Agues, and to make a merry heart, for which purpose some use the flowers, & some the leaves:

Colic: it helpeth also speedily those that are troubled with the Collicke, being boyled in wine and with a little honey taken warme, it doth open the belly; but boyled in red wine and drunke, it stayeth the flux of the belly, &c. it helpeth the Bottes in horses as you heard before;

Sores & ulcers: being outwardly applyed it healeth old Ulcers, that are cancrous or eating, and hollow or fistulous, which many have used and much commended; as also for the sores in the mouth, and secret parts; the leaves when they are full growne being layd upon the skinne, will after a small time, raise blisters thereon as *Tragus* saith:

Distilled water: the water thereof helpeth the heate and inflammation in the eyes: the seede as *Camerarius* saith being taken, causeth paines in the head;

A strewing herb: and because both flowers and herbes are of so pleasing a sweete sent, many doe much delight therein, to have it layd in their Chambers, Parlars, &c. and Queene *Elizabeth* of famous memory, did more desire it then any other sweet herbe to strew her Chambers withall:

In wine: a leafe or two hereof layd in a cup of wine, will give as quick and as fine a rellish thereto, as Burnet will, as I sayd before.

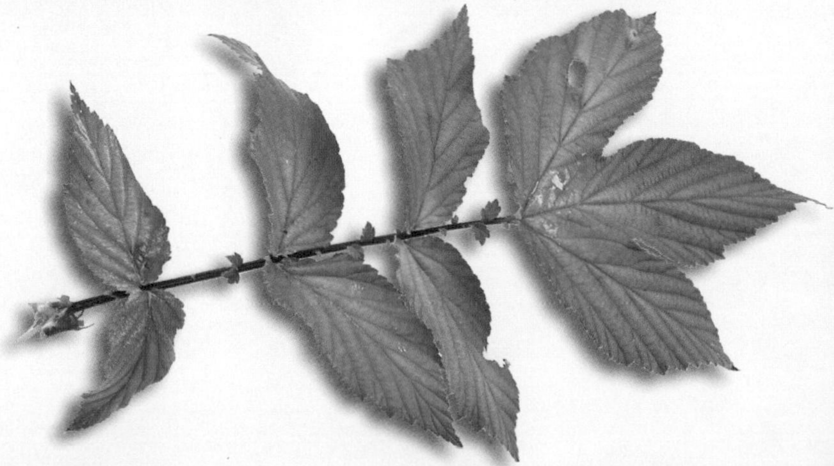

Meadowsweet *Filipendula ulmaria* Rosaceae

Meadowsweet, or medesweete as Parkinson also called it, grows in damp places and by water, and flowers profusely in frothy white masses in high summer. It was Queen Elizabeth I's favourite strewing herb to scent her rooms, as Parkinson mentions in one of our favourite sentences in his whole book. He describes its valuable medicinal use in treating a variety of aches and pains. Today, meadowsweet is mainly a remedy for acidic digestive problems, which Parkinson calls 'flux of the belly'. There is, though, a hint of darker reality within all this summery brightness: the plant grows increasingly astringent as it matures, perhaps mirroring one of its old names: courtship and marriage!

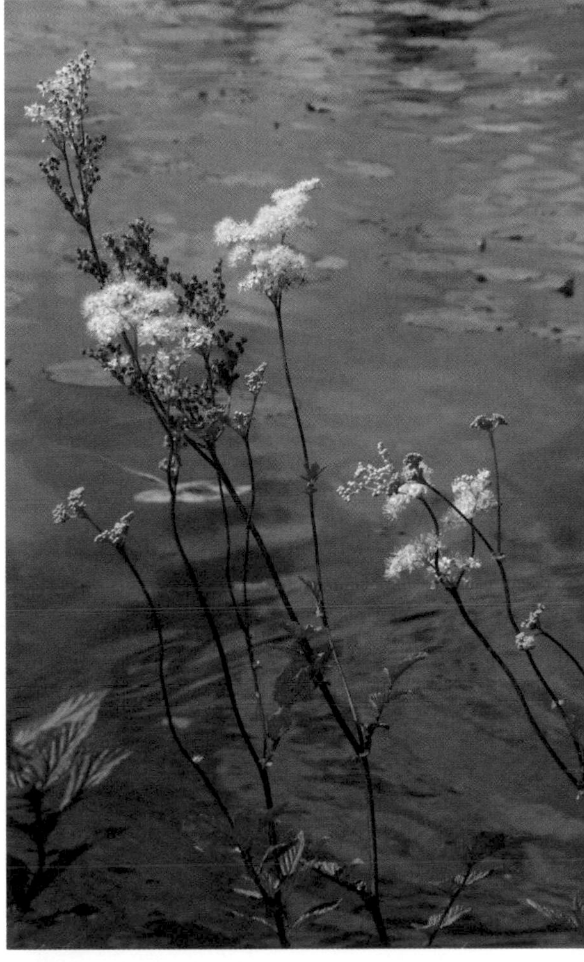

It was 1897 when Felix Hoffmann, a chemist employed by Bayer AG, the German pharmaceutical and agrochemical company, first isolated the salicylates in meadowsweet. This soon led to the possibility of a salicylate-based headache pill suitable for mass production, which Bayer duly patented as aspirin in 1899. The name was based on *Spiraea,* an old Latin term for meadowsweet.

Based on their common origin, meadowsweet has similar properties to aspirin, to alleviate pain and inflammation as well as to lower fevers. However, unlike aspirin, the rawness of which can damage the lining of the stomach, meadowsweet helps the stomach by regulating stomach acid levels. Indeed, meadowsweet can be used to treat stomach ulcers that could well have been caused by aspirin itself.

Astringency: Parkinson describes a more robust range of actions for meadowsweet than current usage would, but his account is indicative of the potential range and strength of meadowsweet to settle digestive and menstrual upsets.

Fever & depression: As he says, it is effective in treating slower-developing forms of fever and is conducive to a 'merry heart', a lightening of the spirit that helps in healing.

Colic: Parkinson notes that boiled with (presumably) white wine it can be 'opening' and lead to diarrhoea, but with red wine it 'stays' or closes down an upset stomach. He points out it also works for botfly gut infection in horses.

Arthritis: Because of its ability to reduce inflammation, acidity and pain, meadowsweet is a useful remedy for arthritis as well as fibromyalgia and other muscle aches and pains. Note his comment that the seed can cause headache and the mature leaves can produce blisters on the skin.

Distilled water: As with other distilled or aromatic waters, that from meadwsweet brings out the milder form of its energetic action, making it soothing for inflamed eyes.

Strewing: Strewing was clever recycling: the dried aromatic herb gave wamth on cold earth floors, masked smells with a pleasing scent of its own, reduced infection, then could be burnt and replaced at no cost. Indeed, a floor covering fit for an eco-queen!

In wine: Meadowsweet's astringency adds an almondy tang to mead, the ancient honey drink, and it serves to give a lively 'rellish' to wine or ale.

Caution: Some people are allergic to meadowsweet pollen in midsummer (Matthew is unfortunately among them), and it can bring on asthma. If you are allergic to aspirin, meadowsweet could cause a similar reaction.

Ladies Thistle

Theatrum Botanicum

Tribe 9, Chapter 8, pp975–77

1. *Carduus Marie vulgaris.*
The common Ladies Thistle.

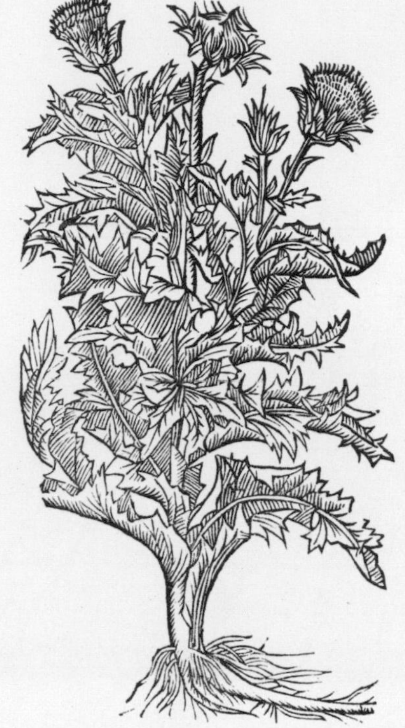

Carduus Marie vulgaris

The Vertues

Fevers & infections: Our Ladies Thistle is thought to be as effectuall as *Carduus benedictus* for all the purposes whereunto it is put, as namely for Agues and for the infection of the Plague, both to prevent and cure it,

Liver & spleen: as also to open the obstructions of the Liver and spleene, and thereby is good against the Iaundies,

Urinary: and provoketh Urine, breaketh and expelleth the stone, and is good for the Dropsie:

Stalks: some doe hold that the young stalkes peeled and dressed as the stalkes of the other Chardons and wilde Artichokes are, and eaten doe helpe to encrease milke in Nourses breasts:

Griping pains: It is effectuall also for the paines in the sides, and many other inward paines and gripings:

Seed & distilled water: the seede is held as powerfull if not more for the purposes aforesaid and so is the distilled water also, and besides is often applied both inwardly to drinke and outwardly with clothes or spunges to the region of the Liver to coole the distemperature thereof, and also to the region of the heart against swownings and passions of it.

Carduus benedictus: holy or blessed thistle
agues: fevers
Iaundies: jaundice
dropsie: dropsy, oedema
doe: do
chardons: cardoon, *Cynara cardunculus*
nourses: nurses
clothes: cloths
spunges: sponges
distemperature: overheating
swownings & passions: fainting and hysteria

Milk thistle is used today as a powerful liver herb, protecting this organ against damage from poisons and inflammation, and helping it to repair and regenerate. It is a tall, very upright prickly thistle with white-veined leaves, which was once considered a sign that it helped breast milk production.

Milk thistle has been very well researched, and has been found to protect the liver. It can even prevent poisoning when death cap mushrooms have been eaten, if taken soon enough. It is used to protect the liver from the damaging effects of some types of chemotherapy and other hepatotoxic drugs, to treat high cholesterol levels, acute and chronic viral hepatitis, alcohol-induced cirrhosis and other chronic liver and gall bladder problems. Milk thistle can be taken whenever the liver is under stress.

Milk thistle appears to have a similar protective effect on the kidneys. It has also been found to help balance blood sugar levels in people with type II diabetes, and research suggests that it may have a role to play in cancer prevention and treatment.

It is still used to increase the supply of breast milk in nursing mothers as Parkinson mentions, but taken today in seed form rather than eaten as young stalks. The distilled water is a remedy worth reviving.

Milk thistle *Silybum marianum*, syn. *Carduus marianum*

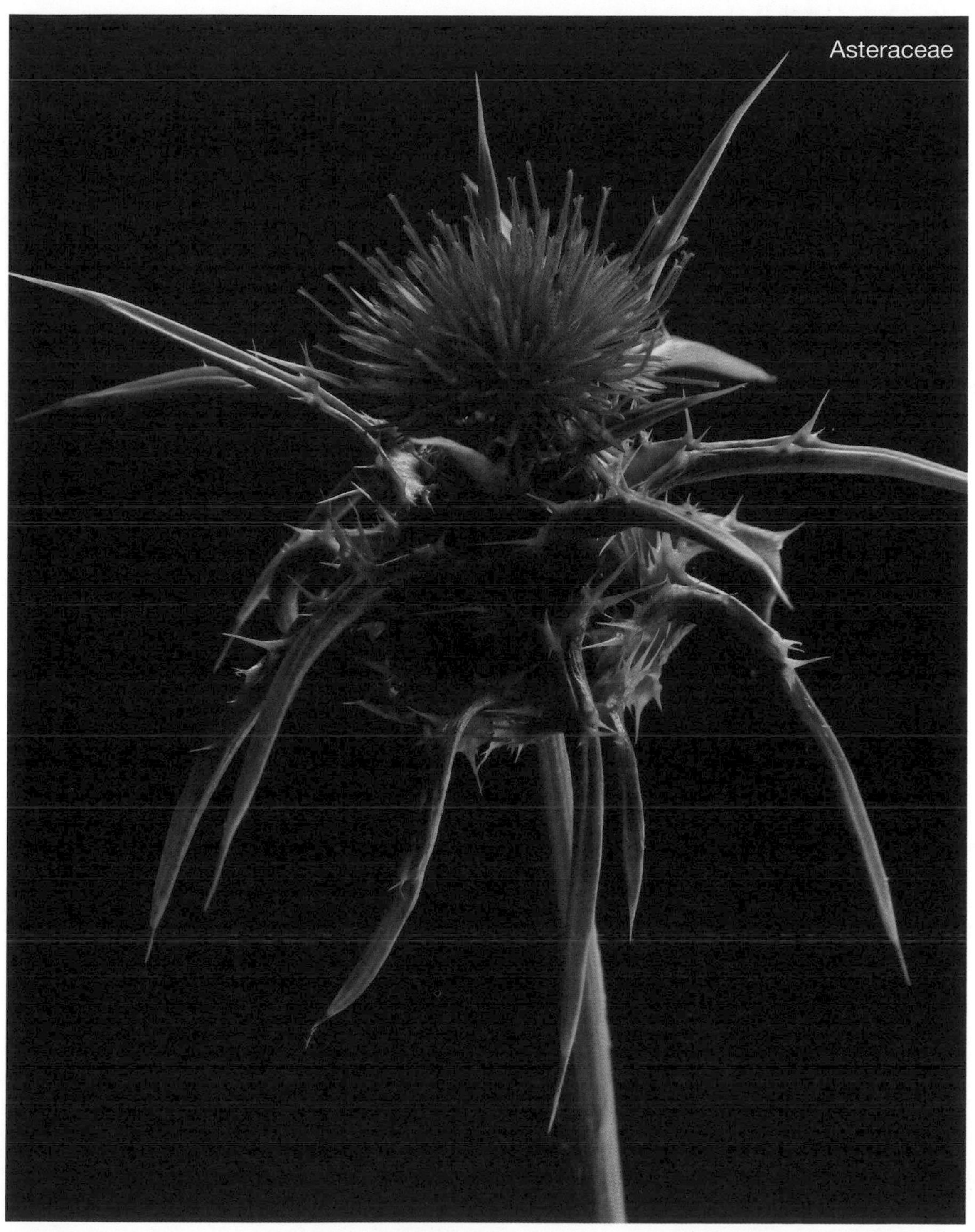

Mintes

Theatrum Botanicum

Tribe 1, Chapter 13, pp31–35

Dioscorides: Greek-speaking Roman physician (mid-first century AD)
stayeth/staieth: stops
round wormes: nematodes
sowre: sour
hickhock: hiccups
choller: choler, one of the four humours; bile
imposthume: purulent swelling
layed to: applied on
barly meale: barley flour
meade: honey drink
profitable: effective
feminine courses: menstruation
whites: leucorrhoea or thrush
breaking out: skin eruption
chaps of the fundament: soreness of anus, buttocks
availeable: beneficial
chimically: chemically

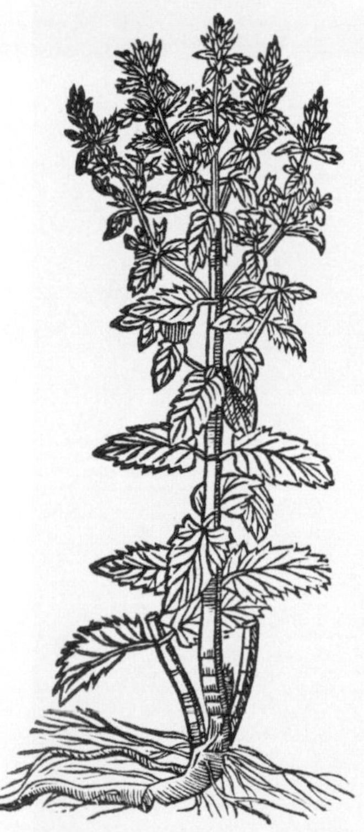

Mentha

The Vertues

The garden Mints in generall, yet the sweeter sorts, that is, the Speare Mint, and Hart Mint, are more usually taken for all the uses whereunto Mints doe serve;

Dioscorides: *Dioscorides* saith it hath an heating, binding, and drying quality, and therefore the juyce taken with vinegar stayeth bleeding. It stirreth up venery or bodily lust, and as hee saith killeth the round wormes, which hath not usually beene knowne to take effect with any, two or three branches thereof taken with the juyce of sowre Pomegranats staieth the hickhock, vomitings, and allaieth choller, it dissolveth impostumes being layed to with barly meale:

Breasts, dogs & ears: it is good to represse the milke in womens breasts when they are swolne therewith, or otherwise, for such as have swollen, flagging, or great breasts, applyed with salt, it helpeth the byting of a mad Dogge, with Meade or honied water it easeth the paines of the eares:

Contraception: applyed to the privie parts of a woman before the act of generation, hindreth conception, which is contradicted as you may read a few lines below,

For the tongue: and rubbed upon the tongue, taketh away the roughnesse thereof.

Milk in stomach: It suffereth not milke to curdle in the stomack, if the leaves hereof be steeped or boyled in it before yee drinke it.

Stomach: Briefly, it is very profitable to the stomack, and in meates is much accepted.

Menstruation: It is of especiall use to stay the feminine courses when they come too fast, as also to stay the whites, for which purpose no other hearbe is more safe and powerfull, for by taking it often it hath cured many.

Head & anus: Applyed to the forehead or the temples of the head it easeth the paines therof. It is also good to wash the heads of young children therewith, against all manner of breaking out therein, whether sores or scabs: and healeth the chaps of the fundament.

Venemous creatures: It is profitable also against the poison of venemous creatures.

Distilled water: The distilled water of Mints is availeable to all the purposes aforesaid, yet more weakely: but if a spirit thereof bee rightly and chimically drawne, it is more powerfull than the hearbe it selfe, in regard the spirit and strength of a greate deale is brought into a small proportion; foure ounces thereof taken as *Matthiolus* saith, doth stay bleeding at the nose, which may be thought incredible to a great many.

Mint *Mentha* spp. *Lamiaceae*

Mint looks like a simple plant: it smells good, it cleans the breath and settles the digestion. Yet it is a botanist's nightmare, with multiple species, cultivars and hybrids. And energetically, as Parkinson found, it offers seeming contradictions in its actions. These days it is classified as both cooling and heating, depending on use, species and form in which it is taken. This dual pattern is recognised in traditional Chinese, Indian and now Western herbalism.

Parkinson says in his introduction that the garden mints for the most part do not set seed, 'but recompence the defect by the increase of the root, which is so plentifull, that being once planted in a garden, they are hardly rid out againe, every small piece thereof being left in the ground increasing fast enough'. This habit of mint to spread will be familiar to any gardener who has grown it and tried to tame it.

He describes 12 different kinds of mint, and illustrates nine. Today we loosely classify mints as belonging to the peppermint group and the spearmint group, but there is a huge range of aromas and varieties, plus hybrids. Peppermint is considered to be a hybrid of watermint and spearmint.

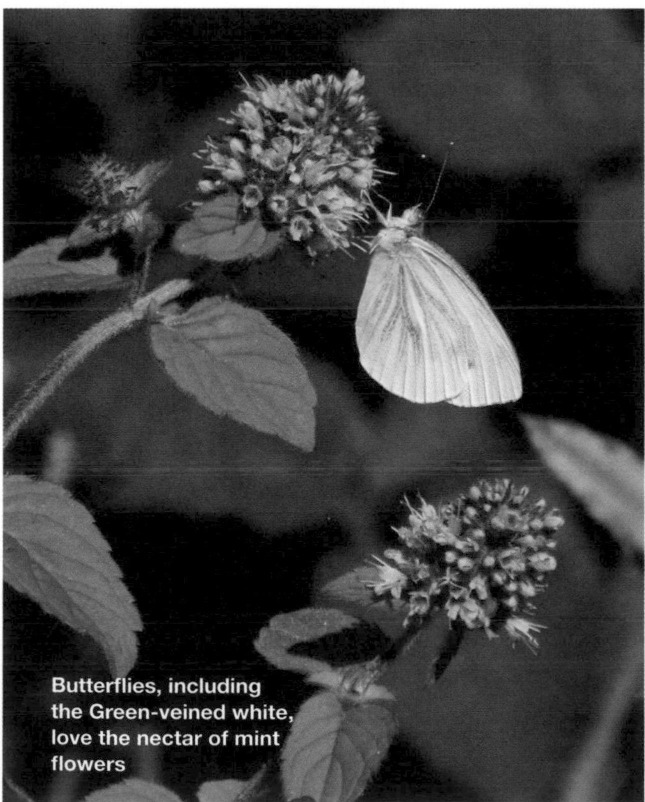

Butterflies, including the Green-veined white, love the nectar of mint flowers

Three of the most popular uses of mint today – to freshen the mouth and breath, to treat headaches, and to soothe the digestive tract – were well known to Parkinson. This chapter in general well illustrates the tension in Parkinson between a desire to accept ancient authority, yet to trust more to his own observation. For instance, is mint an aphrodisiac or a contraceptive, or perhaps both? He wrestles with such issues, without necessarily resolving them.

Dioscorides: He reports Dioscorides as saying that mint is heating, drying and binding, and by humoural theory serves to stop bleeding, stir passion and even kill roundworms. At the same time it sounds as though he doesn't really believe it. The English mints he knew were much more cooling. Today we think of menthol – one of the essential oils in mint – as cool enough to be added to cigarettes.

Breasts, dogs & ears: Websites today offer anecdotal evidence that peppermint tea, cabbage leaf and sage tea can all help to reduce breasts swollen with milk, an idea evidently already current in Parkinson's time.

As for dog bites, this is another area where Parkinson seems to borrow direct from the classics of Greece and Rome. We don't know about mint with honey for ear ache, but expect he has some experience.

Contraception: Here he reports the use of mint leaves as a contraceptive, but at once questions this.

Milk: He notes that mint added to boiled milk will prevent curdling; he says later, in this particularly disjointed chapter, that mint in cheese-milk will stop the solidification process, even if rennet is added.

6. *Mentastrum niveum Anglicum.* White Mints, or Party coloured Mints.

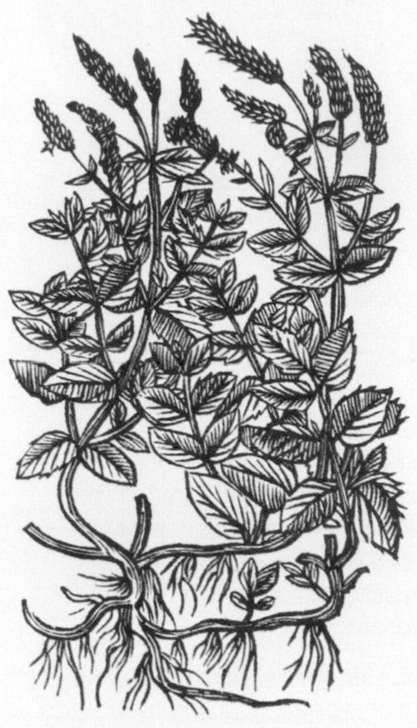

Matthiolus: Pierandrea Mattioli (1501–77), physician and author
Pliny: Pliny the Elder (AD23–79), Roman naturalist
Galen: Claudius Galen (AD130–200), Roman physician and author
simples: healing herbs used singly
Calamintha: calamint
manuring: i.e. garden-grown
digesteth: disperses
long wormes: unidentified intestinal worms
Oxycratum: mix of vinegar and water
sower: sour
Posca: another mix of vinegar and water
tenuity: lack of substance, density
Simeon Sethi: 11th century Jewish doctor, author of *Syntagma*, a study of foods
gnawings of the heart: dull nagging pains
thick and melancholick
cholerick: hot and dry
splenetick: bad-tempered, ill-humoured
bleare: blurry, dim

APHRODISIAC: It is much commended to be available in venereous causes, although *Pliny* in his *lib.* 20 *cap.* 14. doth write to the contrary:

SWEET MINT: but *Galen* in his sixt Booke of Simples, doth render a reason of the faculty hereof very worthily, where he saith, some doe call that *Mentha odorata*, sweet Mint, which by others is called ἡδύοσμος *Hedyosmos*:

CALAMINT: but there is another Mint which is not sweet, which they call *Calamintha*: both of them are sharpe in taste, and hot in quality, yea even in the third degree of heat, but *Mentha odorata* is weaker and lesse heating, so that I may well say that the one seemeth to be as it were the tame, and the other the wild:

APHRODISIAC AGAIN: wherefore by that humidity it hath gained by manuring, it provoketh to Venery, which thing is common to all hearbes that have in them an humidity halfe digested and windy:

ABSCESSES: by reason of which temperature being mingled with Barley meale it is used to ripen impostumes, which you cannot do with *Calamint*, because it heateth and digesteth more, then such things as should ripen impostumes doe require.

WORMS & VOMITING OF BLOOD: It hath also in it a little bitternesse, and some tartnesse, by reason of the bitternesse it killeth the long wormes of the belly, and by the tartnesse it stayeth the vomiting of blood:

THINNING QUALITY: while it is fresh, if it bee taken with *Oxycratum* (which some take to be sower milke, and others to be *Posca*, that is vinegar and water mingled together.) It is of as great tenuity as any hearb whatsoever: these are *Galens* words.

SIMEON SETHI: *Simeon Sethi* saith it helpeth a cold liver, and stregtheneth the stomack and belly, causeth digestion, stayeth vomitings and the hickock, is good against the gnawings of the heart, and stirreth up the appetite, it taketh away the obstructions of the liver, and stirreth up bodily lust;

CAUTION ON DOSAGE: but thereof too much must not be taken, because it maketh the blood thin and whayish, and turneth it into choler, yea, and causeth the blood which is of very thin parts, after it is separated, to become thick and melancholick: and therefore cholerick persons must abstaine from it:

DOGS AGAIN: it is a safe medicine for the byting of a mad Dogge, being bruised with salt and laid on;

DIGESTION & CHILD-BEARING: the powder of it being dryed and taken after meate, helpeth digestion, and those that are splenetick, taken with wine it helpeth women in their hard and sore travels in child-bearing:

FOR EYES, MOUTH & AS A DIURETIC: it is also thought to be good for bleare eyes applyed to them; and that the decoction of them being drunke, doth helpe the bleedings at the mouth speedily, or presently. It is good against the gravell and stone in the kidneys and strangury.

Digestion: Parkinson says mint is 'very profitable to the stomack' and is much used in food. Mint is lovely in green salads and fruit salads, there is mint sauce, of course (Parkinson suggests powdered mint for meat), and mint is used in a variety of Middle Eastern dishes. Peppermint is still used to treat dyspepsia and colic.

Menstruation: Parkinson says that mint is the safest and most powerful herb to treat the discharge known as leucorrhoea ('whites'), as well as to slow down the bleeding of heavy periods.

Head & anus: He notes that mint is versatile enough to ease pain in the head, treat scabs and sores of children while also soothing soreness of the anus.

Distilled mint: We use mint water for digestive upsets, for headaches and as a mouthwash. As Parkinson says, the spiritous water is much stronger, being obtained by distilling the mint in wine or other alcohol instead of plain water. We haven't had occasion to try it for nosebleeds.

Aphrodisiac: Today we don't think of mint as a powerful aphrodisiac, partly because it is too common, in toothpaste, chocolate and biscuits. He notes that Pliny writes against the notion, while later on he relates the story from Aristotle that soldiers were forbidden mint before battle because it reduced their warrior-like energy or promoted 'venery'. In practice, Parkinson doesn't tell us what he thinks, perhaps not knowing himself!

Sweet mint & calamint: Perhaps a solution is found in his next sentence where he draws attention to the differences between different species of mint, instancing sweet mint and calamint. The first is less heating, the tame to the other's wild. Yet he adds that garden-manured plants, mint included, gain 'humidity' and wind, so are bound to be aphrodisiac. This seems counter-intuitive: taming plants in gardens usually reduces their wild strength.

Abscesses: Garden mint mixed with barley flour is good to ripen abscesses, he says, but calamint heats and disperses too much.

Worms & vomiting of blood: He is right that there is some bitterness and tartness, though these days such qualities would not necessarily be used in the same ways as he suggests.

Caution on dosage: Today we would say mint is safe, even for choleric people, but there are cautions with the use of the essential oil as with all essential oils, owing to their strength.

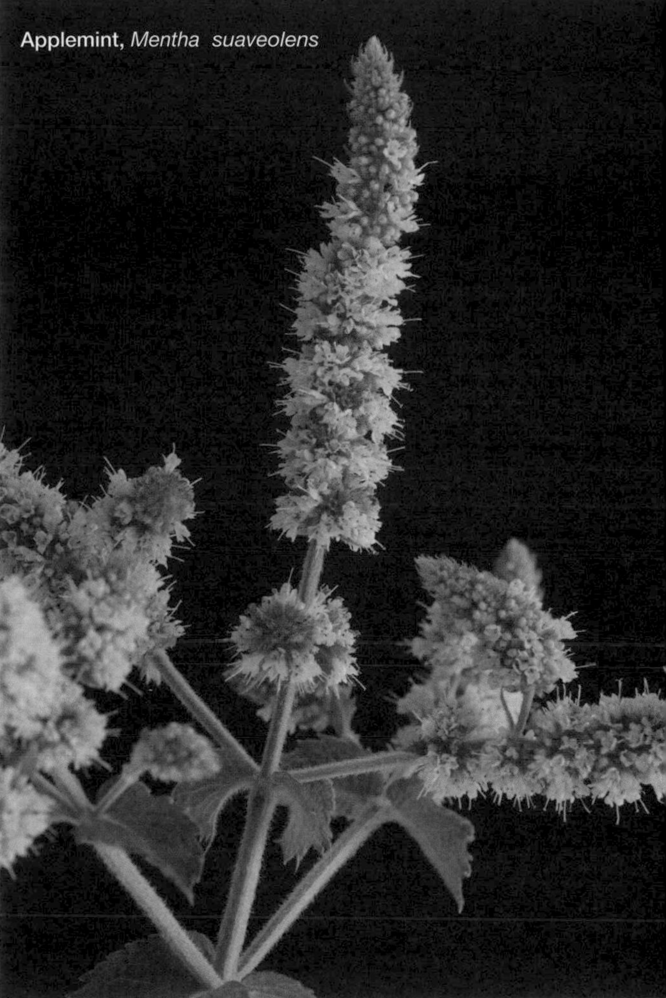

Applemint, *Mentha suaveolens*

Headaches: Peppermint essential oil is sold today in small roller bottles to apply to the forehead or temples to relieve migraines. Fresh spearmint or peppermint tea will often help a headache too. Parkinson says that mint also aids the memory, either by just smelling it or by applying it to the forehead and temples.

For eyes, mouth & as a diuretic: Mint's value to clear the eyes, stop mouth bleeding and to ease gravel and stone in the urinary system is noted. He uses mint as a gargle, to sweeten breath and restore the palate.

Wild mints: Their virtues are explained, he confirms earlier explanations, and restates his earlier concerns.

Dandruff: Combined with vinegar as a hair rinse used after shampooing, mint is an effective treatment for dandruff, and your hair will smell good.

strangury: painful urination
comfortable: relieving
Aristotle: Greek philosopher (384–322BC), student of Plato, writer and teacher
divers: various people
cods: testicles
fume: smoke
Kings-evill: scrofula
kernels of the throat: swollen glands
Great Pompey: Gnaeus Pompeius Magnus (106–48BC), Roman soldier and consul
Lepry: a form of leprosy

For head & memory: It is also comfortable for the head and memory, not onely to be smelled unto, but chiefly to be applyed unto the head and temples, and easeth the head-ach:

Mouth again: the decoction thereof cureth the gums and mouth that is sore, if it bee gargled therewith, and mendeth an ill favoured breath, as also with Rue and Coriander, causeth the uvula or palate of the mouth that is downe, to returne to its place againe, the decoction thereof being gargled and held in the mouth.

Aphrodisiac again: *Aristotle* and other in ancient times forbade Mints to be used of Souldiers in the time of warre, because they thought it did so much incite to Venery, that it tooke away, or at least abated their animosity or courage to fight.

For cheeses: Divers have held for true, that Cheeses will not corrupt, if they be either rubbed over with the juyce or the decoction of Mints, or they laid among them. And some againe, that if the juyce of Mints be put into the milke whereof you meane to make Cheese, that although yee put rennet thereto, it will never draw to curds whereby to become Cheese.

9. *Mentastrum tuberosum Clusij.*
Clusius his knobbed wild Mints.

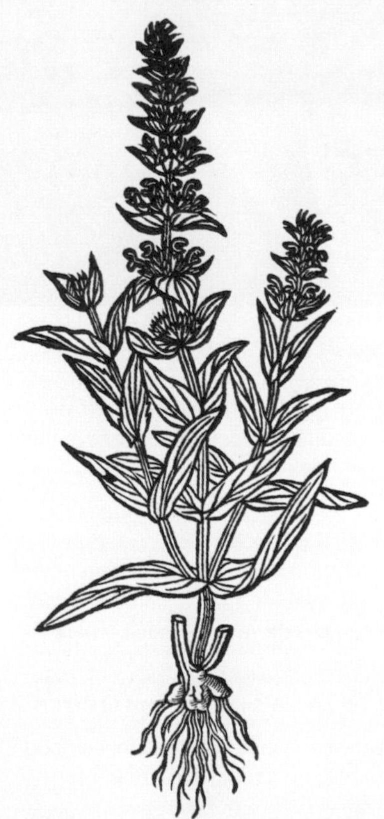

Wild mints: The vertues of the wild Mints are more especially to dissolve winde in the stomack, to helpe the chollick and those that are short-winded, and are an especiall remedy for those that have venerous dreames and pollutions in the night, used both inwardly, and the juyce being applyed outwardly to the testicles or cods;

the juyce therof dropped into the eares easeth the paines, and destroyeth the wormes that breed in them; they are good against the venemous bytings of Serpents, and as it is said, killeth them by the fume thereof, or by the scent of them being layd in any place, the juyce laid on warme helpeth the Kings-evill, or kernels of the throat, the decoction, or the distilled water helpeth a stinking breath, which proceedeth from the corruption of the teeth, and snuffed up into the nose purgeth the head.

Leprosy & dandruff: *Pliny* saith, that in the time of Great *Pompey*, it was found out by experience of one, to cure the Lepry by eating the leaves, and applying some of them to his face, and to helpe the scurfe or dandroffe of the head used with vineger.

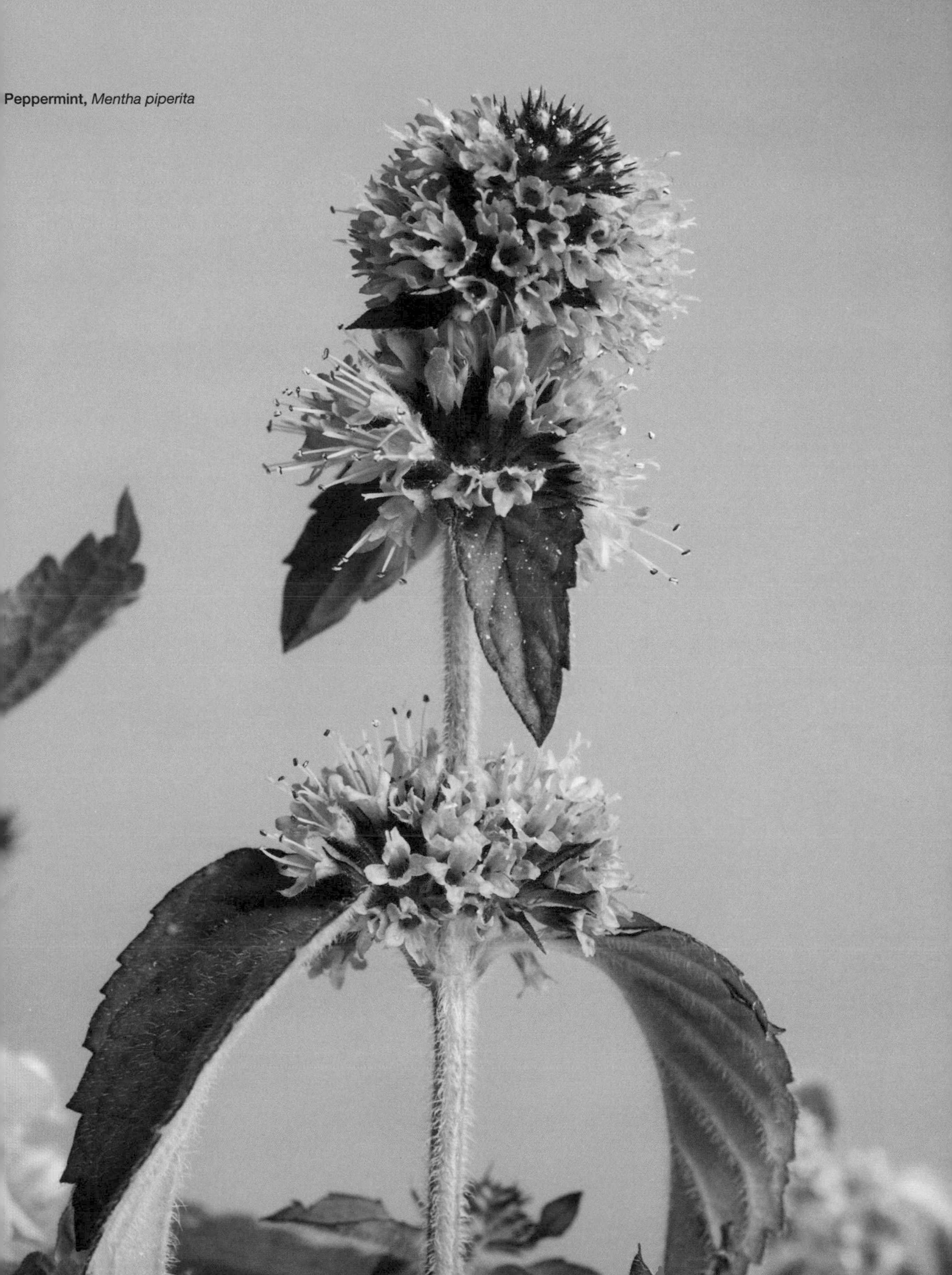

Peppermint, *Mentha piperita*

Missellto

Theatrum Botanicum

Tribe 16, Chapter 3, pp1392–94

subtill: thin, rarefied
acrimony: pungency
birdlime: sticky exudate of mistletoe
mollifie: ease, soften
imposthumes: abscesses
discusseth: disperses
rossin: resin from pines
sandarack: resin of *Tetraclinis articulata*
quick lime: calcium oxide, burnt lime
Matthiolus: Pierandrea Mattioli
pouther: powder
falling sicknesse: epilepsy
Gentilis Fulginas: Italian doctor, d. 1348
Lignum sancta crucis: wood of holy cross
appoplexy: stroke, cerebral haemorrhage
emperickes: unqualified practitioners
divers: various
Tragus: Hieronymus Bock
Pliny: Pliny the Elder (AD 23–79)

Viſcus quercinus.
Miſſellto of the Oke.

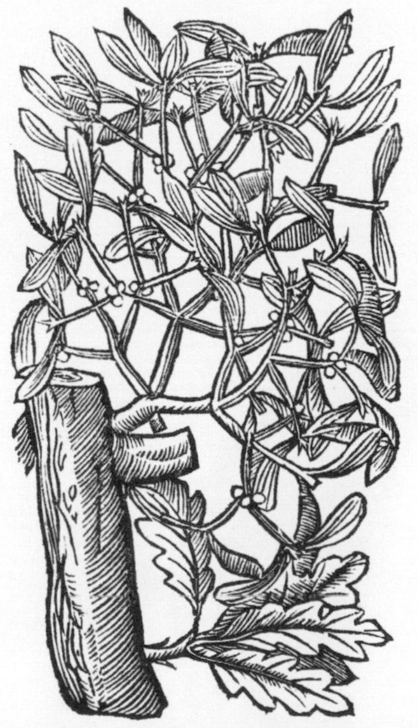

Viscum

The Vertues

ENERGETICS: Missellto is hot and dry in the third degree, the leaves and berryes doe heate and dry, and are of subtill parts, for some acrimony is in them, which overcommeth the bitternesse, the Birdlime doth mollifie hard knots, tumours, and Imposthumes, ripeneth and discusseth them, and draweth forth thicke as well as thinne humours, from the remote places of the body, digesting and separating them:

AS AN OINTMENT: but is not of that property to heate suddainely, but after some time as *Thapsia* doth, and being mixed with equall parts of Rossin and waxe doth mollefie the hardnesse of the spleene, and healeth old ulcers and sores: being mixed with Sandarack and Ortment, helpeth to draw of foule nailes, and if quick lime and Wine lees be added thereunto it worketh the stronger.

EPILEPSY: The Missellto it selfe of the Oke as the best, (or of the Chesnut tree as *Matthiolus* saith to be as good) made into pouther, and given in drinke unto those that have the falling sicknesse, doth heale them as *Matthiolus* saith, and that he had tryed it and healed many assuredly:

TOO SUPERSTITIOUS: but it is fit to use it forty dayes together: and with this caution, that the wood after it is broken from the tree, doe not touch the ground, which is in my minde too superstitious, as is their conceit also, that it hath power against Witchcraft, and the illusion of Sathan, and for that purpose, use to hang a peece thereof at their childrens neckes:

EPILEPSY AGAIN, STROKE & PARALYSIS: *Gentilis Fulginas* and others have so highly esteemed of the vertues hereof, that they have called it *Lignum sanctca crucis*, beleeving it to helpe the falling sicknesse, Appoplexy, and Palsie very speedily, not onely to be inwardly taken, but to be hung at their neckes, and some to hang it at their neckes, or weare it on their arme to helpe them to conceive: and saith *Matthiolus* I have knowne ignorant emperickes, to have given the Birdlime made into pilles to persons to swallow insteade of the wood: and further saith that he knew the Missellto that grew on a Pearetree, given to one that had the parts of his body drawne together, to doe him much good and divers doe esteeme of the Missellto that groweth on Hassell nuts, or Peares, as effectuall as that on the Oke, so it touch not the ground, for the falling sicknesse, to be taken in Wine.

FOR EARS: *Tragus* saith that the fresh wood of any Missellto bruised, and the juyce drawne forth, and dropped into the eares that have Imposthumes in them, doth helpe and ease them within a few dayes:

FOR CATTLE: the leaves are often given to cattell saith *Pliny*, to fatten them and purge them first: but if they be diseased they cannot continue long, this manner of curing them lasteth for forty dayes in Summer.

Mistletoe *Viscum album* Santalaceae

Mistletoe is the best-known evergreen parasitic among European plants, and everyone is familiar with the pleasant tradition of kissing beneath it at Christmas. The Latin name *Viscum* refers to the sticky juice of the white berries, which are poisonous to some people, though not all. The leaves and twigs are used medicinally, and it has a reputation as a powerful herb in treating nervous and heart conditions, and various tumours. The identity of the host plant can affect its complex chemistry, and correct dosage is vital.

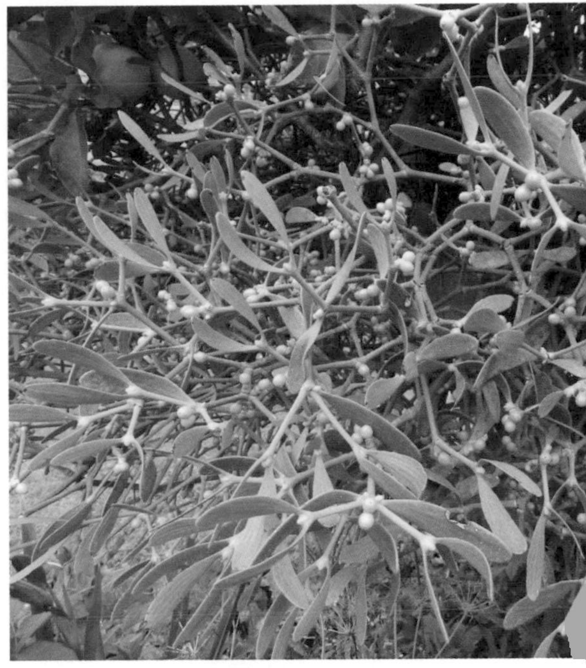

Energetics: In his opening sentences Parkinson demonstrates how precisely he employs humoural theory. He says the leaves and berries of mistletoe are 'of subtill parts', and their pungency overcomes bitterness, while the exudate, birdlime in his term, is effective for dispersing tumours and both thick and thin bodily fluids from the body's extremities.

What is fascinating is how well these findings, traditional in Parkinson's day, parallel modern descriptions of mistletoe's energetics. For example, American herbalist Peter Holmes calls mistletoe an 'antidyskratic detoxicant' for depositions and enlargements, as in cysts, arthritis and benign tumours. He notes that extracts of European mistletoe have been used and clinically researched for malignant tumours in all stages of cancer. He concludes: 'At the very least, Mistletoe preparations should become standard for aftertreatment of anticancer chemotherapy and radiation therapy' (*Energetics of Western Herbs* (Berkeley, CA, 1983), pp515–16).

As an ointment: Again Parkinson refers to a specific quality in mistletoe of slow heating, which in an ointment works to reduce the swelling and ease the pain of a diseased spleen, as also 'old ulcers and sores', and which with strong resins can be used to draw out pus from 'foule nailes'.

For epilepsy: The powder of oak or chestnut mistletoe taken in liquid is found by experience, he reports, to ease epileptic conditions. Modern herbalism would say 'antispasmodic', and mistletoe carries a continuing reputation for treating convulsive nervous disorders, though these would usually be referred to orthodox medicine rather than be treated at home. Mistletoe was once a specific for St Vitus Dance (Sydenham's chorea).

Too superstitious: This paragraph and the next frame Parkinson's priorities: he wants readers to see mistletoe as a medicinal, without added 'superstition'; indeed, the practices he mentions have long disappeared.

Epilepsy again, stroke & paralysis: Here, he touches on mistletoe as a heart and circulatory herb, uses that were as prominent in his day as in our own. It has been used to treat hardening of the arteries, for staunching blood, such as nose bleeds, and for normalizing blood pressure and the circulation. It is known as a heart *qi* circulation herb in Chinese medicine; and the Austrian herbalist Maria Treben writes in *Health through God's Pharmacy* (Steyr, Austria,1980), p33: 'I cannot emphasize Mistletoe enough for circulatory problems.'

Caution: Mistletoe is a powerful and still largely clinically unexplored medicinal; dosage is key to successful, safe use. If in doubt, consult your herbal practitioner.

Kissing cousins: The American mistletoe (*Phoradendron flavescens*) is a close relative of European mistletoe, sharing with it the ability to ease nervous tension and act as a vasoconstrictor. It does increase blood pressure, though, and is not to be taken by those with hypertension. As a strong uterine stimulant, it was used by both Native American and settler women as an aid to childbirth; by the same token it should be avoided in pregnancy itself.

Mugwort

Theatrum Botanicum

Tribe 1, Chapter 33, pp90–92

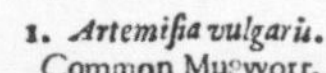

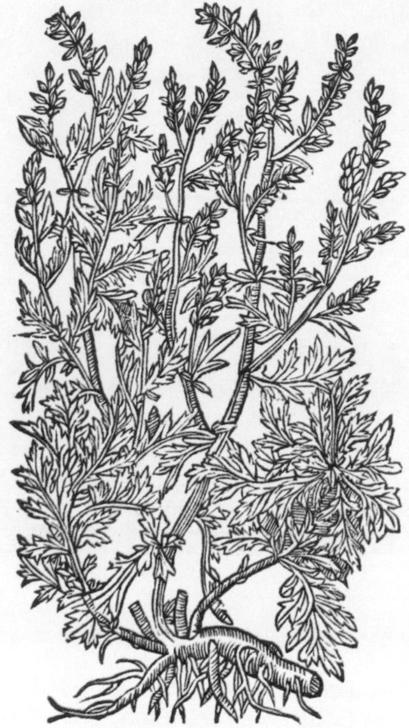

Dioscorides: Greek-speaking Roman physician (mid-first century AD)
extenueth: reduces the seriousness
the mother: the uterus
Axungia: soft animal fat, goose fat
Wens: sebaceous cysts
kernels: hard swellings or swollen glands
Daisies: *Bellis perennis*
Opium: drug prepared from *Papaver somniferum*
three drammes: ⅜ oz, 11.67g
Camomill: chamomile
Agrimony: *Agrimonia* sp.
Pliny: Pliny the Elder (AD23–79), Roman naturalist
Bauhinus: Gaspard Bauhin (1560–1624), Swiss botanist
Saint John's eve: 23 June
falling sickness: epilepsy

Artemisia

The Vertues

Dioscorides saith, it heateth and extenuateth.

Gynaecological uses: It is with good successe put among other hearbes, that are boyled for women to sit over the hot decoction, to draw downe their courses, to helpe the delivery of the birth, and to expell the secondine or afterbirth, as also for the obstructions and inflammations of the mother;

Urinary: it breaketh the stone, and causeth one to make water where it is stopped: the juyce thereof made up with Myrrhe, and put under as a pessary, worketh the same effect, and so doth the roote also,

Neck & throat: being made up with Axungia into an oyntment, it doth take away Wens and hard knots, and kernels that grow about the necke and throat, as also to ease the paines about the necke, but especially and with more effect, if some field Daisies be put with it.

Opium antidote: The hearbe it selfe being fresh, or the juyce thereof taken, is a speciall remedy, upon the overmuch taking of *Opium*:

Sciatica: three drammes of the powder of the dryed leaves taken in wine, is a speedy, and the best certaine helpe for the Sciatica.

Cramp & sinews: A decoction thereof made with Camomill and Agrimony, and the place bathed therewith while it is warme, taketh away the paines of the sinewes, and the crampe.

Superstitions: It is said of *Pliny*, that if a Traveller binde some of the hearbe about him, he shall feele no wearinesse at all in his journey: as also that no evill medicine or evill beast shall hurt him that hath this hearbe about him.

Many such idle superstitions and irreligious relations are set downe, both by the ancient and later Writers concerning this and other plants, which to relate, were both unseemely for me, and unprofitable for you.

I will onely declare unto you, the idle conceit of some of our later dayes concerning this plant, and that is even of *Bauhinus*, who glorieth to be an eye witnesse of this foppery, that upon Saint *Johns* eve, there are coales to be found at mid-day, under the rootes of Mugwort, which after or before that time, are very small or none at all, and are used as an Amulet to hang about the necke of those that have the falling sicknesse, to cure them thereof. But Oh the weak and fraile nature of man! which I cannot but lament, that is more prone to beleeve and relye upon such impostures, than upon the ordinances of God in his creatures, and trust in his providence.

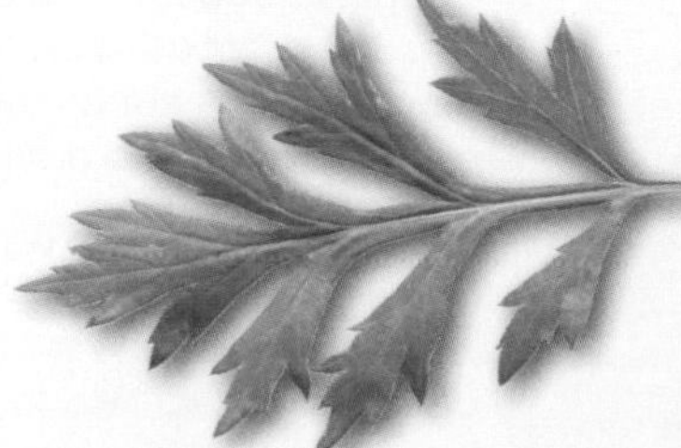

Mugwort *Artemisia vulgaris* Asteraceae

Mugwort has beneficial effects on digestive problems and the nervous system, and is a valuable warming tonic that improves health and well-being. It is an important woman's herb for use from puberty through to menopause, is helpful for stress and anxiety, and has a history of association with magic and protection.

Mugwort grows in Europe, northern Africa and Asia and has been introduced to North America. Like woodruff, it becomes more aromatic when dried.

It was considered a herb of Artemis, protector of women, by the Greeks, and in the Christian era became associated with St John. It is still used in St John's day mid-summer celebrations on the Isle of Man, but Parkinson had little sympathy for the 'idle superstitions' written about by Pliny and others. He gets particularly irate with Bauhin, who claimed to be an eyewitness to finding coals upon the roots of the plant at midday on St John's eve.

Gynaecological uses: Mugwort regulates the menstrual cycle, and is particularly useful where the period is absent. It is useful for difficult or delayed puberty and also for menopausal problems, including anxiety.

Urinary: Mugwort is rarely used as a urinary herb nowadays, but it is diuretic and its use for stones deserves another look.

Addiction: Mugwort is used with other herbs in treating alcohol addiction, as well as withdrawal from heroin and opium. It is helpful for anorexia and other eating disorders as it also gently improves digestion.

Sciatica: Mugwort's affinity for the nervous system and relaxing tension makes it a good candidate for treating sciatica.

Cramp & sinews: Agrimony and chamomile also relax tension, and applying the mixture warm increases its effectiveness for cramps.

Other uses: Mugwort is used as moxa in Chinese medicine, burned to heat and stimulate acupuncture points.

Mugwort is considered protective, and, like other members of the genus, is burned in smudge sticks to clear stuck energies. Some people find it gives them very vivid dreams, either just used as a pillow or else smoked or ingested.

It was one of the herbs often used in making ale, before hops was introduced for beer-making.

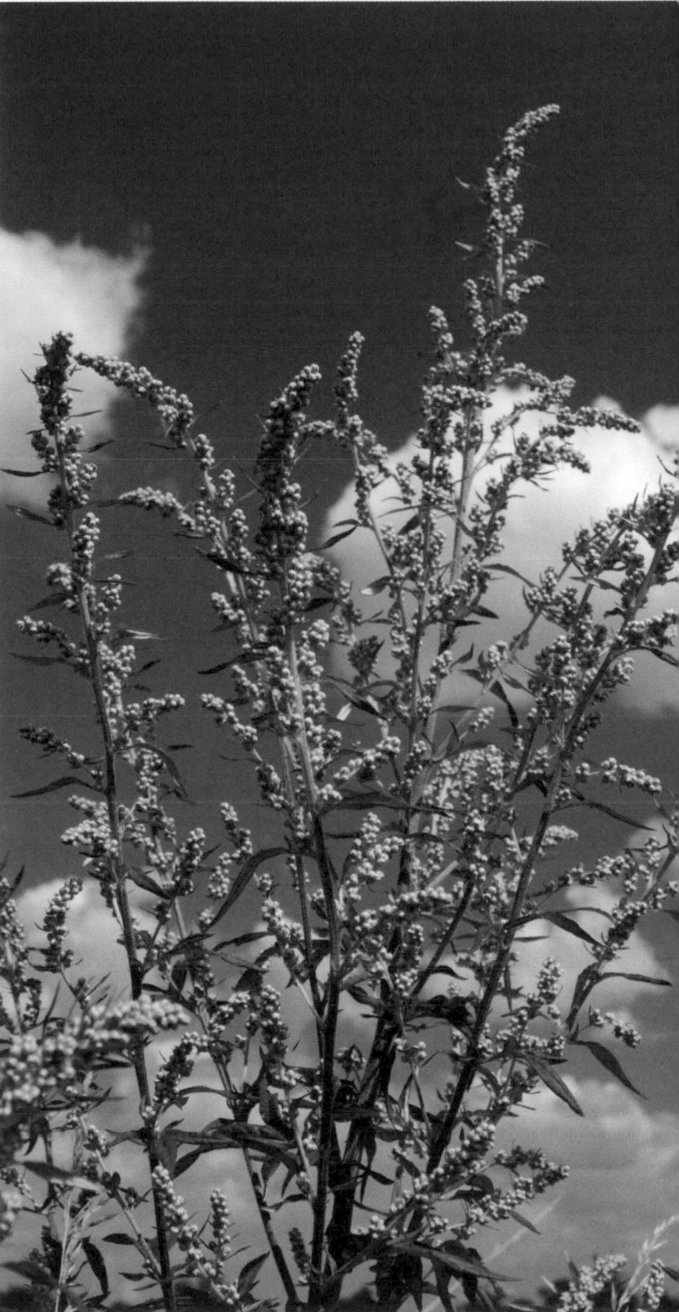

Mullein

Theatrum Botanicum

Tribe 1, Chapter 21, pp60–63

1. *Verbascum album vulgare sive Tapsus barbatus communis.* Common Mullein.

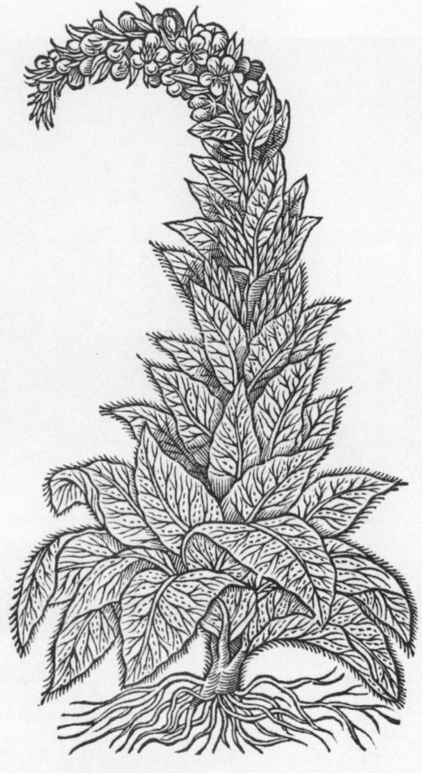

Dioscorides: Greek-speaking Roman physician (mid-first century AD)
laskes: dysentery
fluxes: flows
bursten: ruptured
Camomill: chamomile
Venice Turpentine: larch resin
chafing-dish: portable heating dish
Close-stool: enclosed cabinet for chamber pot
fundament: bowel
bloody flixe: bloody dysentery
oyle: oil
ague: fever
reines: kidneys
Marjerome: marjoram
stark: standing out
gowt: gout
Arnaldus de Villanova: Catalan physician, alchemist (c.1235–1311)

Verbascum

The Vertues

Mullein is commended by *Dioscorides* against laskes and fluxes of the belly, if a small quantity of the root be given in wine: the decoction thereof drunke is profitable for those that are bursten, and for those that have crampes and convulsions; and likewise for those that are troubled with an old cough: the decoction thereof gargled, easeth the paines of the toothache.

Fumes: If the seed and flowers hereof, together with the flowers of Camomill, and the powder of dryed Venice Turpentine, be cast upon a few quick coales in a chafing-dish, or such like other thing set into a Close-stoole, and the party sitting bare over the fumes, that is troubled with the piles or falling downe of the fundament, or any the paines of that place, doth give much ease and helpe: as also for those that have a great desire to go3 often to the stoole and can doe nothing, especially to such as have the bloody Flixe.

Oil & decoction: An oyle made by the often infusion of the flowers, is of very good effect for the piles also. The decoction of the roote in red wine, or in water, if there be an ague, wherein red hot steele hath beene often quenched, doth stay the bloody flixe. The same also openeth the obstructions of the bladder and reines when one cannot make water. A decoction of the leaves hereof, and of Sage, Marjerome, and Camomill flowers, and the places bathed therewith, that have their veines and sinewes starke with cold, or with crampes, doth bring them much ease and comfort.

Distilled water: It is said that there is not a better remedy found out for the hot gowt then to drinke three ounces of the distilled water of the flowers every morning and evening for some dayes together.

Fevers: *Arnaldus* saith, that if two drams of the juyce of the rootes of Mullein before it beare stalke, be taken in a draught of Muscadine at every time, for three or foure times one after another, an houre before the fitt of the quartane ague commeth upon any, it shall surely helpe them.

Warts: The juyce of the leaves and flowers being laid upon rough warts, as also the powder of the dried rootes rubbed on, doth easily take them away, as *Matthiolus* saith, although it will doe no good to those that are smooth:

Aches, tumours & other uses: and that the powder of the dryed flowers is an especiall remedy for those that are troubled with belly aches, or the paines and torments of the collick. The decoction of the root hereof, and so likewise the leaves is of great effect to dissolve the tumors or swellings, as also the inflammations of the throat. The seed and leaves boyled in wine, and after laid to any place that is prickt with a thorn, hath a splinter, or such like thing got into the flesh, draweth the forth speedily, easeth the paines, and healeth them also. The leaves

Mullein *Verbascum* spp. Scrofulariaceae

Mullein has a long history of use in its southern European and Asian home, and has been naturalized in parts of North America and Australia. The spires of yellow flowers can be 7 feet (over 2 metres) tall and are unmistakable in summer. Its special affinity is the respiratory system, but it also calms and strengthens the nerves, digestive and urinary systems; it is good for swollen glands and to relieve pain.

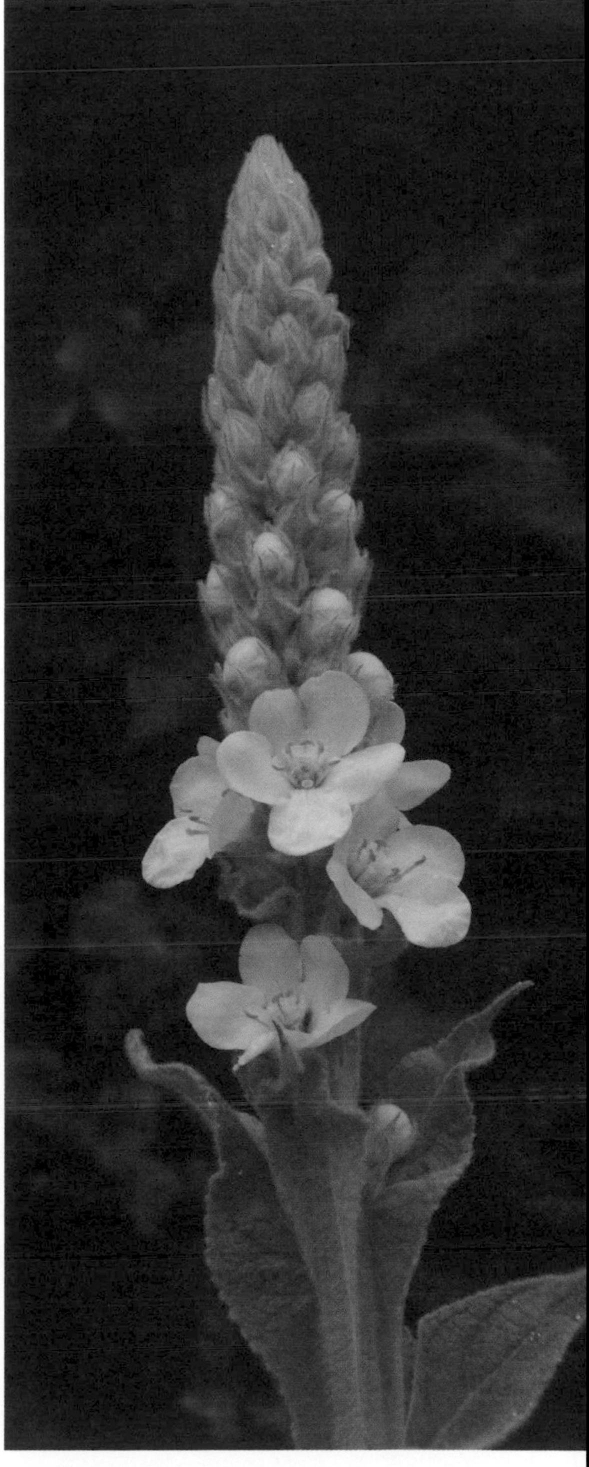

Mullein is a fine example of the wide range of applications Parkinson brought to his herbalism. He differentiates between the plant's seed, root, leaf and flower, while his preparations include the juice, decoctions in wine, water or vinegar, heated herbs to be applied as poultices or to provide healing smoke, infused oils, distilled waters and ointments.

Diarrhoea: His first recommendation, based on the classics, is using a decoction of the root in wine for diarrhoea, upset stomach, ruptures, cough and toothache.

Old coughs: Mullein is still used frequently by herbalists to treat coughs, and is especially soothing for dry coughs. It is interesting that Parkinson also mentions mullein broth as a country remedy for cattle suffering with coughs.

Toothache: Mullein is a pain-relieving herb, and Parkinson suggests gargling with the decoction to ease the pain of toothache.

Haemorrhoids: Parkinson describes several different methods of using mullein to treat piles. The first is to sit or squat over the fumes of mullein seed and flowers heated with chamomile and dried Venice turpentine. He also recommends a strong infused oil made with the flowers (which we still use for earache) to apply on the haemorrhoids. The third recommendation is an interesting ointment recipe, using bruised mullein flowers, leek juice, egg yolk and bread crumbs.

Fevers: Parkinson recommends a decoction of the root in red wine for fevers. He also quotes Arnaldus, who prescribes the juice of mullein root to be taken in Muscadine wine an hour before the quartain fever is due to return.

Warts: He supports Matthiolus' treatment of rubbing the juice of fresh leaves or flowers, or the powder of dried mullein roots on warts, but states clearly that it will only work for rough warts and not for smooth ones.

Dysentery: For bloody diarrhoea, he recommends the decoction of the root in water that has been used frequently to quench hot steel, and the same preparation for obstructed urine. Blacksmiths traditionally quenched hot steel in cold water to make it much harder. Blacksmith's water was a

5. *Verbascum nigrum vulgare.*
Ordinary blacke Mullein.

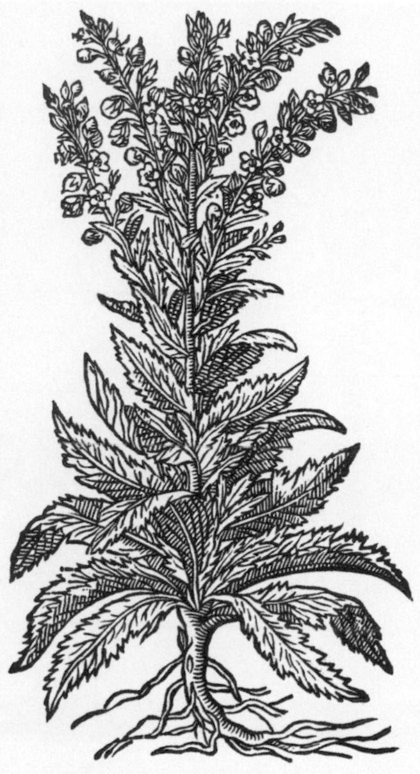

Muscadine: sweet Muscat wine
fitt of the quartan ague: chills of a four-day fever
Matthiolus: Pierandrea Mattioli (1501–77), physician and author
prickt: pricked
double papers: double wrapped
botch: blemish
boyle: boil
hapneth: occurs
gowt: gout
Gutta Rosacea: acne rosacea
Camphire: camphor
crummes: crumbs
Cattell: cattle
shooing: shoeing
Dioscorides: Greek-speaking Roman physician (mid-first century AD)
lapped: wrapped
figges: figs
lye: caustic solution obtained by leaching wood ash

being bruised wrapped in double papers, and covered with hot ashes and embers, to bake a while, and then taken forth and laid warme upon any botch or boyle that hapneth in the groine or share, by filthinesse or otherwise, doth dissolve and heale them. The seed hereof bruised, boyled in wine, and laid upon any member out of joynt after it is set in againe, taketh away all swellings and paines thereof. The leaves and toppes of the lesser white Mullein boyled in water, and laid upon the places pained with the gowt, doth wondrously ease them.

Distilled water 2: The distilled water of the flowers hereof dropped into the eyes, taketh away the watering in them, as also taketh away that rednesse of the face, is called in Latine *Gutta Rosacea* and in English, the Rose, if it bee washed therewith often, having a little Camphire dissolved in it. The water is likewise used against running or creeping sores, or any other deformity of the skin.

Haemorrhoids: The flowers bruised and made up into an oyntment with the yolke of an egge, a few crummes of bread, and the juyce of leekes laid upon the painefull piles when they swell, doth ease the paines exceedingly, and helpe to bring them into their right place.

Veterinary uses: Country men doe often give their Cattell that are troubled with coughes, the broth of the hearbe to drinke with good successe, as also to those that by casualty, or through loosenesse and weakenesse, void out their guts behind them. The leaves also a little bruised, and laid or bound to a Horse foote that is grievously prickt with shooing, doth wonderfully heale it in a short space

Preservative, rouge, hair dye: *Dioscorides* saith it was a report in his time that if dryed figges were lapped in the leaves of female Mullein, which is that with large and white flowers, they will not putrifie at all. The golden flowers of the blacke Mullein boyled in lye, dyeth the haires of the head yellow, and maketh them faire and smooth. The leaves boyled in wine and a little honey put to it, is fit to wash and clense foule ulcers, and boyled in vineger, doth helpe greene wounds. Taken also with Rue it is a remedy against the stinging of Scorpions.

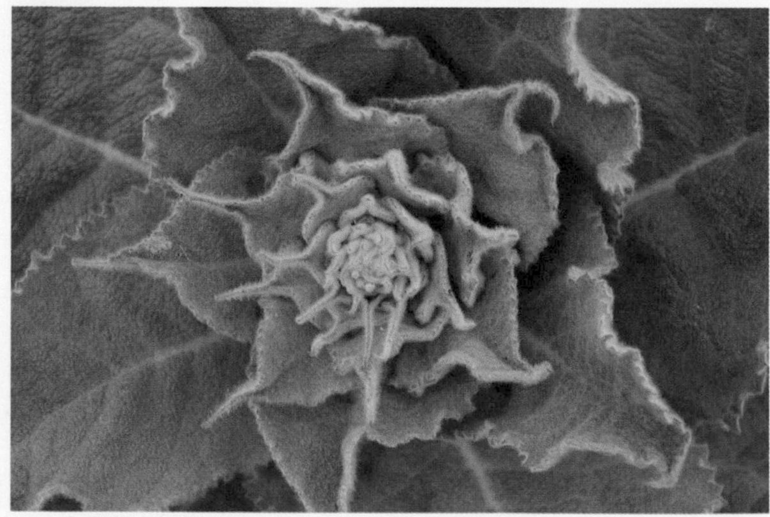

popular ingredient in medical treatments, presumably because it would have a high mineral content.

Gout: Distilled mullein flowers are recommended as one of the best remedies for gout, with three ounces being drunk morning and evening. Parkinson also advises using the leaves and tops of lesser white mullein, boiled in water and then applied as a poultice to the parts affected by gout, saying it 'doth wondrously ease them.'

Distilled water: Apart from gout, Parkinson suggests the distilled water for bathing watery eyes, and for clearing any deformities of the skin, including weeping sores and acne rosacea.

Throat problems: Mullein works on the lymphatic system, and is still much used by herbalists for swellings and inflammations of the throat. Mullein is a member of the Scrofulariaceae, a plant family named for its use in treating scrofula or tubercular swellings in the neck and throat.

Thorns & splinters: Parkinson says to boil the seed or leaves of mullein in wine, and then use the liquid as a poultice for splinters and thorns. He promises it will relieve the pain, draw out the splinter and then help the wound heal. He also recommends the bruised leaf as a poultice for horses whose feet have been injured by the blacksmith's nails during shoeing.

Preservative & hair dye: Mullein leaves have long been used to wrap and store fruit; other uses have been for baby nappies, a natural toilet paper and soothing insoles for shoes, especially for plantar fasciitis.

Black mullein flowers make a yellow hair dye, Parkinson says.

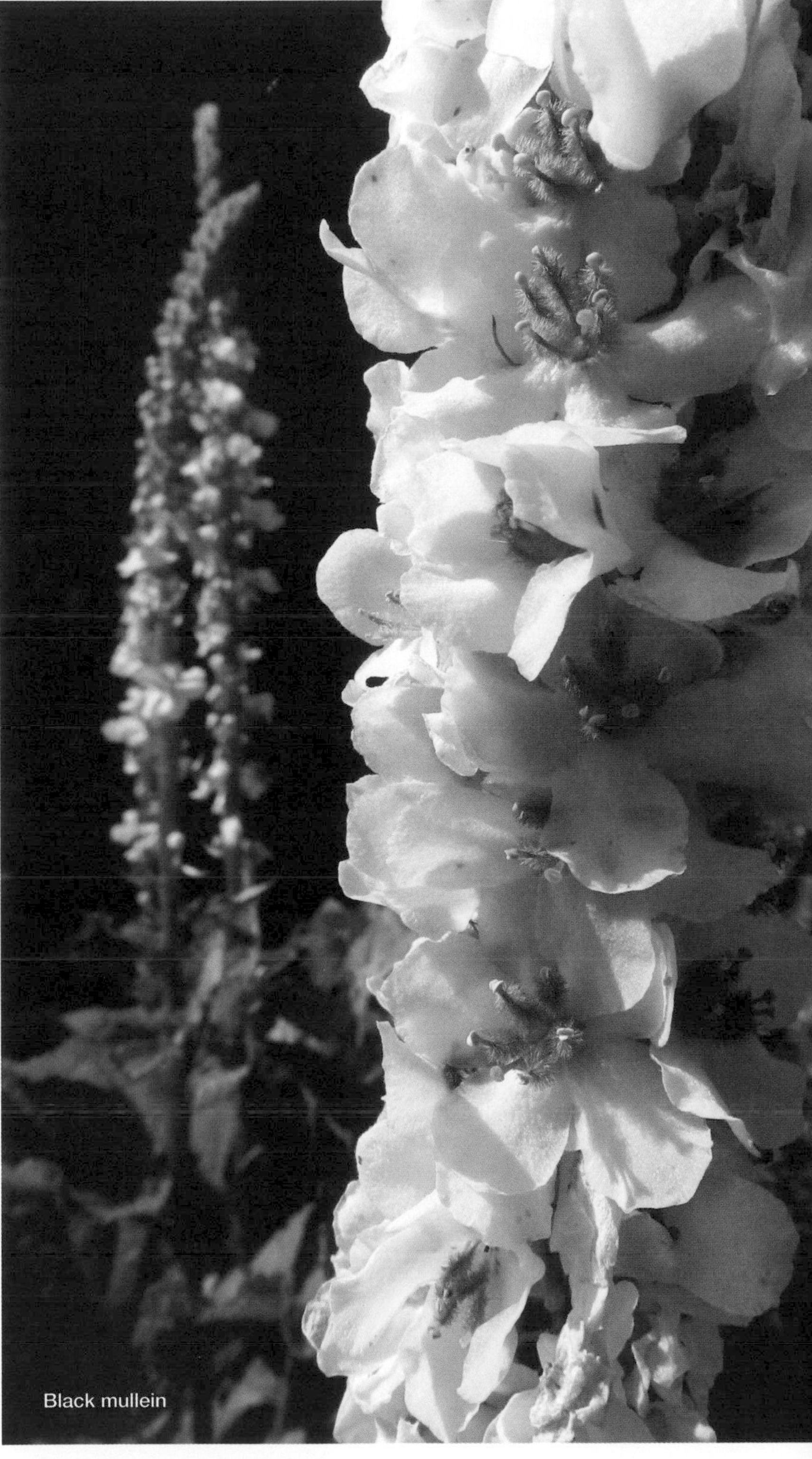
Black mullein

Nettles

Theatrum Botanicum

Tribe 4, Chapter 13, pp440–42

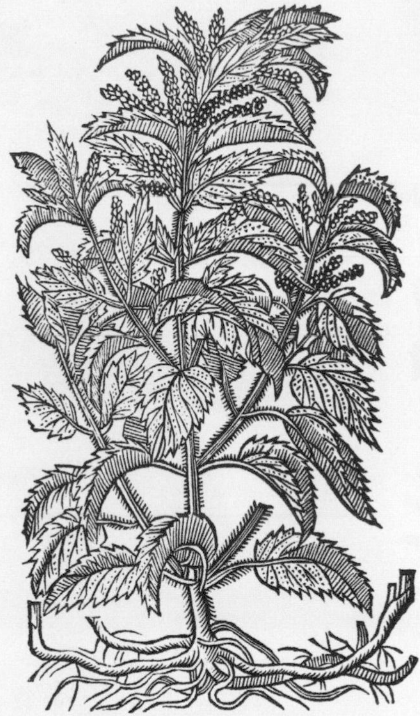

causticke, exulcerating: hot, inflaming
open belly: remove obstructions to
soluble: liquid, moveable
Electuary: powder in honey
expectorate cold phlegme: spit out cold mucus
raise the impostumated Pleurisie: clear abscesses on the lung
spend by spitting: expel by spitting
Almonds of the throate: tonsils
provoke womens courses: stimulate menstruation
suffocation or strangling of the mother: constriction of womb
Myrrhe: resin of *Commiphora* tree
gravel, stone: calculi in urinary tract
provoke Venery: incite to lust
stayeth: prevents, stops
poysonfull: toxic
Lethargy: torpor or chronic fatigue

Urtica

The Vertues

The sting: Although Nettles doe hurt and sting the skinne and flesh, while they are greene, which is caused by the haire or rough downe upon them, and might be thought to be causticke or exulcerating being otherwise applyed, yet it is not so, being found to be hot and dry in the second degree;

Opening the belly & lungs: the leaves boyled in wine and drunke, is said to open the belly and make it soluble: the rootes or leaves boyled, or the juice of either of them, or both, made into an *Electuary* with Honey or Sugar, is a safe or sure medicine to open the pipes and passages of the Lungs, which is the cause of wheesings and shortnesse of breath, and helpeth to expectorate tough cold flegme sticking in them, or in the chest or stomacke, as also to raise the impostumated Pluresie, and spend it by spitting:

Opening the throat: the same also helpeth the Almonds of the throate when they are swelled, to gargle the mouth and throate therewith, the juice also is effectuall to settle the pallate of the mouth in its place, and to heale and temper the inflammations and sorenesse of the mouth and throate:

For women: the decotion of the leaves in wine and drunke, is singular good to provoke womens courses, and to settle the suffocation or strangling of the mother, and all other the diseases thereof, as also applyed outwardly with a little Myrrhe:

As a diuretic: the same also or the seed provoketh urine, and expelleth gravel and the stone in the reines or bladder; often prooved to be effectuall in many that have taken it;

For worms & wind: the same decoction also of the leaves or seede, or being beaten and drunke in that decoction, killeth the wormes in the bellies of Children, and is said to ease the paines in the sides, and to dissolve or breake the windinesse in the spleene, as also in the body;

Provoking venery: but others doe think that it being somewhat windy of it selfe, is not so powerfull or availeable to expell wind, but onely to provoke Venery;

Bleeding of the mouth: the juice of the leaves taken two or three dayes together, stayeth bleeding at the mouth, which riseth from the stomacke:

For stings, bites & poisons: the seed being drunke is a remedy against the stinging of venemous creatures, the bitings of madde dogs, the poysonfull qualities of Hemlocke, Henbane, Nightshade, Mandrake, or other such like herbes, that stupify and dull the senses, as also the Lethargy, but especially to use it outwardly to rubbe the forehead and temples in the Lethargy, and the places bitten or stunge with beasts,

Nettles *Urtica* spp. Urticaceae

Nettle is one of the world's great herbs, and has been recognized throughout history as such wherever it grows. It was an important medicinal in Parkinson's time, and his account of the virtues of nettle is exemplary in its thoroughness and exact, experimentally observed applications. We should heed his work.

The sting: By dying in 1650 Parkinson missed by only 15 years the first publication of microscopic images of nettle by Robert Hooke, but it was a revelatory new world away. While Parkinson could talk of 'rough downe' causing the sting, Hooke in 1665 could actually see the syringe of silica that a nettle sting really is, and postulate the hypodermic explanation of pressure gradients and the poison (formic acid) moving from the nettle into the pierced place.

Yet Parkinson also observed that when applied in a medicinal content it was not caustic but rather moderately hot and dry. He did not write that simple heating was enough to neutralize the toxicity of the sting, and perhaps did not know it as such.

Opening the belly & lungs: Here Parkinson is highly specific: boiling the leaves in wine (and who does that today?) is opening for the belly, while boiling and sweetening either leaves or the more powerful roots as an electuary opens the 'pipes and passages' of the lungs. Nettle prepared in this way is decongestant and clearing, effectively unsticking glutinous mucus, which can then be expectorated and spat away.

Opening the throat: The same preparations work similarly for the throat, he says, in tonsillitis and to settle the palate, in fact for any inflammatory conditions in the mouth. A modern way to extend this understanding is to say nettle is anti-allergenic, being effective in treating allergies such as asthma and hay fever.

For women: Nettle's older reputation as a 'woman's herb' is confirmed here, with its capacity to stimulate menstruation and to treat a number of malfunctionings of the womb; it can be applied externally with myrrh, he says. He does not mention here nettle's reputation for increasing breast milk.

A modern application of nettle root, unknown to Parkinson, is for treating prostate problems in men, and nettle is now generally described as a blood restorative and as nutritive, as well as containing bio-available iron useful in treating anaemia.

As a diuretic: Again he confirms common knowledge of nettle roots, leaves or seed as diuretic, hence promoting urination and helping dissolve and clear smaller and larger calculi (gravel and stones) from the kidneys and bladder.

For worms and wind: Nettle kills worms in the belly, especially of children, and reduces windiness in the body, he says.

Provoking venery: Parkinson invariably associates 'wind' with 'venery', and does so

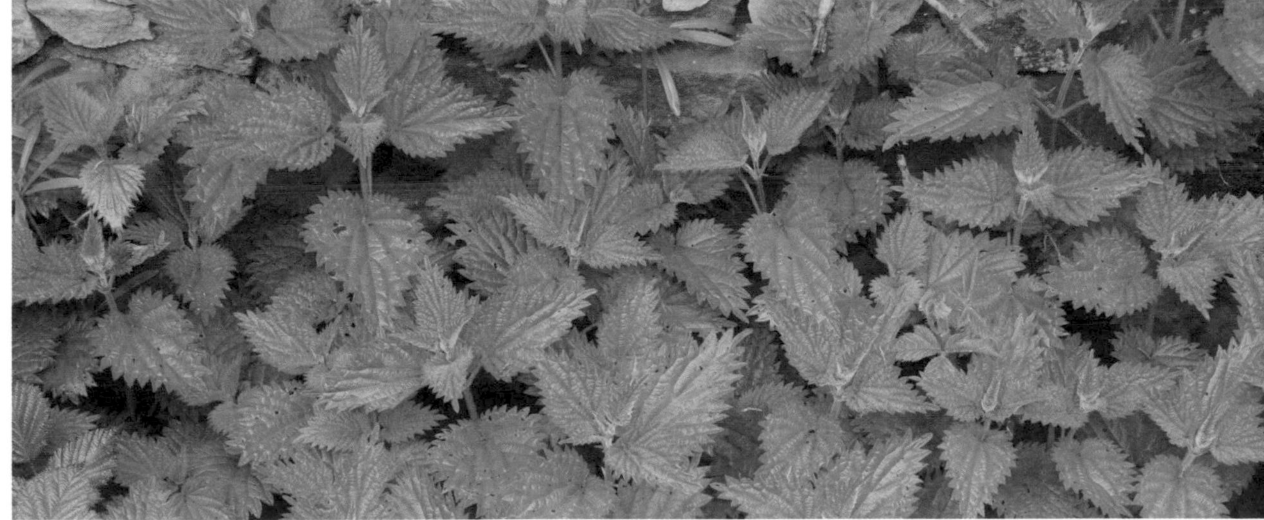

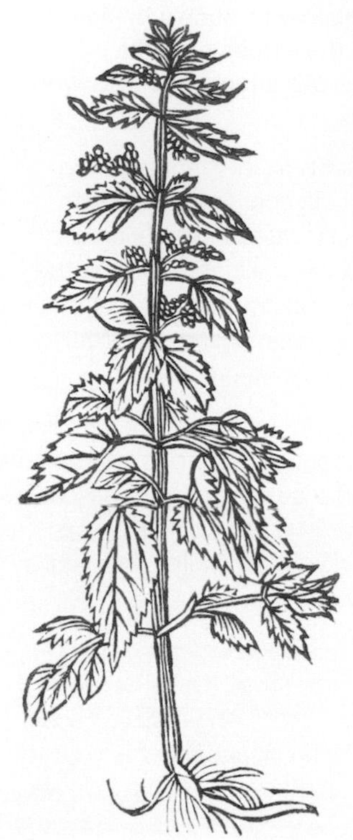
4. *Vrtica minor.*
The lesser wild Nettle.

Nicander: Greek poet and physician (2nd century BC)
surfet: excess
Morphew: discoloration of skin
Lepry: form of leprosy
Polypus: polyps
fistulaies: fistulas, tube-like openings
manginesse: with bare spots, mange
greene wounds: fresh wounds
members: limbs
discusseth the defluctions: dilutes flow
benummed: stiff, arthritic
Wallwort, Danewort: *Sambucus ebulus*
lyen: remained
hennes: chickens
meate: their food
privities: private parts
cover: mate
Roman nettle: *Urtica pilulifera*
the least: i.e. small nettle, *U. urens*
availeable: effective

For other toxins: used with a little salt, *Nicander* saith, it helpeth them that have taken Quicksilver, and those that have eaten evill Mushromes, or surfet of the good;

For the skin & nose bleeds: the distilled water of the herbe is very effectuall, (although not so powerfull,) as well for all the diseases aforesaid, as for outward wounds, and sores, to wash them, and to clense the skinne from Morphew, Lepry, and other discolourings thereof; the seede (and some also use the leaves) being bruised, and put into the nostrils, doth stanch the bleeding of them, and taketh away the flesh growing in them, called *Polypus*:

For sores & scabs: the juice of the leaves or the decoction of them or of the rootes, is singular good to wash either old rotten and stinking sores, or fistulaies and Gangrenes also, and such as are fretting eating or corroding scabbes, also manginesse and itches in any part of the body, as also greene wounds, by washing them therewith, or putting the juice into the sores or wounds, or applying the greene herbe bruised thereunto, yea although the flesh were separated from the bones;

For joint pain: the same also applyed to overwearied members refresheth them, or to places out of joynt, after the joynt is set in its right place, it strengtheneth, dryeth, and comforteth them, as also to those places troubled with aches and goutes, and the defluction of humours upon the joynts or sinewes, it easeth the paines, and dryeth or discusseth the defluctions:

Ointment: an ointment made with the juice, oyle and a little wax, is singular good to rubbe cold and benummed members, to bring them to their proper activity againe;

A recipe for gout: a handfull of the greene leaves of Nettles, and another of Wall-wort or Dane-wort, bruised and applyed simply of themselves to the Gout, Sciatica, or joynt aches, in any part, hath beene found to be an admirable helpe thereunto: it is said that if greene Nettles be put into the urine of a sicke body, if it be fresh and greene, after it hath lyen foure and twenty houres therein, the party shall recover of that sicknesse, but if it doe not abide greene, it signifieth death or great danger;

For birds & animals: if you give hennes some dry Nettles broken small, with their meate in winter, it will make them lay egges all the winter more plentifully; it is said also, that if the herbe be rubbed on the privities of female beasts, that will not suffer the males to cover them, it will cause them the more willingly to suffer them to doe it:

For stinging nettles themselves: the oyle of roses or sallet oyle boyled with the juice, or the juice of the leaves themselves, is a present remedy to take away the stinging of the Nettles:

The Roman nettle: to all the purposes aforesaid, the Romane Nettle is held the most effectuall, yet where it cannot be had, the other are in a degree next to it, as effectuall, yet the least is thought of some to be lesse powerful, and of others to be as availeable as any of the other two.

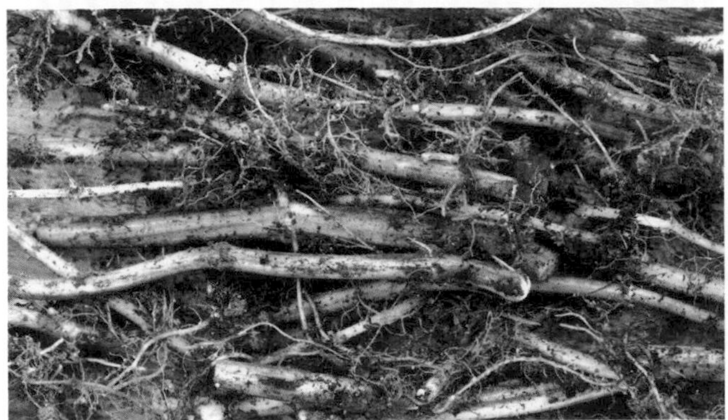

here. Dried nettle seed has had a reputation as an aphrodisiac in many cultures and times, and 'sado-masochism' is the name given to the habit of beating another or oneself with nettle leaves for gratification.

Energizing seeds: We have had experience of the 'speedy' effect of nettle seed. Friend A had dried a bottle of the seed, and visiting Friend B was feeling tired. Friend A suggested a spoonful. Friend B took this to mean a dessertspoon full, while Friend A had intended a teaspoon full. After half an hour Friend B was whizzing around a supermarket, returned home to Friend A and proceeded to vacuum her whole house, ask where the paints were so she could do the walls, and kept going at high revs for hours.

Not only is taking the seed a guarantee of the housework being done, it is valuable against narcotic herbs, says Parkinson, and the mad dogs that worry him so much.

For other toxins: He reports the Greek poet and physician Nicander as writing that nettle will counter the effects of mercury, poisonous fungi or a surfeit of mushrooms. Nicander was a respected expert on antidotary, writing two long poems, *Theriaca* and *Alexipharmica*, that Parkinson evidently knew.

For the skin & nose bleeds: He now suggests nettle distilled water for all the foregoing conditions and to wash outward sores; he adds that the seed or leaves can staunch nasal bleeding (much as yarrow does) and remove nasal polyps.

For sores & scabs: Similarly, the leaves or roots, in decoction, are 'singular good' for sores, fistulas and gangrene, scabs and itches on the skin. This applies to old or fresh sores, and even when flesh is separated from the bones.

For joint pain: Continuing with the many virtues of this most virtuous herb, he mentions how decoction of nettle will confirm reset joints in position, relieve aches and gout, and dry or dilute descending mucus.

Ointment: A nettle ointment, he says, will heat and relax cold and stiff limbs, restoring a more normal range of action.

Urine test: Parkinson suggests a urine test using nettle leaves. He says that nettle mixed with healthy urine will stay green after 24 hours, but in morbid urine will lose its greenness and indicate a very poor prognosis for the patient.

For stinging nettles themselves: He observes the commonly known fact that nettles can be used in an oil or juice to treat nettle rash.

The Roman nettle: In his introduction Parkinson mentions the story of Roman nettle *Urtica pilulifera*, popularized in William Camden's *Britannica* (1586). Camden said it was introduced by Julius Caesar's invading army in 55BC and that the Roman soldiers rubbed their limbs with it for warmth (urtication). Roman nettle survived into Parkinson's time but was lost to the British plant list many years ago.

Other uses of nettle: He does not mention nettle's already known value, in composts and spring soups. Modern research is looking at nettle for assistance as a diabetes medicine.

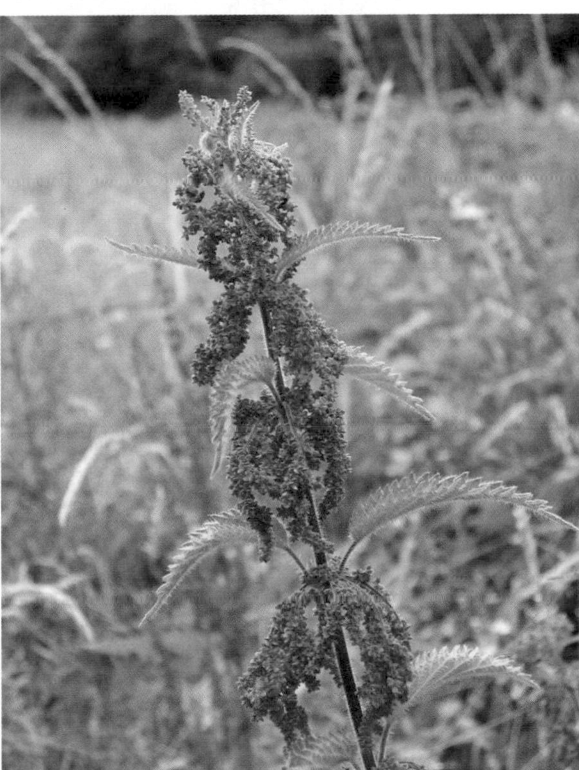

Onion, Leek & Garlic

Theatrum Botanicum

Tribe 7, Chapter 29, pp870–74

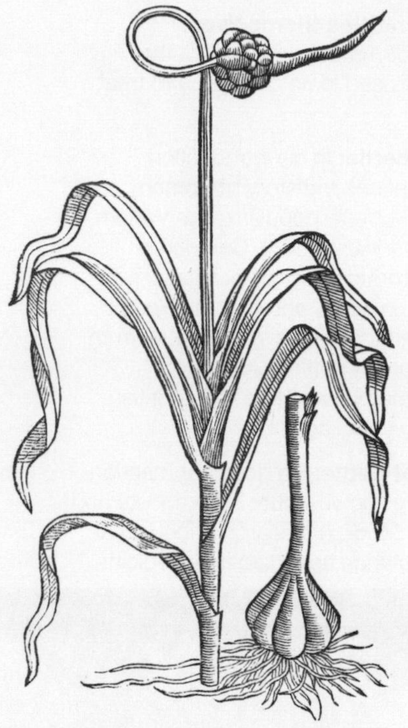

Cepaceum genus

The Vertues

ONIONS: Onions are flatulent or windy, yet doe they somewhat provoke the appetite encrease thirst and ease the belly and bowells, provoke urine and womens courses, helpe the biting of a mad Dog, and of other venemous creatures, to be used with a little Hony and Rue, and encrease Sperme, especially the seede: they also kill the Wormes in children if they drinke the water fasting wherein they have beene steeped all night: being roasted under the Embers, and eaten with Hony or Sugar and Oyle, they much conduce to helpe an inveterate Cough, by cutting the tough flegme and causing it the easier to bee expectorate: the juice being snuffed up into the Nostrills, purgeth the Head, and helpeth the Lethargie, yet the often eating of them is said to procure paines in the Head: it hath beene held with divers country people a good preservative against infection to eate Onions fasting with bread and salt, as also to make a great Onion hollow, filling the place with good Treakle, and after to roast it well under Embers, which after taking away of the most outermost skinnes thereof, being beaten together is a soveraigne salve for eyther Plague sore, or any other putred Ulcer:

JUICE: the juice of Onions is good for scalding or burning by fire, water or Gunpouther, and used with Vineger taketh away all blemishes, spots, and markes in the skinne, and dropped into the eares easeth the paines and noyse in them: applyed also with Figges beaten together helpeth to ripen and breake Impostumes and other sores.

LEEKS: Leekes are much about the same propertie that Onions be, yet not altogether so effectuall; they are a remedy against a Surfet of Moshromes being baked under the Embers and taken, and helpeth the Piles boyled and applyed warme; to avoyd tautologie I referre you to what hath beene saide before of Onions.

GARLIC: Garlicke the garden kinds as the best, and the other as meaner are hotter then Onions or Leekes, and is more effectuall to all the purposes aforesaid, being anciently accounted the poore mans Treakle, for that it is a remedy for all diseases or hurts, for besides the properties whereunto Onions are conducible, it hath a speciall qualitie to discusse the inconveniences by corrupt agues or minerall vapours, or by drinking corrupt and stinking waters as also by taking off Woolfesbane, Henbane, Hemlocke, or other poisonfull or dangerous herbes: it is held good also in hydropick diseases, the Iaundise, Falling sicknesse, Crampes, Convulsions, the Piles or hemorrhoides and other cold diseases: but to alter the strong sent thereof and cause it to be lesse offensive, divers have set downe divers things, as some to eate Rue, or herbe Grace, some to eate a raw Beane after it, others to take of a Beete roote roasted under the Embers and others say by eating a few Parsley leaves.

womens courses: menstruation
Hony: honey
Rue: *Ruta graveolens*, herb of grace
fasting: without eating
steeped: soaked
conduce: tend to
inveterate: chronic
Lethargie: tiredness, chronic fatigue
divers: various
Treakle: medicinal antidotal mixture
sovereign salve: supreme ointment
Gunpouther: gunpowder
noyse: roaring, tinnitus
Figges: fig, *Ficus carica*
Impostumes: cysts, abscesses
Surfet of: too many
avoyd tautologie: avoid repetition
poor mans Treakle: theriac, panacea
discusse: dispel
corrupt agues or minerall vapours: feverish infections, poisonous gases

Woolfesbane: *Aconitum lycoctonum*
Henbane: *Hyoscyamus niger*
Hemlocke: *Conium maculatum*
hydropick: watery swellings
Falling sicknesse: epilepsy
Parsley: *Petroselinum crispum*

Onion, leek & garlic

Allium spp.

Parkinson's comments here reflect a time when bulbs, and other growing parts, of the *Allium* family were in widespread use for medicine as well as food. He regards leeks, onions and garlic as medicinal in ascending order, much as we do today, while his account is a fascinating insight into lost medicinal possibilities.

Onions: In *A Dictionary of Plant-Lore* (Oxford, 1995), p267, plant folklorist Roy Vickery records a saying from Cambridgeshire in 1952: 'If an onion is eaten every morning before breakfast, all the doctors might ride on one horse.' Among the many common plants used by our grandparents as hedgerow medicine, onion was one of the last to go, reflecting its enduring value for everyday mishaps.

Parkinson gave it a much stronger role, against bites from venomous creatures or intestinal worms, to increase appetite – and sperm – and to keep infection away, even at the cost of headache. The hollowing out of a large onion, filling it with 'good Treakle' and baking it was an important external dressing for sores and ulcers. It is likely some rural families in Europe and North America still use onion similarly today.

Garlic: Parkinson comments matter-of-factly in the *Paradisi* that you need a strong constitution to eat garlic, which 'will not brooke in a weake and tender stomacke'. But he knows well that the pungency and heat is what makes garlic such a good medicinal; he explains how garlic was 'poor man's treacle', treacles in his day being complicated and expensive formulae made up as electuaries to antidote poisons.

He specifies its value as a protective against poisonous plants and gases, infectious fevers, and various serious 'cold' conditions; today's practitioner might look at garlic as part of a remedy to treat thrombosis, high blood sugar, bronchitis, catarrh, intestinal worms, ear infection, candida, MRSA and allergies such as hay fever.

The 'strong sent' – from sulphur compounds – was a problem in Parkinson's time too. The unavoidable fact is the useful active parts of the plant are the smelly ones; deodorized garlic isn't so effective. Parsley was a standby deodorizer in his day as it is for ours.

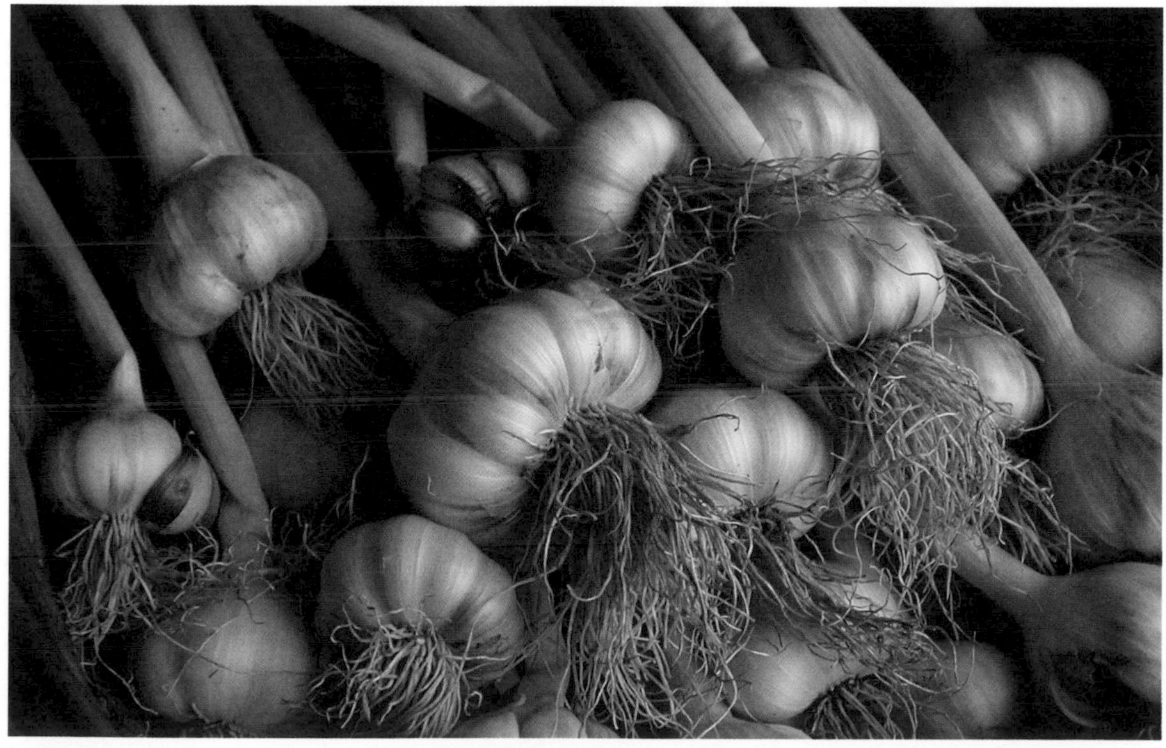

Paritary of the Wall

Theatrum Botanicum

Tribe 4, Chapter 11, pp436–38

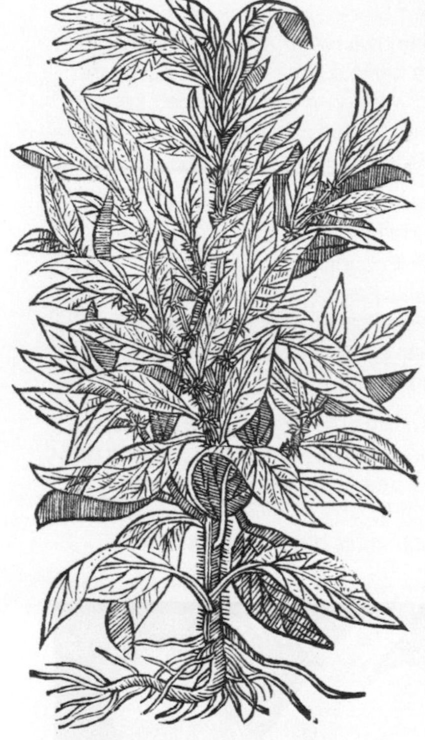
1. *Parietaria vulgaris.* Common Pellitory of the Wall.

Electuarie: electuary, herb and honey
hony: honey
continuall: persistent
suppression: cessation
gravell: gravel, urinary crystals
glisters: enema or rectal injection
stoppings: prevention
Muskadine: wine of Muscat grapes
tyle: tile
quick coales: burning embers
Chaffing dish: portable heating dish
mother: womb
bringeth down courses that are staied: stopped
purples: purplish rash
whcales: pimples or pustules
morphew: discolouration of skin
noise: tinnitus
prickings: smarting

Helxine sive Parietaria

The Vertues

Electuary for coughing & wheezing: The dried herbe Paritary made up with hony into an Electuarie, or the juice of the herbe, or the decoction thereof made up with Sugar or Hony, is a singular remedy for any old continuall or dry cough, the shortnesse of breath and wheezings in the throate:

Juice as diuretic: the juyce thereof taken to the quantie of three ounces at a time doth wonderfully ease those that are troubled with the suppression of their urine, causing them very speedily to make water, and to expell both the stone and gravell that are engendred in the kidnies and bladder, and therefore it is usually put among other herbes that are used in glisters, to mittigate paines in the backe, sides, or bowells, proceeding of winds or the like stoppings of urine, or the gravell and stone:

Warmed herb for belly: it worketh the like effect also, if the bruised herbe sprinkled with some Muskadine be warmed upon a tyle, or in a dish upon a few quicke coales in a Chaffing dish, and applied to the belly:

Decoction for female conditions: the decoction also of the herbe being drunke, easeth the paines of the mother, and bringeth downe the courses that are staied;

Decoction as diuretic: the same also easeth those griefes that arise from the obstructions of the liver, spleene, and reines:

Decoction as bath: the same decoction also may serve in stead of a bath for men and women to sit in, for the foresaid purposes:

Decoction as gargle: the same decoction also with a little hony added thereto, will serve to very good purpose to gargle the throate when it is swollen and pained;

Juice for teeth: the juice held a while in the mouth easeth the paines in the teeth:

Distilled water for the skin: the distilled water of the herbe drunke with some Sugar to make it the more pleasant, worketh the same effects, and moreover clenseth the skinne from spots, freckles, purples, wheales, sunburne, morphew, &c. and leaveth the skinne, cleare, smooth and delicate:

Juice for the ears: the jouce dropped into the eares caseth the noise and hummings in them, and taketh away the prickings and shooting paines in them:

Pellitory of the wall *Parietaria judaica* Urticaceae

Parkinson was on something of a mission to change the common name of pellitory to the more correct *paritarie*, from the Latin, but he was not heeded, and pellitory of the wall it still is. We have a mission too: to persuade people that this plant, a common weed growing on old buildings and walls in much of the temperate world, but too ordinary to be noticed, is a wonderful kidney tonic with many other virtues. It is a forgotten herb, thriving in plain sight, and we are pleased to present Parkinson's encyclopaedic coverage.

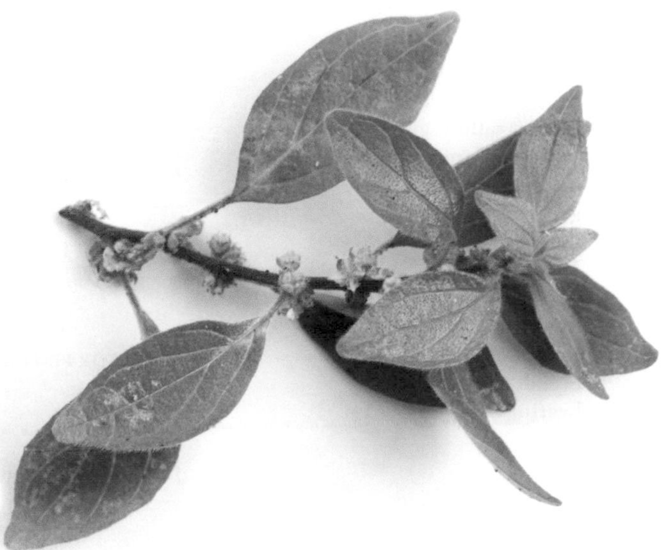

Electuary for cough & wheezing: Electuaries, made by mixing a powdered form of herb with honey, are a good way to get bad-tasting things down your throat. In the case of pellitory, which is rather greeny-bland, it is more a matter of giving it a pleasant taste. Parkinson offers variations, using the juice of the fresh plant or a sweetened decoction, and calls it a 'singular remedy' for persistent or dry coughs and shortness of breath.

Juice as diuretic: Pellitory still maintains a reputation as a diuretic that began with the ancient Greeks. It was once named '*officinalis*', i.e. used in orthodox medicine for this purpose. Contemporary English herbalist Julian Barker puts it well, saying that any ancient plant with a broad reputation, especially one honoured as '*officinalis*', is "By Appointment To Mankind" (*Medicinal Flora*, West Wickham, Kent, 2001, p84).

Parkinson proposes the juice or glisters for difficulty or pain in urination and for expelling stone or gravel from the kidneys or bladder. Nicholas Culpeper, writing a few years after Parkinson, went so far as to offer his readers free treatment if they took pellitory syrup daily or even once a week and failed to observe improvement in their dropsy (i.e. oedema, water retention). Modern usage would add cystitis and kidney-related oedema, for both of which pellitory is a leading herbal application.

Warmed herb for belly: Parkinson also suggests an informal recipe for applying the heated herb externally on the belly to ease pain.

Decoction for female issues: A decoction or infusion of pellitory is the most usual form for the herb today, as evidently in Parkinson's. Here he outlines its use for pains of the womb or for restarting menstruation.

Decoction as diuretic: The decoction is also recommended for diuretic problems. Mrs Grieve's famous *A Modern Herbal* (1931, p624) says of pellitory: 'its action upon the urinary calculus [stone] is perhaps more marked than any other simple agent at present employed'.

Decoction as bath: Adding the decoction to the bath is another option for the same conditions.

Decoction as gargle: It also works well as a gargle, Parkinson says.

Juice for teeth: Meanwhile the juice is again mentioned for easing tooth pain.

Distilled water for the skin: A milder way to take the plant is as a distilled or aromatic water. As with other diuretics, what is good for the urinary system is also good for the skin, both drunk and applied externally.

Juice for the ears: This use for inner ear pain or tinnitus is probably long forgotten, but is worth trying if the need arises.

Juice or the water for hot inflammations: Parkinson advises cloths soaked in pellitory juice or the distilled water for any sort of hot inflammations and skin eruptions. In these and other applications pellitory has a remineralizing effect, restoring potassium especially, which is necessary for cellular health.

Liniment for ulcers & scabs, hair care, piles & gout: Parkinson proposes a pellitory liniment for all these conditions.

asswage: allay
imposthumes: cyst or swelling
Saint Anthonies fire: erysipelas
liniment: embrocation
Cerussa: a white mineral, lead carbonate
anointed: smeared
rotten: decayed, putrid
creeping: growing gradually
fundament: anus, buttocks
Goates tallow: goat fat
Cyprian Cerote: wax from Cyprus
fistulaes: fistulas, hollow ulcers
greene: fresh
pultis: poultice
Mallows: mallow, *Malva sylvestris*
branne: husk
flower: flour
tendone: tendon
bloud: blood
beatings: blows

JUICE OR THE WATER FOR HOT INFLAMMATIONS: the said juyce or the distilled water, doth asswage hot and swelling imposthumes, burnings or scaldings by fire or water, as also all other hot tumours or inflammations, be it Saint *Anthonies* fire, or any other eruptions of heate, being bathed often with wet cloths dipped therein;

LINIMENT FOR ULCERS & SCABS: or the said juice made into a linament with *Cerussa* & oyle of Roses, & anointed therewith, which also doth clense foule rotten ulcers, and staieth spreading or creeping ulcers, and the running scabbes or sores in childrens heads:

LINIMENT FOR HAIR CARE: the same also helpeth to stay the falling of the haire of the head;

LINIMENT FOR PILES & GOUT: the said ointment or the herbe applied to the fundament, openeth the piles, and easeth their paines, and being mixed with Goates tallow, or the *Cyprian Cerote*, doth helpe the gout:

JUICE FOR FISTULAS: the juyce is very effectuall to clense fistulaes, and to heale them up safely, or the herbe it selfe bruised and applied with a little salt:

JUICE TO HEAL FRESH WOUNDS: it is likewise so effectuall to heale any greene wound, that if it be bruised and bound thereto for three dayes, you may afterwards take it away, for you shall not neede any other salve or medicine to heale it further:

POULTICE FOR BRUISES: a pultis made hereof with Mallowes, and boyled in wine with Wheate branne, and Beane flower, and some oyle put thereto, and applied warme to any bruised sinew, tendone, or muscle, doth in a very short time restore them to their strength, and taketh away the paines of the bruises, and dissolveth the congealed bloud of any beatings, or falls from high places.

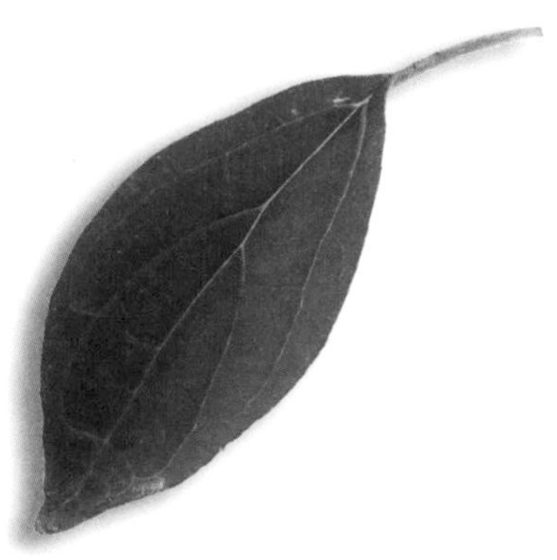

Juice for fistulas & fresh wounds: In this comprehensive inventory of pellitory's medicinal virtues, Parkinson adds use of fresh juice or a mixture with salt for fistulas and fresh wounds. He is very confident: binding a wound with pellitory for three days will heal it, he says.

Poultice for bruises: Parkinson's poultice, made with mallow, and stiffened by boiling in wine with added wheat and beans, is applied on bruising of muscles, sinews or tendons, even if the cause is a beating!

Other uses: Pellitory has been used in Europe to treat *Herpes zoster* infections and has promise for other viral infections.

Caution: For most people pellitory is good for asthma, but for some it aggravates hay fever and allergic rhinitis. In Australia it is called 'asthma weed', and has been declared noxious, which means it must be destroyed if occurring on your property.

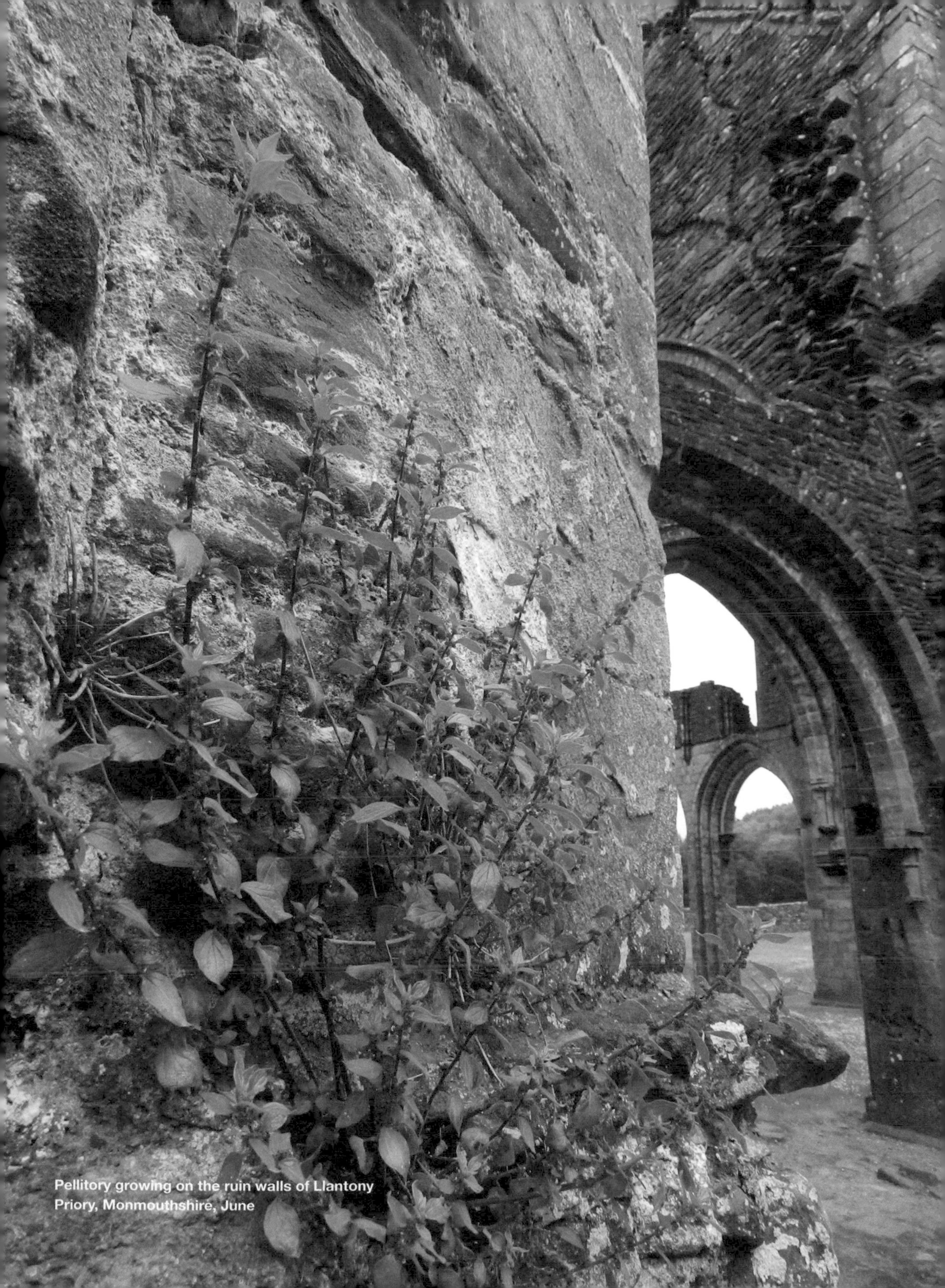

Pellitory growing on the ruin walls of Llantony Priory, Monmouthshire, June

Pimpernell

Theatrum Botanicum

Tribe 5, Chapter 41, pp557–59

1.2.3.4. *Anagallis floribus phæniceis, cæruleis, obsolete purpureis & carneis.* Pimpernell of foure sorts of colours in the flowers. that is, red, blew, sullen red, and blush colour.

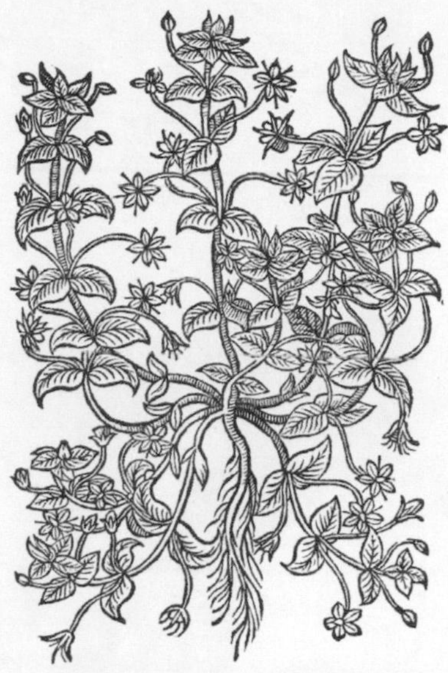

Galen: Claudius Galen (AD130–200), Roman physician and author
faculties of simples: the qualities of herbs
attractive: expelling or drawing, as in splinters
soder the lippes: fuse the edges
French Dames: fashionable French ladies
mervailous: wonderful
venemous beasts: Parkinson's usual list of snakes, scorpions and mad dogs
availeable: beneficial
raines: kidneys
stone and gravell: larger and smaller concretions
conduceth: helps
fretting and running: seeping
fluxe of humours: flowing liquids in body
drive forth the fundament: rectal prolapses

The Vertues

Cleansing and drying: Pimpernell as *Galen* saith, in his sixth booke, of the faculties of simples, of both sorts with red or blue flowers, are of a clensing faculty, they have also an attractive heate, whereby they draw forth thornes or splinters, or other such like things fastneth in the flesh, and therefore the juyce put up into the nostrils, purgeth the head; briefely also they have a drying faculty without sharpenesse, whereby they are good to soder the lippes of wounds, and to clense foule ulcers; thus saith *Galen*;

Skin & plague remedy: whereby it is plaine, that they erre greatly, that make Pimpernell, to be cold and moyst, when as they are quite contrary hot and dry, and of such a clensing quality, that the distilled water or juyce, are by the *French* Dames accounted mervailous good to clense the skinne from any roughnesse, deformity or dicolouring thereof, and to make it smooth neate and cleere: being boyled in wine and given to drink, it is a good remedy against the Plague, and other Pestelentiall Fevers, and contagious diseases, so as after the taking thereof warme, they lye in their beds, and sweate for two houres after, and hereby the venome of the disease would bee expelled, yet so as that bee used twice at the least:

Venemous beasts: the same also helpeth all stingings and bitings of any venemous beasts, be they of Serpents, as the Viper, Adder, or Scorpion, or madde dogges, or any other, used inwardly, and applyed outwardly:

Liver & kidney, & wounds: the same also openeth the obstructions of the Liver, and is very availeable against the infirmities of the raines, provoketh urine, and helpeth to expell the stone and gravell out of the Kidnies and Bladder, and conduceth much in all inward wounds, and ulcers. The decoction or the distilled water, is no lesse effectuall, to be outwardly applyed to all wounds, be they fresh, to consolidate them, or old filthy or fretting and running ulcers, venemous also, or infected, by clensing their corruption, by restraining their malignant corroding, and infectious qualities, by drying up their fluxe of humours, which hindreth their cure, and quickly bringing them to healing:

Eyes & teeth: a little honey mixed with the juyce, and dropped into the eyes, clenseth them from cloudy mistes, or filmes growing over them, which hinder and take away the sight; it helpeth the toothach being dropped into the eare, on the contrary side of the paine:

Haemorrhoids & prolapse: it is effectuall also to ease the paines of the hemorrhoides, or piles: the male Pimpernell is sayd to drive forth the fundament, and the female to repell it, and drive it into his place againe, whereby it is found that the male is more powerfull in expelling, and the female in repelling.

Pimpernel *Anagallis arvensis* Primulaceae

The scarlet pimpernel is a stirring sight in summertime gardens and fields, with, as Parkinson writes, 'a fine pale red colour, tending to an Oreng'. He does not mention the folklore that bestowed the name Poor man's weatherglass on the plant for its habit of opening only when there is strong sunlight and warmth: if the flowers were open it meant good weather ahead, and also the converse. Nor does he refer to the meaning of *Anagallis* – 'laughter bringer' – but he has serious matters, like plague and fevers, to bring to his readers.

Cleansing & heating: Parkinson refers at once to Galen, who spoke of red and blue forms. Gerard (1597) took this further, calling the red pimpernel male and the blue female. Parkinson followed him, as we will see below. Using the plant to draw splinters, to clear the head or as an antiseptic to close wounds are practical examples of its 'attractive heate'.

Skin & plague remedy: Parkinson gives an example of this drying heat, with a distiiled water or the juice used externally as a skin wash, in France and elsewhere. A stronger preparation, made by boiling pimpernel in wine, brought out its sweat-inducing (diaphoretic) qualities, thought beneficial in treating fevers, including plague.

Venemous beasts: We find Parkinson often mentions 'venemous beasts', which may partly reflect borrowing from his classic Greek and Roman sources, but we can at least note that pimpernel makes a good first-aid remedy for garden stings, thorns and the like.

Liver, kidney, wounds: Internal use of pimpernel is currently discouraged, and few herbalists currently adopt it, but clearing liver obstructions and stones with it was routine in Parkinson's day. He makes a strong case for its effectiveness in outward wound treatment.

Eyes & teeth: These remedies are from Dioscorides, but we have not tested them.

Haemorrhoids & prolapses: Here Parkinson differentiates the red (male, in his terms) and blue pimpernels in dealing with haemorrhoids and prolapse. There is a fascinating specificity in his account, and we hope someone will research it. Indeed, overall this is a plant with overlooked potential that would repay further investigation, including its older reputation for relieving depression.

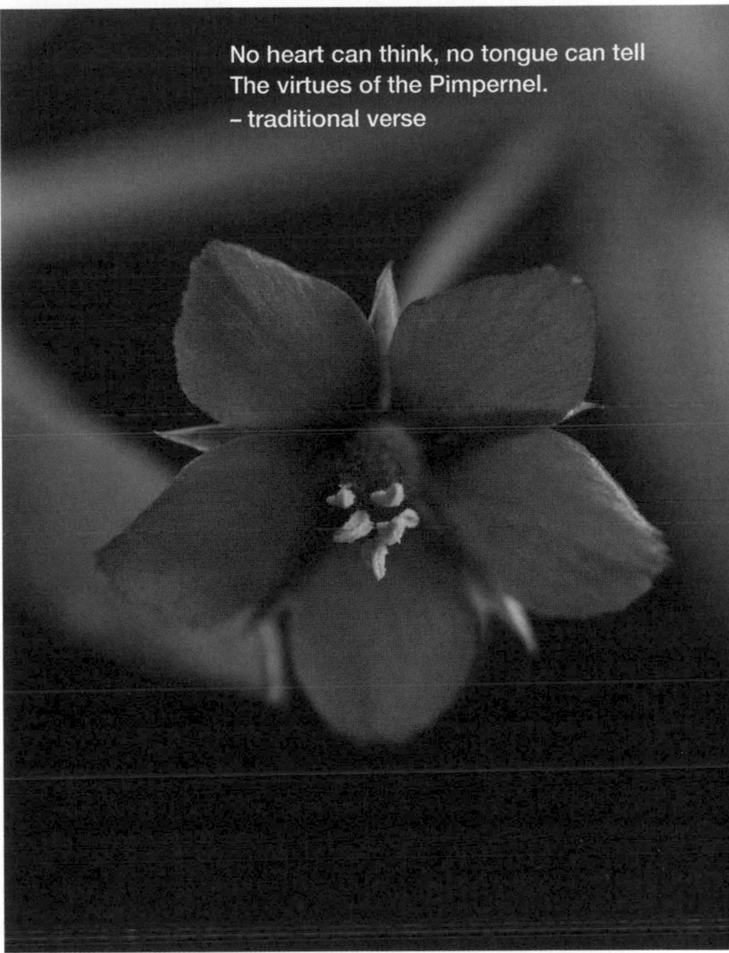

No heart can think, no tongue can tell
The virtues of the Pimpernel.
– traditional verse

Parkinson is a modest writer, but he is not shy to point out his own opinions or discoveries where appropriate. The pimpernels offer a small example. He describes five species, including a pale bluish form, which he names *Anagallis flore carneo*, distinct from the blue pimpernel (now called *A. foemina*) that was already known. He says this plant 'is not remembered or spoken of by any other but my selfe'. What is interesting is that very recent DNA research seems to confirm his idea of a separate species.

Poppie

Theatrum Botanicum

Tribe 3, Chapter14, pp365–69

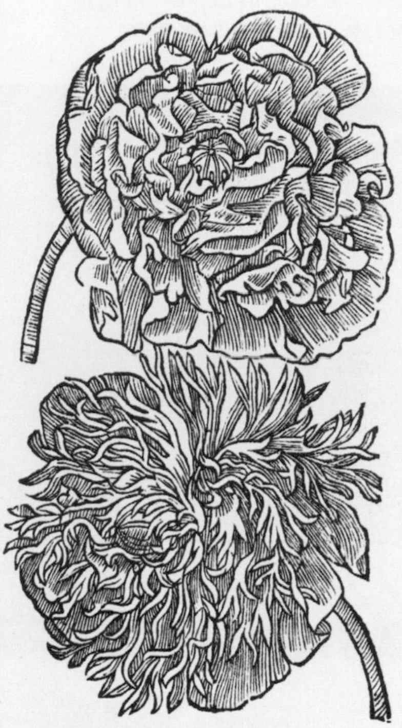

Papaver multiplici flore.
Double Garden Poppies.

Papaver

The Vertues

Cold or hot? All the sorts of Poppyes are cold in the fourth degree, but especially *Opium* or the condensate juice, as *Galen* and divers other authours doe affirme, yet *Matthiolus* sticketh thereat, thinking it rather to be hot, by the sharpnesse and bitternesse thereof, and is *Anodinum medicamentum*, that is such a medicine, that by procuring sleepe, easeth many paines of the present, which indeede it doth but palliate or cause to be quiet for a time;

Narcotic: The continuall use whereof, bringeth very often more harme, and a more dangerous disease then it hath allayed, that is an insensiblenesse or stupefaction of a part or member, which commeth to be the dead palsie, for although *Dioscorides, Galen,* and others write, that the white seed is familiarly taken in bread, and made into cakes and eaten with pleasure, and *Matthiolus* and divers others have observed that in our dayes, the white Poppy seede, is sowen in *Italy* and other places, and much used, yea and the black seede also, although they all agree, it is stronger in operation, and onely medicineable, or onely to be used in Physicke to helpe diseases;

Black & white seed: for *Matthiolus* writeth that the inhabitants about *Trent,* doe sow the blacke seede in their fields and grounds, among Beanes and other pulse, which they familiarly eate, being made into cakes, that are made of many foldes, the seede being cast in betweene the folds, and so kneaded together, and yet hee saith, they are no whit more sleepy or drowsie, then those that eate none of them: as also that in *Stiria* and the upper *Austria*, the inhabitants doe eate the oyle pressed out of the blacke seede in their meates familiarly, in the stead of Sallet oyle, and finde no inconveniency of drowsinesse at all thereby; which made him as he saith, venture to give the creame of the seede made up with Barly water oftentimes, and in great quantity, in the hot fits of agues, and burning feavers, both to aswade thirst, and to procure rest, and hereby as he saith, he shooke of that feare of Poppy, that his wise Masters had by their grave admonitions, seasoned him withall in former times:

Garden poppy: the Garden Poppy heads with seedes made into a Syrupe, is both frequently used in our dayes, and to very good effect to procure rest and sleepe in the sicke and weake, and to stay catarrhes, and defluxions of hot and thinne rheume, from the head into the stomacke, and upon the lungs, causing a continuall cough, the forerunner of a consumption; but hath not halfe that force in those that are stronger, for the strength or debility of nature worketh divers effects, as you see, as well in this, as in all or most other things; the same also helpeth the hoarsenesse of the throate, and when one hath lost their voyce, which the oyle of the seede doth likewise:

Black seed: the blacke seed boyled in wine and drunke, is said also

Opium: *Papaver somniferum*
Galen: Claudius Galen (AD130–200), Roman physician and author
Matthiolus: Pierandrea Mattioli (1501–77), physician and author
Anodium medicamentum: pain-relieving medicine, anodyne
dead palsie: catatonia
Dioscorides: Greek-speaking Roman physician (mid-first century AD)
Trent: area of Trento, northern Italy
foldes: folds, layers
Stiria, Upper Austria: areas of northern Austria
familiarly: frequently
Sallet oyle: salad oil, usually olive oil
Barly: barley
fits of agues: attacks of high fever
aswade: assuage
stay: stop

Poppies *Papaver* spp. Papaveraceae

This is a fascinating chapter by Parkinson, where you can feel him stretching the limits of classic Galenic medicine, as did Matthiolus before him: was poppy an extremely cold plant, as tradition dictated, or actually also hot, as observation revealed? Parkinson opts to sit on the fence, but is very careful to distinguish the types of poppy and their uses, guiding his reader towards a safe and responsible relationship with this important pain-relieving plant.

Cold or hot: Parkinson states the accepted position of poppy, and especially opium ('or the condensate juice') as the coldest of elements. But straightaway he mentions that his predecessor, the Italian physician Matthiolus, argued that it was hot. The reason, and the sticking point, is the acridity and bitterness of opium, which by one reading of classic humoural theory meant it must promote digestive fire, hence be hot. Today's herbalism tends to distinguish cooling bitters (e.g. lettuce) and heating bitters (e.g. wormwood), but this gradation was not easily accepted while Galenism had such a hold on practice and thought.

Parkinson refers here to the value of opium as an anodyne, the inducer of a sleep that allows the body to recover while also easing pain. Even in today's medicine there are no better pain-relievers than codeine and morphine, the purified extracts of opium poppy, a fact that would not have surprised Parkinson.

Narcotic: He is very aware of the narcotic effects of prolonged and addictive use of poppy, as indeed Dioscorides and Galen had been 1,500 years before. But this raises another question in his mind: how can white poppy seed be used in everyday bread and cakes, eaten for pleasure, and not give the same result?

Black & white seed: He mentions that even the stronger black poppy seed, made into a folded cake, or squeezed into an oil, does not cause tiredness, let alone stupor. This observation led Matthiolus to mix poppy seed with barley water for treating fevers, to 'procure rest' and assuage thirst. Experience had let Matthiolus lose his inculcated fear of poppy.

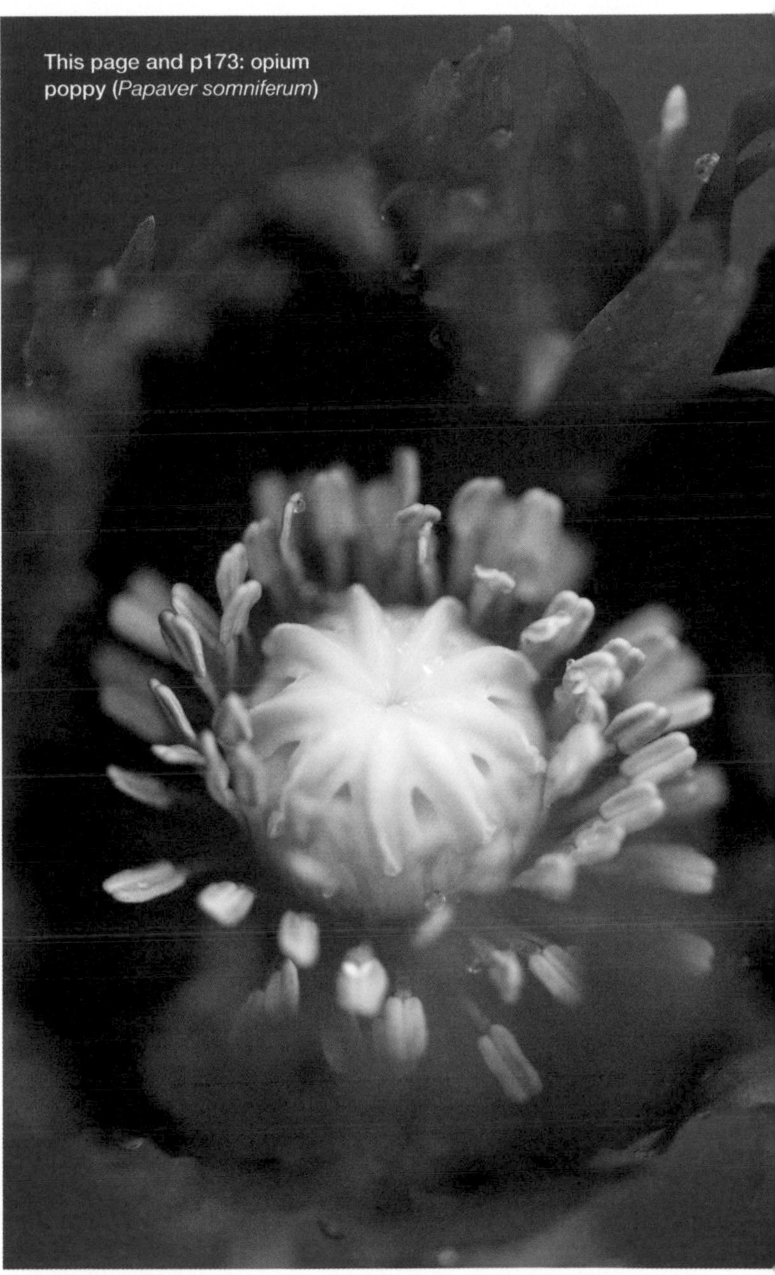

This page and p173: opium poppy (*Papaver somniferum*)

defluxions of hot and thinne rheume: dropping of clear mucus from the head
consumption: tuberculosis
voyce: voice
fluxe of the belly: upset stomach
immoderate course: heavy menstruation
pultis: poultice
Axungia: soft animal fat, often goose
Saint Anthonyes fire: erysipelas
accessory: acquired
Glaucium: horned poppy
milke: white sap
ancients: the old authorities
descant: discourse
Treakle: theriac, antidote compound
Mithridatum: mithridatium, antidote compound
frensies: wild behaviour
ocular: of the eyes
auricular: of the ears
falling sicknesse: epilepsy
Theophrastus: Greek philosopher (c.371–c.287BC)
Plurisie: pleurisy
cephalicall: of the head
pectorall: of the chest

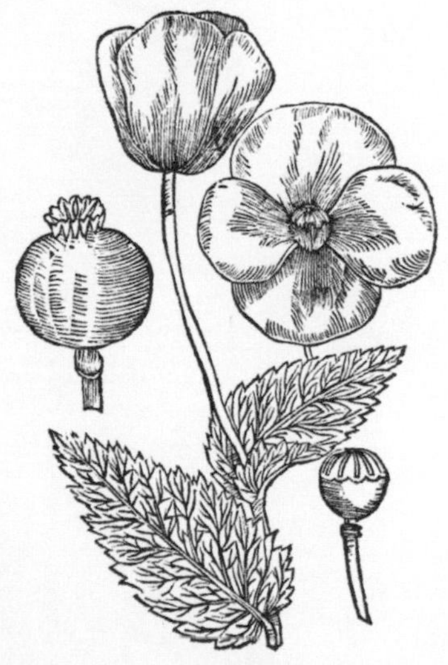

to stay the fluxe of the belly, and the immoderate course of womens sickenesse:

Seed heads: the empty shels of the Poppy heades, are usually boyled in water, and given to procure rest and sleepe: so doe the leaves in the same manner, as also if the head and temples be bathed with the decoction warme, or with the oyle of Poppyes, the greene leaves or heads bruised, and applyed with a little vinegar, or made into a pultis with Barly meale and *Axungia*, cooleth and tempereth all inflammations, as also that disease called Saint *Anthonyes* fire.

Opium/Meconium: The *Opium,* but I may rather say *Meconium,* (which is the juice of the Poppy thickned) that is commonly used in the Apothecaries shops, and is much weaker by the judgement of all, both moderne and ancients, then the true *Opium,*) is much colder, and stronger in effect, than any other part of the plant, but if we may know the temperature and qualities of things, by their taste and effect, we may rather judge *Opium* to be hot then cold, or at the least, to have very hot parts in it, witnesse the bitternesse thereof, the heate and sharpenesse that is felt in the mouth, upon the tasting, and keeping it in the mouth a while, that it is ready to blister both tongue and pallate; as also the grievous or heady heavy smell, as well in it, as in the whole plant: but it may be saith *Mattiolus,* the bitternesse, heate, and sharpenesse in *Opium,* or *Meconium*, is rather accessory then innate, and is therein by the mixture and adulterating of it with *Glaucium,* and to give a yellow juice, for our *Opium* if it be dissolved doth shew a brownish yellownesse;

A fence to sit on: yet by his leave I may say, that even the fresh milke with us, is bitter and strong in smell like the *Meconium* or *Opium*, but because our ancients, who have found out the qualities of things and left them for our knowledge, have so found and judged of *Opium,* I must as *Matthiolus* saith, leave it for others to descant theron, as reason and experience shall direct them:

Basics: It is generally used as I said before in *Treakle* and *Mithridatum,* and in all other medicines that are made to procure rest and sleepe, and to ease paines in the head, as well as in other parts, as I said before, or rather to palliate them, it is used also both to coole inflammations, agues, or frensies, and to stay defluctions, which cause a cough or consumption, as also other fluxes of the belly, or womens courses, and generally for all the properties that the seede or any other part of the plant is used: it is also put into hollow teeth to ease the paine:

Eyes & ears: it is used in both *ocular* and *auricular* medicines with some, and to stay fluxes and to ease paines, but *Galen,* and divers others in the former as well as in our times, have forbidden such medicines, as too dangerous for the eyes, and even any other wayes used inwardly, it is not to be taken, but with good correction and great caution, yet divers have found that applyed to the gout, it hath given much ease of paine:

Red poppy: The wild or red Poppy that groweth in the corne, while it is young, is a Sallet herbe in *Italy*, in many places, and in the territory of *Trent* especially, as *Matthiolus* saith, as also to prevent the falling

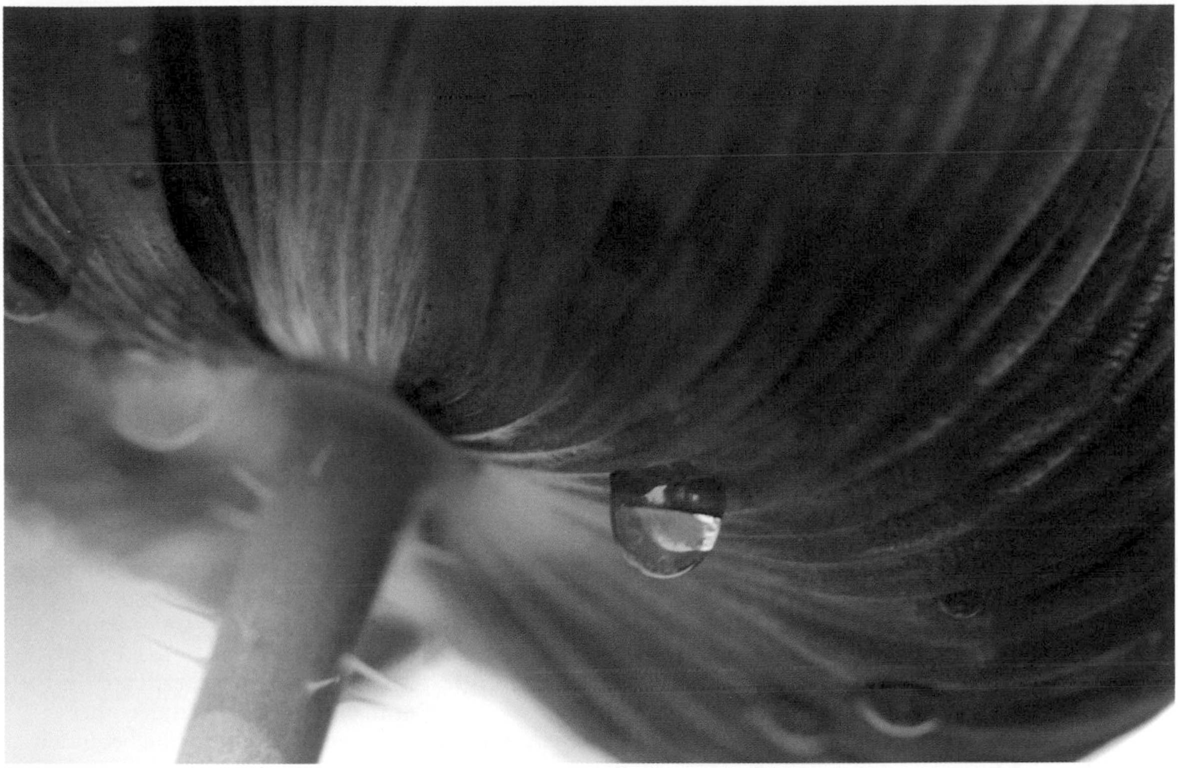

2. *Papaver ſativum ſimplex nigrum.*
Single garden blacke Poppie.

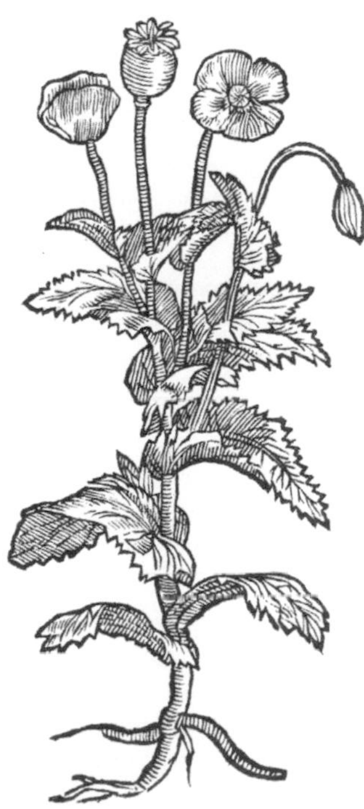

Garden poppy: Parkinson now turns to garden (white) poppy and the syrup made from its seeds. This is commonly beneficial for rest and sleep, he says, but also to reduce catarrh and the downward flow of mucus from the head, which can lead to a continual cough and consumption, and for hoarseness.

Black seed: Being more powerful in its effect, he says, the black poppy seed, made into a hot tincture (with wine), can calm the most upset of stomachs or irregular menstruation.

Seed heads: Here he deals with the uses of garden poppy, with dried seedheads or the leaves boiled in water, as a decocted rub for the head or made into a poultice with barley meal and an oil to apply to any inflammation or the angry red outbursts of erysipelas.

Opium & meconium: He explains that meconium is an apothecary's syrup (it is in the *London Pharmacopoeia* of 1618) of white and black poppy seed, steeped and boiled in water and then in sugar. But he soon returns to the conundrum of bitterness and heat, which applied to opium and meconium alike. He now brings in Matthiolus' argument that these qualities are added rather than innate to poppy. Perhaps adulteration with *Glaucium* or horned poppy is the reason, he muses.

A fence to sit on: His final position is to leave this awkward issue to others, trusting both the judgement of the ancients and the experience of his peers.

Return to basics: He is on safer ground by rehearsing the general benefits of generic poppy treatment, including its part in poison antidotes such as treacles and Mithridatium.

4. Papaver Rhœas.
Wild Poppie or corne Rose.

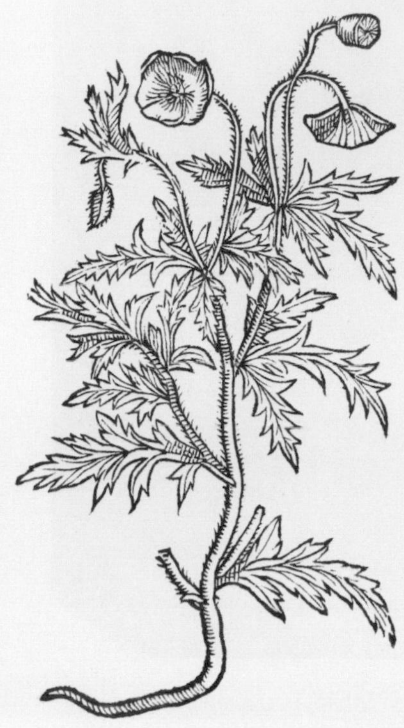

sicknesse, which *Theophrastus* also saith in his 9. Booke and 13. Chapter, was common in his time:

RED POPPY SYRUP: the Syrupe made of the flowers is with good effect, given to those that have Plurisie, and the dryed flowers also, either boyled in water made into a powder and drunke, either in the distilled water of them, or in some other drinke, worketh the like effect; the same also is availeable, in all other cephalicall or pectorall griefes:

RED POPPY WATER: the distilled water of the flowers of the wilde red Poppyes, is held to be of much good use against surfets, to drinke it evening and morning: it is also more cooling in quality then any other Poppy, and therefore cannot but be as effectuall in hot agues, frensies, and other inflammations, either inward or outward, the Syrupe or water to be used therein, or the greene leaves used outwardly, either in an ointment as it is in *Populeon*, a cooling ointment, or any other wayes applyed, *Galen* in 7. *facultatum simplicium medicamentorum,* saith the seede is dangerous to be used inwardly.

GERARD: *Gerard* was much mistaken, to thinke that this wilde Poppy should be that, which should be used in the composition called *Diacodium* and citeth *Galen* for his authour, as if he had taught him that opinion, not understanding what kinde of Poppy *Galen* doth meane by wild Poppy, for he according as *Dioscorides* afore him hath done, accounteth onely the great white Poppy, whose heads are somewhat long, to be the garden or manured kinde, and the other blacke kind to be wild, and doth not meane this red Poppy, because it is onely wild with us, and not sowen, as whosoever shall observe the places throughly shall finde.

The thorny Poppy being but of late invention, hath not beene applyed to any disease by any, that I can heare of.

surfets: excesses
Populeon: black poplar, *Populus nigra*, ointment
facultatum simplicium medicamentorum: 'knowledge of simples and their power'
Diacodium: syrup of poppy
garden or manured: synonyms for Parkinson
thorny Poppy: named *Papaver spinosum* by Parkinson; he also refers to the Italian name 'Figge of hell'

Eyes & ears: He repeats the warning by Galen and others that poppy is not permitted for the eyes, or inward use, yet he is also right to point out that with great caution and attention to dosage poisons can be used with benefit. He instances the relief of gout pain, as he had mentioned toothache before.

Red poppy: Among the benefits of wild red poppy, *Papaver rhoeas*, are a syrup of the fresh flowers for pleurisy or the dried flowers for easing pain in the head or chest; a distilled water (the coolest poppy form of all, he adds) for all hot conditions and inflammations; and an ointment, similar to populeon, an ointment of black poplar.

Gerard: He ends by chiding Gerard for misidentifying the kind of poppy used in the poppy syrup called diacodium. Gerard recommended the wild red poppy, the only wild form in Parkinson's time, but what the ancients had meant was the garden poppy.

The physician Thomas Sydenham (1624–89), 'the English Hippocrates', was a near contemporary of Parkinson. Sydenham wrote of opium: 'Of all the remedies it has pleased almighty God to give man to relieve his suffering, none is so universal and so efficacious as opium.' He should have declared an interest, though: he developed his own form of opium tincture, which he called laudanum. It would be a blessing and a curse.

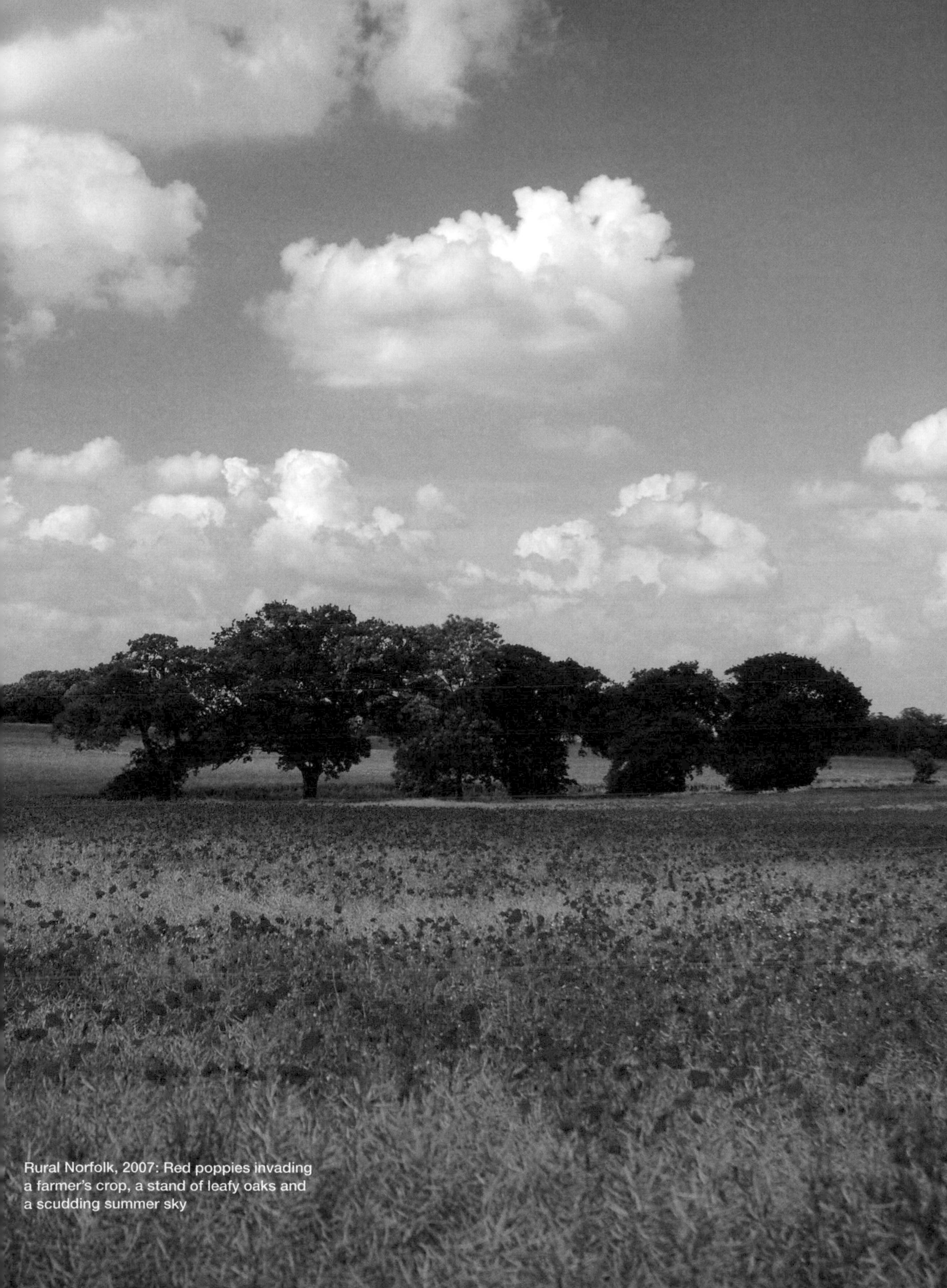

Rural Norfolk, 2007: Red poppies invading a farmer's crop, a stand of leafy oaks and a scudding summer sky

Primroses & Cowslips

Theatrum Botanicum

Tribe 5, Chapter 29, pp534–38

Primula veris vulgaris.
The ordinary field Primroſe.

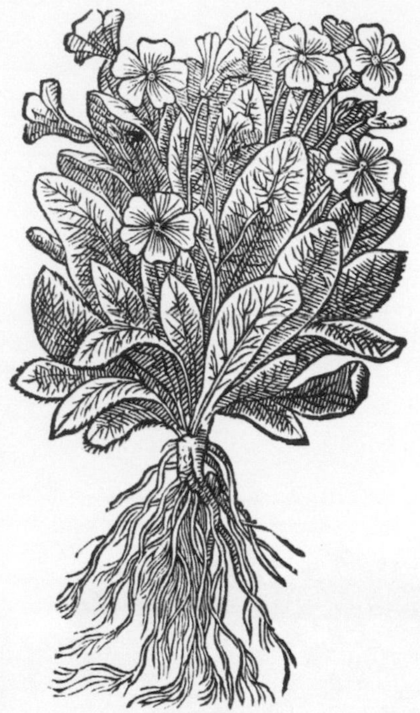

Primula veris pratensis & sylvestris

The Vertues

Head & joint pain: Primroses and Cowslips are much used to be eaten in Tansies Sallets, &c. by those beyond Sea, and are accounted very profitable for paines in the head, and are accounted the best for that purpose next unto Betony, they are excellent good against any joynt aches as the palsie and to ease the paines of the sinewes, as the names doe import.

Skin treatment: Of the juice or water of the flowers of Cowslips, divers Gentlewomen know how to clense the skin from spots or discolourings therein, as also to take away the wrinckles thereof, and cause the skinne to become smooth and faire,

Back, bladder & wounds: the rootes made into decoction and taken, easeth the paines of the backe and bladder, opening the passages of urine which was the cause thereof; they are likewise often used in wounds either greene or old, and that to very good purpose.

Palsy & vertigo: The Beares eares according to their name Sanicle, are no lesse powerfull in healing then the common, as also for the palsie and trembling of the joynts, *Clusius* saith that the mountainers that hunt after wilde beasts doe use the rootes of Beares eares to helpe either paines in the head, or the giddinesse that may happen thereto, by the sight of such fearfull *precipices* or steepe places, that they must often passe by in following their game, and are admitted as good Wound herbes as the former Cowslips.

tansies: puddings made with egg, cream, breadcrumbs and herbs
sallets: salads
beyond Sea: in mainland Europe and elsewhere
profitable: effective as a remedy
Betony: wood betony (*Stachys officinalis*)
as the names doe import: i.e. older names *arthritica* for primrose and *paralysis* for cowslip (*Paradisi*, p247)
divers Gentlewomen: various ladies
greene: fresh
Beares eares: Mountain cowslip or auricula (*Primula auricula*); also confusingly known as sanicle
Clusius: Charles de l'Ecluse (1526–1609), French botanist and author
giddinesse: vertigo

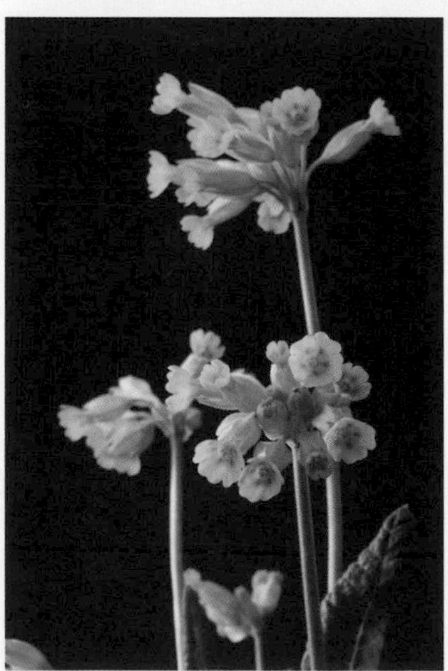

Primula veris flore purpureo Turcica.
The Turkie purple Primroſe.

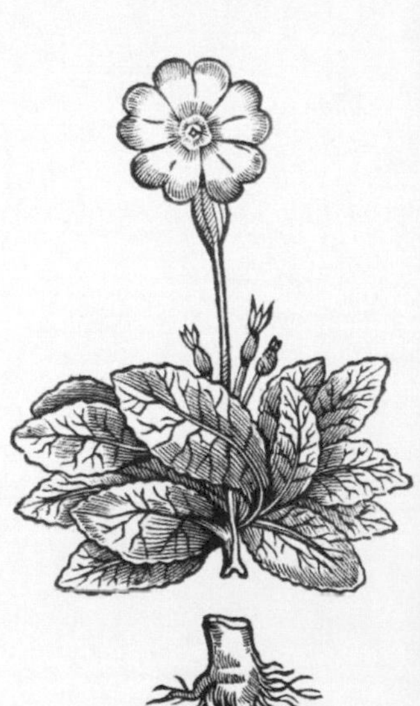

Primroses & cowslips

Primulaceae

Primroses (*Primula vulgaris*) are a strong symbol of spring and Easter; the word means 'first rose', and among its delightful old names are ladies of the spring and darling of April. It was a former cash crop, picked for sale in London and transported by train. Cowslips (*Primula veris*) (shown against black background, opposite), less fortunately, were named for cow dung, probably because they grow where cows graze; they are, however, the more effective medicinal.

Head & joint pain: In the *Paradisi* (p247), Parkinson calls these Primulas 'Cephalicall', and writes there, as he does here, that they are almost as effective as betony for treating headaches and 'paines in the head'. Primroses were once called *arthritica*. In modern terms both plants are nervines, which calm and soothe the nervous system. Their flowers are sedative, and the tea, which looks like liquid gold and smells of honey, is effective for stress and insomnia, especially in children. Cowslip wine too is tonic and sedative.

Skin: The juice or distilled water of cowslips – the more medicinally used of the two plants – is a traditional remedy as a skin toner. Its gentle astringency was applied to wrinkles and left a smooth-feeling skin. A cowslip ointment works similarly. A friend likes to use primrose water against stomach pains.

Back, bladder & wounds: The roots of both plants boiled up as a decoction make a strong expectorant to relieve catarrh and spasmodic coughing. Parkinson's uses, to treat back and bladder pain by cleansing the urinary tract, are worth further research. The external wound use could also be revisited.

Palsy & vertigo: The roots have a traditional history of treating inner ear dysfunction as evident in vertigo and some types of palsy. Auriculas share this usage, to which Parkinson makes a rather picturesque reference. The old names of palsywort and paralysis for cowslip no doubt refer to this same quality.

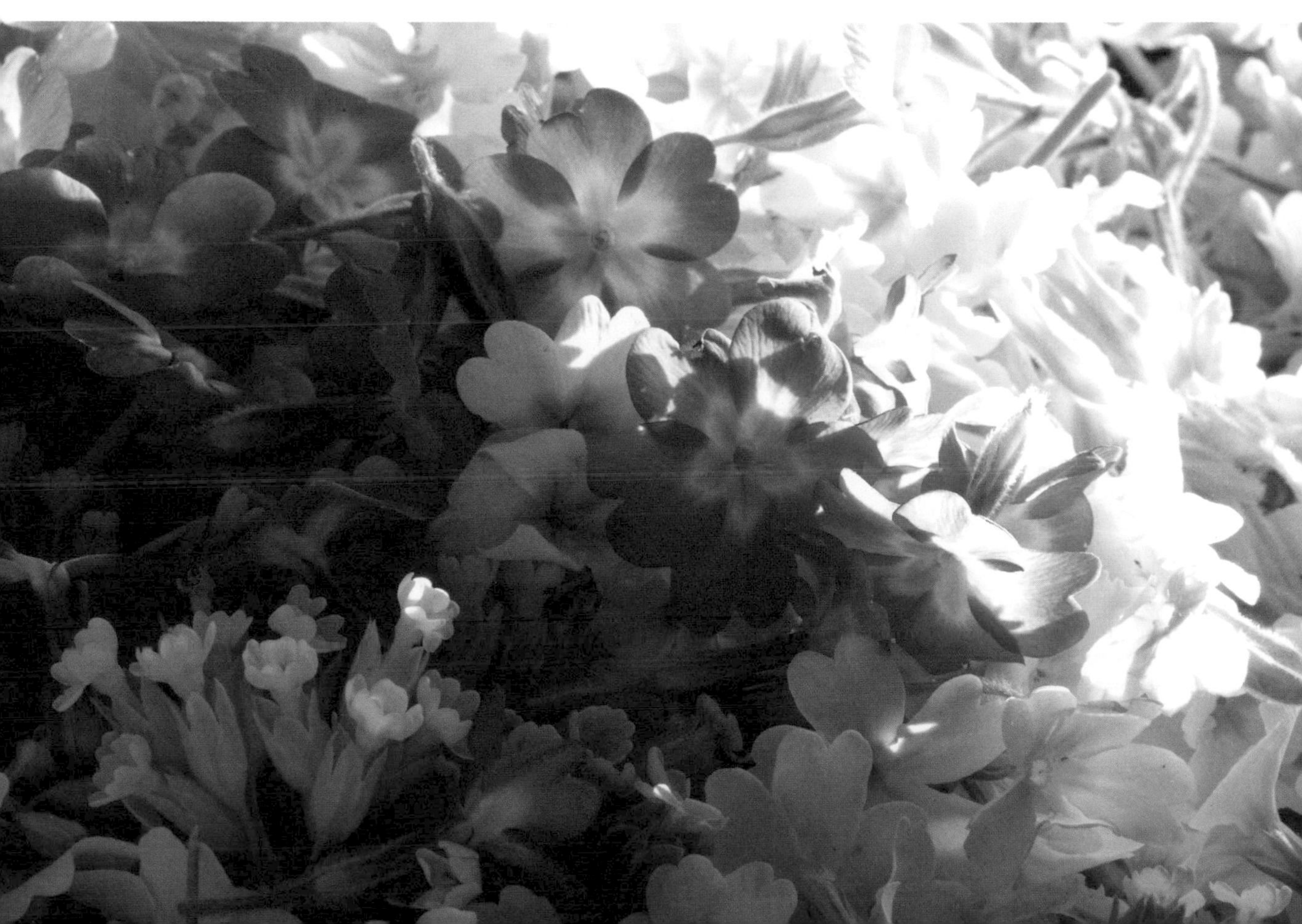

Rosemary

Theatrum Botanicum

Tribe 1, Chapter 25, pp74–77

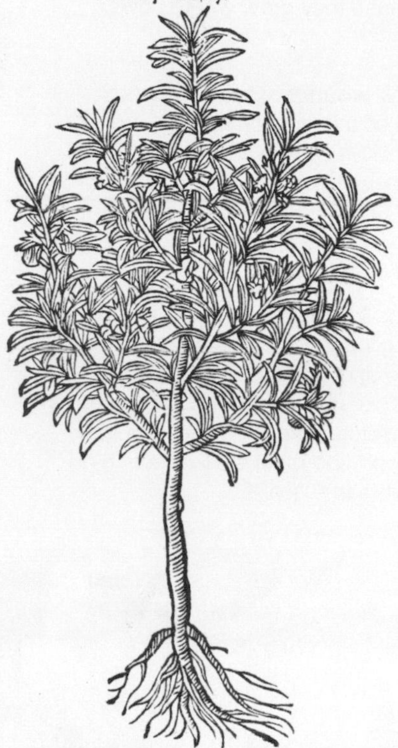

Physicall: i.e. in physic, medicine
civill: i.e. non-medical
distillations: thin mucus dripping from the head
giddinesse, swimming: faintness, vertigo
stupidnesse: slow-wittedness
dumb palsie: paralysis with loss of speech
lethargie: tiredness, chronic fatigue
falling sicknesse: epilepsy
rheume: watery discharge
quickning: enlivening
comfortable: agreeable
stay: prevent, stop
casting: vomiting
windinesse: gassiness
hypochondriack passion: melancholic or hysterical state
liver-grown: swollen liver
extenuating the grossnesse: spreading the heaviness

Rosmarinum

The Vertues

Civil purposes: Rosmary is an hearbe of as great use with us in these dayes, as any other whatsoever, not only for Physicall, but civill purposes: the civill uses as we all know, are at Weddings, Funerals, &c. to bestow upon friends:

Physical remedies: the Physicall remedies, both for inward and outward diseases are many and worthy, for by the warming and comforting heate thereof it helpeth all cold diseases, both of the head, stomack, liver, and belly: the decoction thereof in wine helpeth the cold distillations of the braine into the eyes, &c. and all other cold diseases of the head and braines, as the giddinesse or swimming therein, drowsinesse or dulnesse of the minde and senses like a stupidnesse, the dumbe palsie, or losse of speech, the lethargie and falling sicknesse, to be both drunke, and the temples bathed therewith:

Mouth: it helpeth the paines in the gummes & teeth by the rheume falling into them, or by putrefaction causing an evill smel from them, or a stinking breath:

Memory: it helpeth also a weake memory by heating and drying up the cold moistures of the braines, and quickning the senses:

Stomach: it is likewise very comfortable to the stomack in all the cold griefes thereof, and to stay the pronenesse to casting, causing the stomack the better to containe and to digest the meate, either the decoction or powder taken in wine:

Windiness: it is a remedy for the windinesse in the stomacke or bowels, and expelleth it powerfully, as also the hypochondriack passion, and winde in the splene:

Liver: it helpeth also those thot are liver-grown, by opening the obstructions thereof, by warming the coldnesse extenuating the grossnesse, and afterwards binding and strengthening the weaknesse thereof:

Flowers: it helpeth dimme eyes, and to procure a cleare sight, if all the while it is in flower, one take of the flowers fasting with bread and salt: both *Dioscorides* and *Galen* say, that if a decoction be made thereof with water, and they that have the yellow jaundise, doe exercise their bodies presently after the taking thereof, it will certainely cure it, the flowers and the conserve made of them, is singular good to comfort the heart and to expell the contagion of the pestilence, to burne the hearbe in Houses and Chambers in the time of the infection to correct the aire in them:

For women: both the flowers and the leaves are very profitable for women that are troubled with the whites, if they be daily taken:

Rosemary *Rosmarinus officinalis* Lamiaceae

Rosemary is an old Mediterranean native herb that has spread around the temperate world. It is perhaps best known today in cooking, but also deserves a place as a medicine. Its very name of '*officinalis*' means it was an approved medicinal for doctors and apothecaries in the past. We should use its pungent aromatic oils to bring warmth to the circulation, tonify the whole body and stimulate the head, stomach, heart and nervous system.

Civil purposes: Rosemary is an important herb of his day, Parkinson confirms, for both 'civill' and 'physicall' use. He disposes of the first rapidly, saying that everyone knows of rosemary's ritual presence at celebrations. Parkinson's near contemporary, the poet Robert Herrick, expressed this neatly: 'Grow for two ends, it matters not at all, / Be't for my bridal or my burial.' Interestingly, Parkinson neglects to mention the culinary value of rosemary, but he is eager to get to the main item on the menu.

Physical remedies: Rosemary, he says, is warming and comforting, which means it can counteract 'all cold diseases', especially of the head and digestive system. He recommends drinking hot a decoction of rosemary leaves boiled in wine or bathing the temples with this fluid once cooled for any stage of a head cold and to stimulate a variety of poorly functioning mental states.

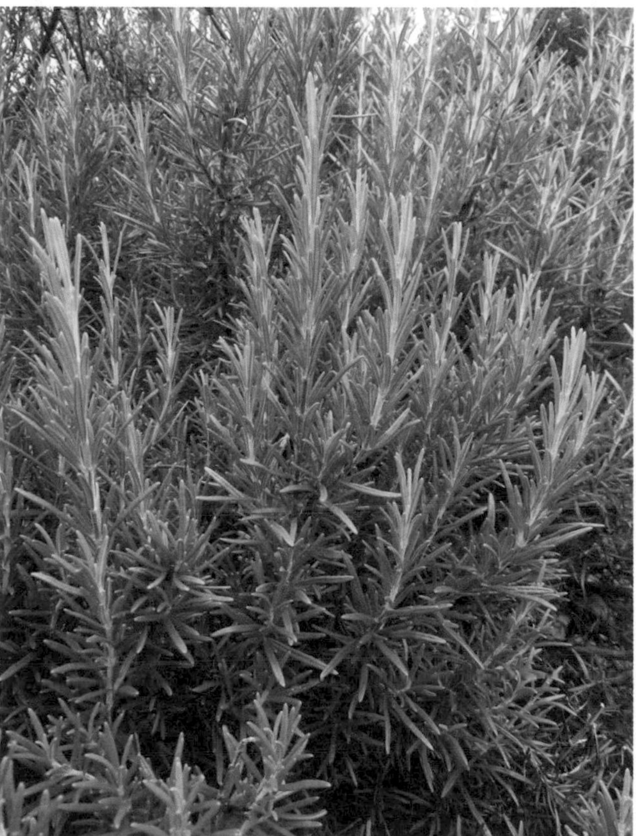

The key in a rosemary preparation, as he knew, is to release its locked-in volatile oils, which is best achieved by heat, such as boiling it in water as a tea or using it in the bath; another way is to slow-release the oils into a maceration of wine, ale or vinegar over a period of about two weeks. As a warming circulatory stimulant rosemary promotes sweating and opens the sinuses, enabling it to clear catarrh and deep-seated colds.

The rosemary smell is distinctive: moderately pungent, aromatic and camphor-like yet still pleasant. It is highly therapeutic, strongly antidepressant and lifts the spirits. When he drank rosemary wine, the Strasbourg herbalist Walther Ryff (1500–48) said: 'The spirits of the heart and entire body feel joy from this drink, which dispels all despondency and worry.'

Mouth: Rosemary makes an effective pain-reliever for tooth and gum pain and freshens the breath, Parkinson reports.

Memory: 'Rosemary, that's for remembrance,' says Ophelia in Shakespeare's *Hamlet* (published 1603), as had been common knowledge for centuries. What was not known until recent times was how this happened. Parkinson's explanation is that rosemary heats and dries cold moistures of the brain and enlivens the senses.

In modern biomedical terms rosemary helps maintain the brain chemical acetylcholine. Low or decreased levels of this neurotransmitter in the memory area are an indicator of memory dysfunction. The effect can range from Alzheimer's disease at one extreme to mere forgetfulness or lethargy.

Research from 2012 tested rosemary's traditional reputation for reducing cognitive

fasting: on an empty stomach
Dioscorides: Greek-speaking Roman physician (mid-first century AD)
Galen: Claudius Galen (AD130–200), Roman physician and writer
pestilence: plague, infectious disease
the time of the infection: during a plague year
correct the aire: purify the air
profitable: advantageous
whites: leucorrhoea or thrush
Tisick: cough
consumption: pulmonary tuberculosis
bathings: the bath
cold benummed joynts: stiff or arthritic joints
members: limbs
chymicall oyle: essential oil
soveraigne: supreme
inward griefes: any internal malady
quick and piercing: stimulating and penetrative
insolation: in the sun
digest: steep
close stopped: sealed
Baulme: balm
Rosemary of Silesia: known as *Rosmarinum sylvestre Bohemicum*
sit often: i.e. as in a bath

Cough: the dried leaves shred small and taken in a Pipe like as Tobacco is taken, helpeth those much that have any Cough or Tisick, consumption, by warming and drying the thinne distillations, which cause those diseases:

Leaves: the leaves are much used in bathings, and made into oyntments or oyles, is singular good to helpe cold benummed joynts, sinewes or members.

Essential oil: The chymicall oyle drawne from the leaves and flowers, is a soveraigne helpe for all the diseases aforesaid, to touch the temples and nostrils with a drop, two or three for all those diseases of the head and braines, spoken of before, as also to take a drop two or three, as the cause requireth for the inward griefes, yet it must be taken with discretion, lest it doe more harme than good, for it is very quick and piercing, and therefore but a little must be taken at once.

Sun-infused oil: There is another oyle made by insolation in this manner: take what quantity you will of the flowers and put them into a strong glasse close stopped, and digest them in hot Horse dung for 14. dayes, which then being taken forth and unstopped, tye a fine linnen cloth over the mouth, and turne the mouth downe into another strong glasse, which being set in the Sunne, an oyle will distill downe into the lower glasse, to be preserved as precious for divers uses, both inward and outward, as a soveraigne Baulme to heale the diseases before spoken of, to cleare a dimme sight, and to take away spots, markes and scarres in the skin.

The Rosmary of *Silesia* is by often experience found to bee good for the shrinking of the sinewes, for the Patient to sit often in the decoction thereof, and to bathe the affected parts.

Essential oil: Another way of taking rosemary internally is the essential oil. The oil was brought into widespread European use by successful steam distillation in Spain in 1330. The oil is still used in perfumery and medicinally.

To Parkinson it was superb: 'a soveraigne helpe for all the diseases aforesaid'. He proposes small drop doses and urges caution in administration, because it is 'very quick and piercing', and it can 'doe more harme than good'. Modern research supports his discretion.

Sun-infused oil: His recipe can be modified for today's use: we suggest a warming room, such as an airing cupboard, is adequate to replace his horse dung regimen.

Other uses: Australian research in 2011 confirmed that rosemary suppressed tumour growth in several kinds of cancer, including in breast, colon, liver and stomach, as well as controlling melanoma and leukaemia cells.

decline in the elderly. A full randomized, double-blind, placebo-controlled test of a sample of older people showed low doses of rosemary were statistically beneficial against placebo but higher doses impaired cognitive function. The study recommended low dosages over long periods for best results.

We think of rosemary as the 'head herb'. In addition to cognitive support – students in both ancient Greece and Elizabethan England wore strands of rosemary leaves in their hair to help them concentrate – it helps relieve migraines and headaches, sharpens the eyesight ('helpeth dimme eyes', says Parkinson), freshens the breath and is one of the best shampoos, face washes, skin rubs and gargles. John Evelyn's *Acetaria* (1699) summarized: 'Soverainly Cephalic, and for the Memory, Sight and Nerves, incomparable' (p39).

Stomach: Parkinson says rosemary is 'very comfortable to the stomack', assisting in digestion of food and reducing a propensity to vomiting.

Liver: In modern terms, rosemary is a stimulating bitter tonic for the liver, which promotes the free flow of bile and improves fat digestion. This supports its primary digestive action in the stomach. Parkinson adds a role for rosemary in jaundice treatment, deriving this from the ancients.

Flowers: Parkinson advocates using the flowers for the heart, for the sight, as a plague remedy and specifically with exercise for jaundice.

Heart: Rosemary is an important heart herb. Herbalist Juliette de Baïracli Levy (1971) explains it well: 'Rosemary herb has all of the three medicinal properties necessary in heart treatment: it is tonic, cleansing, and also a nervine' (*The Complete Herbal Book for the Dog* (1971), p144). This combination is unusual, and because it warms and stimulates sluggish circulation – being 'singular good to comfort the heart', says Parkinson – rosemary offers whole-body activation. This explains its excellence for mental function, eyesight, digestion, liver support and for pain relief in arthritis and rheumatism.

For women: Both flowers and leaves taken daily relieve leucorrhoea, Parkinson says. We should add a note of caution too. Rosemary is a uterine stimulant, making it aphrodisiac in some women but also bringing on heavy menstruation or early contractions in others. Accordingly, it is best avoided during pregnancy.

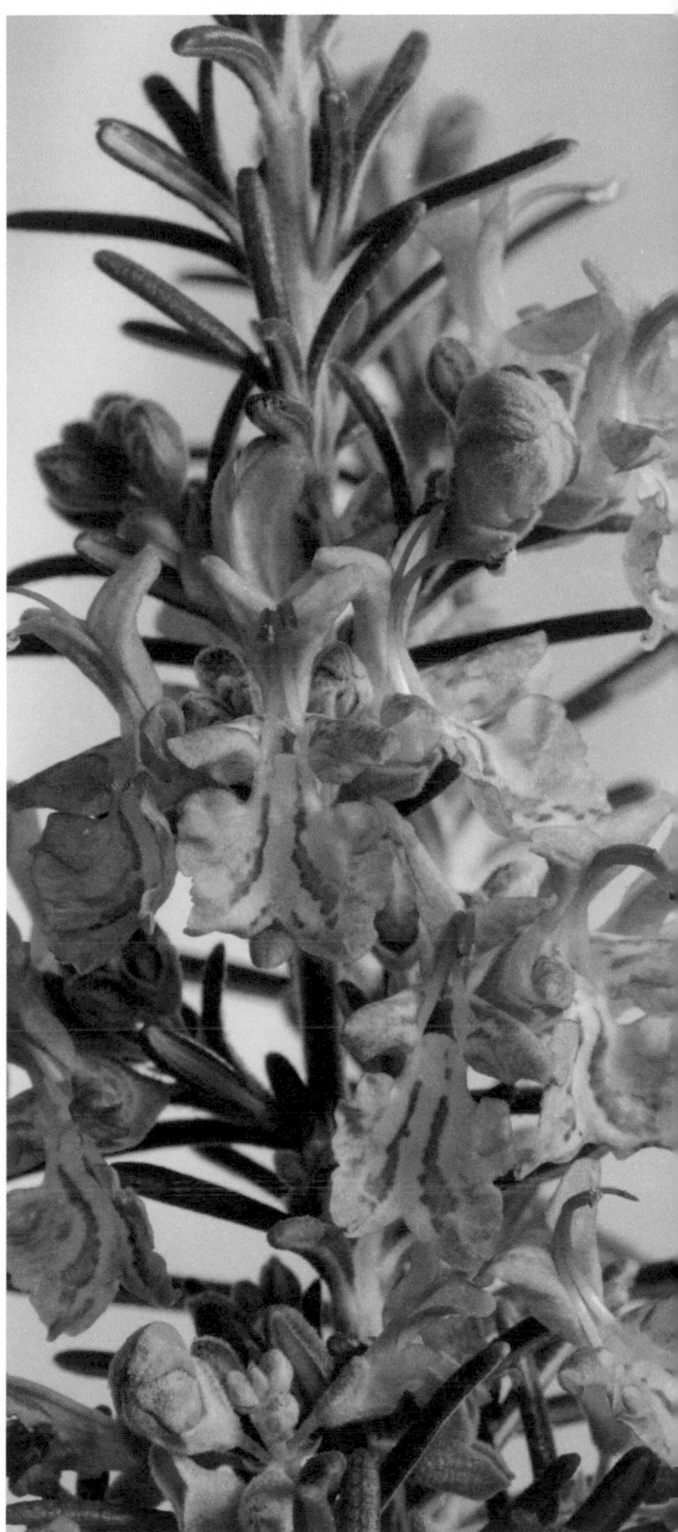

Sage, Salvia

Theatrum Botanicum

Tribe 1, Chapter 19, pp49–54

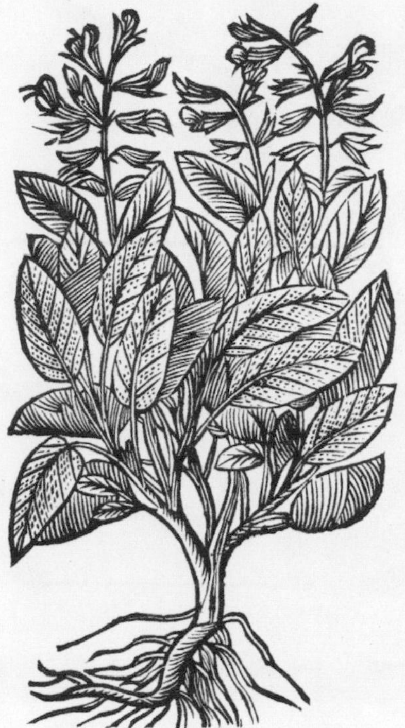
1. *Salvia major vulgaris.* Ordinary Garden Sage.

Dioscorides: Greek-speaking Roman physician (mid-first century AD)
feminine courses: menstruation
Puffen or Forkfish: puffer fish
cods: scrotum
Gallen: Claudius Galen (AD130–200), Roman physician and writer
Ætius: Aetius of Antioch, 4th century theologian and doctor
Agrippa: Heinrich Cornelius Agrippa (1486–1535), German occult scientist
Orpheus: [unknown]
Taken fasting: on an empty stomach
consumption: pulmonary tuberculosis
Spiknard: spikenard, *Nardostachys grandiflora* or nard
dramme: apothecary's weight, ⅛ oz
long pepper: pippali, *Piper longum*
Matthiolus: Pierandrea Mattioli (1501–77), physician and author
falling sickness: epilepsy
lethargie or drowsie evill: extreme tiredness or narcolepsy
palsie: paralysis, trembling

Salvia major vulgaris

The Vertues

Dioscorides: A decoction of the leaves and branches of Sage made and drunke, saith *Dioscorides*, provoketh urine, bringeth downe the feminine courses, helpeth to expell the dead child, and is a remedy against the prickes of the Puffen or Forkfish, and causes the haires likewise to become black: it stayeth the bleeding of wounds, and clenseth foule ulcers or sores: the decoction of the leaves and branches made with wine, doth take away the itching of the cods, if they be bathed therewith.

Galen & Aetius: *Gallen* saith it is of manifest heating quality, and a little binding, and *AEtius* saith the same also, but he further saith, that some report that the fumes thereof being taken when it is burnt, doth stay the immoderate fluxe of womens courses, and all other fluxes of theirs:

Agrippa: *Agrippa* saith that if childing women whose wombes be too moist and slippery, not able to conceive by reason of that default, shall take a quantity of the juyce of Sage with a little salt, for foure dayes before they company with their Husbands, it will helpe them to conceive, and also for those that after they have conceived, are subject often to miscarry upon any small occasion, for it causeth the birth to be the better retained, and to become the more lively: therefore in *Cyprus* and *AEgypt*, after a great plague, women were forced to drinke the juyce of Sage, to cause them to be the more fruitfull.

Orpheus: *Orpheus* saith, that three spoonefuls of the juyce of Sage taken fasting with a little honey, doth presently stay the spitting or casting up of blood:

Consumption: For them that are in a consumption, these Pills are much commended. Take of Spiknard and Ginger of each two drammes, of the seed of Sage a little tosted at the fire eight drammes, of long pepper twelve drammes, all these being brought into fine powder, let there bee so much juyce of Sage put thereto, as may make it into a masse, formable for pills, taking a dramme of them every morning fasting, and so likewise at night, drinking a little pure water after them.

Matthiolus: *Matthiolus* saith, that it is very profitable for all manner of paines of the head, comming of cold, and rheumaticke humours, as also for all paines of the joynts, whether used inwardly or outwardly, and therefore it helpeth such as have the falling sicknesse, the lethargic or drowsie evill, such as are dull and heavie of spirit, and those that have the palsie, and is of much use in all defluxions or distillations of thin rheume from the head, and for the diseases of the chest or brest.

Sage *Salvia officinalis, Salvia* sp. Lamiaceae

Just as in Parkinson's time, herbalists today regard the combination of warming and drying qualities as underlying sage's medicinal actions. Its aromatic oils can stimulate the pituitary gland, the adrenals, the reproductive hormones and the body's immune system. Its tannins help dry excess mucus in the respiratory tract, reduce sweating and can prevent lactation. Sage also promotes circulation and can help the memory. It is too multifaceted to be relegated to the status of occasional culinary herb.

Hair rinse: Sage is traditionally used as a hair rinse for dark hair, often combined with rosemary. It helps keep the hair thick and shiny.

Tuberculosis, coughs & sore throats: Herbalists are not likely to treat tuberculosis (consumption) in our age of antibiotics, but Parkinson's remedies would still be of use in conjunction with standard medicial treatment, especially as so many antibiotic-resistant bacterial strains now occur.

Today, sage seed is little used, and we tend to stick to the leaves and flowers only. Sage tea with lemon and honey is particularly good for wet phlegmy coughs.

Warm sage tea is an excellent gargle for sore throats. Some salt or a little cider vinegar can be added.

Consumption pills: The pills Parkinson advocates would be of use for any chronic cough or lung congestion, and would also be warming to the digestion.

Abscesses/sage & nettle poultice: A poultice of bruised sage and nettle leaves does work well on abscesses and boils. Simply crush the fresh leaves in roughly equal amounts, and apply to the affected area.

For rheumatic pains: Being warming and drying by nature, sage is ideally suited to treat rheumatic pains caused by cold, damp weather, again as a tea or poultice.

For menstrual problems: Sage affects hormone balance by its action on the pituitary and adrenal glands. It is particularly valuable where there are heavy periods, but it can be used in moderation for any kind of irregularity of the menstrual cycle.

These days, it is particularly used for menopausal symptoms. A cool glass of sage infusion drunk several times a day can make a dramatic reduction in hot flushes and night sweats.

For memory: Sage has a strong reputation to this day of helping the memory, as is indicated by its name.

The most pleasant way to take sage to help your memory is a cup of sage tea daily. Use a sprig of fresh sage or a rounded teaspoon of dried leaves per cup of boiling water, cover and allow to brew for up to a minute. Traditionally, a few leaves of sage were eaten in a daily sandwich.

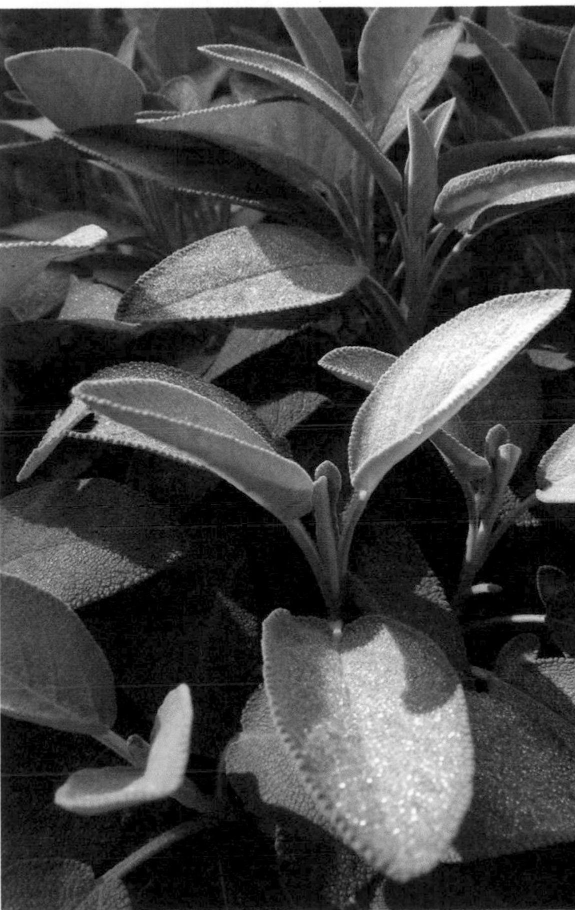

Our conserve of sage flowers

To make a conserve of sage flowers, take fresh flowers of sage and an equal weight of sugar. Grind them together in a mortar, then put them in a glass jar, and set thom in the sun. Stir daily.

If it is very hot and sunny, the conserve will be ready in a few days. If the weather is cooler, allow a few weeks – taste it to see.

6. *Salvia Cretica angustifolia non aurita.*
Small Candy Sage without eares.

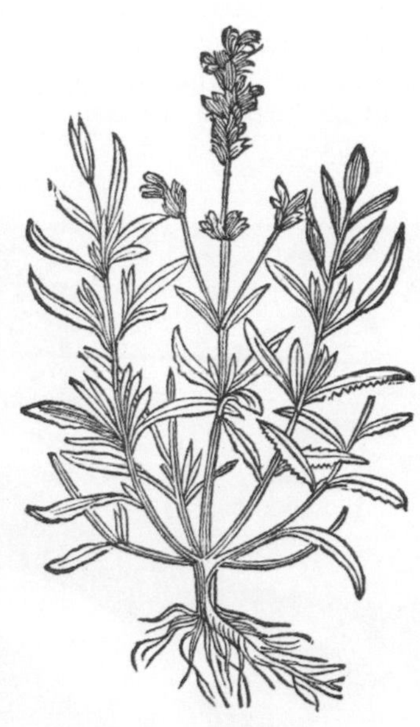

Abscesses: The leaves of Sage and Nettles bruised together, and laid upon the impostume that riseth behind the eares, doth asswage and helpeth it much:

Coughs & throat: also the juyce of Sage taken in warme water, helpeth an hoarsnesse and the cough: the leaves sodden in wine and laid upon any place affected with the Palsie, helpeth much, if the decoction be drunke also. Sage taken with Wormewood is used for the bloody fluxe;

Pliny: *Pliny* saith it procureth womens courses, and stayeth them comming downe too fast; helpeth the stinging and bytings of Serpents, and killeth the wormes that breed in the eares, and also in sores.

Memory: Sage is of excellent good use to helpe the memory, by warming and quickning the sences, and the conserve made of the flowers is used to the same purpose, as also for all the former recited diseases:

Toads & snakes: they are perswaded in *Italy* that if they eate Sage fasting with a little salt, they shall be safe that day, from the danger of the byting of any venemous beast: they use there also never to plant Sage but with Rue among it, or neare it, for feare of Toades and other Serpents breeding under it, and infecting it with their venemous spittle, &c. the danger whereof is recorded in *Boccace*, of two Friends or Lovers, that by eating the leaves of that Sage under which a Toade was found to abide, were both killed thereby, and therefore the Poet joyneth them both together to have wholesome drinke, saying; *Salvia cum ruta faciunt tibi pocula tuta.*

Plague: Sage hath beene of good use in the time of the plague at all times, and the small Sage more especially (which therefore I thinke our people called Sage of Vertue) the juyce thereof drunke with vineger.

Sandwiches & ale: The use of Sage in the Moneth of May, with butter, Parsley, and some salt, is very frequent in our Country to continue health to the body: as also Sage Ale made with it, Rosemary, and other good hearbes for the same purpose, and for teeming women, or such as are subject to miscary, as it is before declared.

Gargles: Gargles likewise are made with Sage, Rosemary, Honisuckles, and Plantaine boyled in water or wine, with some Honey and Allome put thereto, to wash cankers, sore mouthes, and throats, or the secret parts of man or woman as need requireth.

Baths: And with other hot and comfortable hearbes to be boyled, to serve for bathings of the body or legges, in the Summer time, especially to warme the cold joynts or sinewes of young or old, troubled with the Palsie or crampe, and to comfort and strengthen the parts.

Stich: It is much commended against the stitch or paines in the side comming of winde, if the grieved place be fomented warme with the decoction thereof in wine, and the hearbe after the boyling be laid warme also thereto.

defluxions: flow of liquid
thin rheume: thin phlegm
imposthume that riseth behind the eares: abscess behind the ears
sodden: soaked
bloody fluxe: dysentery
Pliny: Pliny the Elder (AD23–79), Roman naturalist
Boccace: Giovanni Boccacio (1530–75), author of *The Decameron*
Salvia cum ruta faciunt tibi pocula tuta: saying recorded by Boccacio, 'plant rue among sage to keep away noxious toads', i.e. make it safe
Sage of Vertue: Small sage, *Salvia minor,* which Parkinson writes about in another chapter
teeming: pregnant
allome: alum, usually a potassium aluminium sulphate
cankers: mouth ulcers
palsie: palsy
fomented warme: application of cloth soaked in warm sage tea as a poultice

Toads & snakes: Parkinson here reports a story that he obviously doesn't believe, as there is so much superstition involved. It may be that sage does have some power to protect against toxins and poisons.

For plague: Thankfully, this is something we do not have to deal with in our times. However, Parkinson's recommendation of drinking sage with vinegar would be effective in helping prevent a range of infections, from the common cold to influenza.

Sage sandwich: It was traditional in England to eat sage in May to ensure good health throughout the year. Chop up fresh sage and parsley and mix with butter and salt. This can be tried on bread or in baked potatoes or on other cooked vegetables.

Sage ale: We believe Parkinson means ale actually brewed with sage, as in his day many people made their own ale as a matter of course.

Sage ale can be made the short way by putting sage, rosemary and any other herbs you are using in a pan of ale and warming gently on the stove, covered by a lid, for an hour to infuse the liquid. Strain and drink.

Sage gargle: Warm or cool sage tea makes a wonderful gargle for sore throats. It's also useful for mouth infections and gum disease. We would make Parkinson's recipe with the herbs and honey but without the alum, because of its aluminium content. However, it is FDA-approved in the US, so is regarded as safe. Alum has a styptic and antibacterial effect.

Chewing sage brings relief to a sore throat, and rubbing leaves on the teeth whitens them and eases gingivitis in the gums, leaving the mouth feeling clean.

Baths: We like to use sage in footbaths and handbaths. Make a strong infusion, brewing for about 3 minutes. Add to a small basin of warm water and sit with your feet or hands soaking in it for 15 minutes.

We find hand and footbaths wonderfully relaxing, as you are adding stillness and repose to the therapeutic action of the herbs. How often in a normal day do we just sit still for quarter of an hour?

A poultice for stitch & colic: Make a decoction of sage in wine, heating it to simmering in a pot on the stove for about 15 minutes. Strain and lay the sage on the stitch or cramp, then soak a cloth in the liquid and place over the leaves, replacing with a warm one as it cools, or use a hot water bottle to keep it warm. Repeat as necessary until relief is obtained.

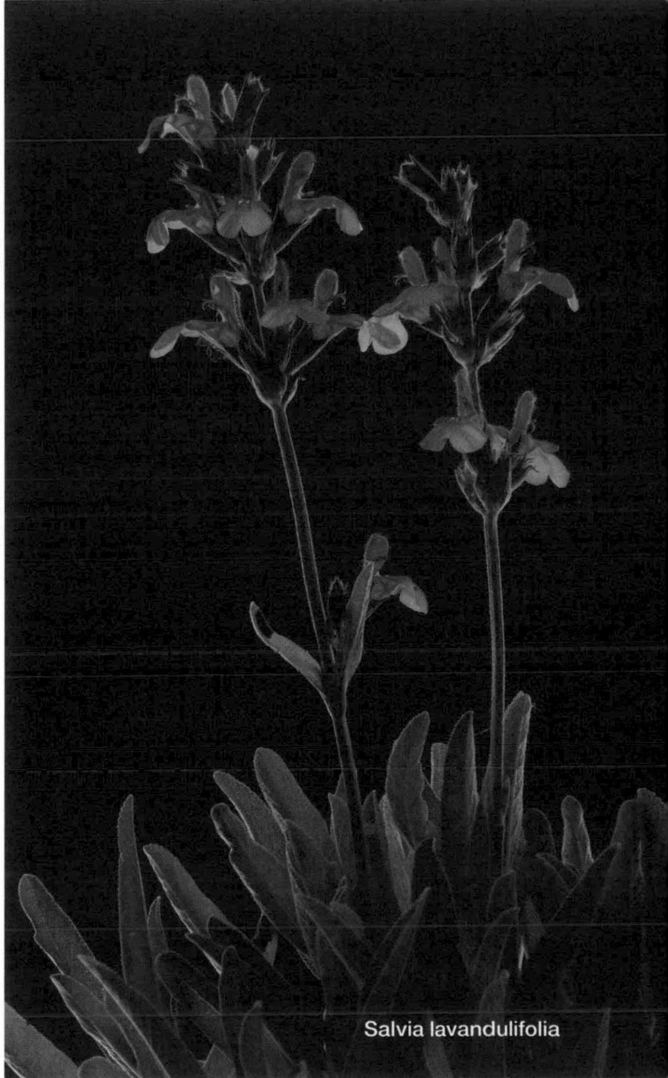

Salvia lavandulifolia

Rosemary & sage infused wine

Take a bottle of red wine (or white wine if you prefer) and drink a glassful to make room in the bottle, then put into the bottle 4 sprigs rosemary, 2 sprigs sage, an aril of mace, a few slices of fresh ginger root and a small cinnamon stick.

Steep for two weeks in a warm dark place, then strain through muslin, into a sterilised bottle.

A wineglassful a day is a tonic after illness and is a traditional drink to help improve memory and poor circulation. Also good for itchy cods!

Sanicle

Theatrum Botanicum
Tribe 5, Chapter 28, pp532–34

1 *Sanicula vulgaris sive Diapensia.* Ordinary Sanicle or Selfe heale.

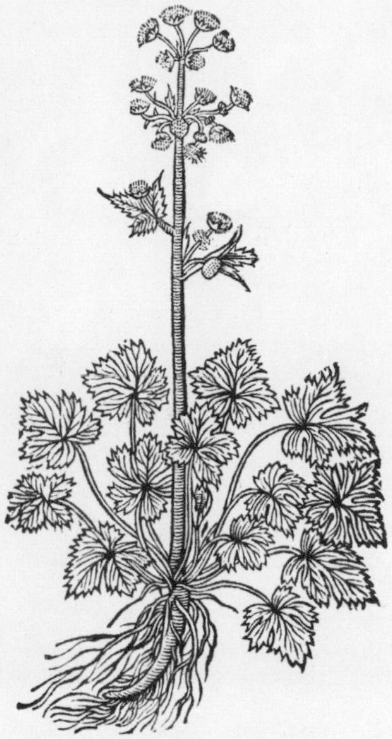

greene wounds: fresh or raw wounds
imposthumes: abscesses
represseth the humours: dries up moisture
privities: sexual organs
stay womens courses: stop menstrual bleeding
fluxes: flowings
laskes of the belly: griping or diarrhoea
reynes: kidneys
Consound: a wound-healing herb
Kines Udders: cows' udders
rist: swollen
Physitians: physicians

The Vertues

Sanicle is bitter in taste, and thereby is heating and drying in the second degree, it is astringent also, and therefore exceeding good to heale all greene wounds speedily, or any ulcers, imposthumes, or bleedings inwardly;

Tumours: it doth wonderfully helpe those that have any tumour in their bodies in any part, for it represseth the humours, and dissipateth them, if the decoction or juice thereof be taken, or the powder in drinke, and the juice used outwardly;

Lungs, mouth & throat: for there is not found any herbe that can give such present helpe, either to man or beast, when the disease falleth upon the lungs or throate, and to heale up all the maligne putride or stinking ulcers of the mouth, throat, and privities, by gargling or washing with the decoction of the leaves and roote made in water, and a little hony put thereto;

Bleeding: it helpeth to stay womens courses, and all other fluxes of blood, either by the mouth, urine, or stoole, and laskes of the belly, the ulceration of the kidneyes also and the paines in the bowels, and the *gonorrhea* or running of the reynes, being boyled in wine or water and drunke, the same also is no lesse powerfull, to helpe any ruptures or burstings used both inwardly and outwardly:

Wound healing: and briefely it is as effectuall in binding, restraining, consolidating, heating drying, and healing, as Comfrey, Bugle, or Selfe-heale, or any other of the Consounds or vulnerary herbes whatsoever.

Butterwort: Butterwort* is as one writeth to me a vulnerary herbe, of great esteeme with many, as well for the rupture in Children as to heale greene wounds; the Country people that live where it groweth; doe use to annoint their hands when they are chapt by the winde, or when their Kines Udders are swollen by the biting of any virulent worme, or otherwise hurt, chapt or rist, the poorer sort of people in *Wales* make a Syrupe thereof, as is of Roses, and therewith purge themselves and their children: they put it likewise into their broths for the same purpose which purgeth flegme effectually: they also with the herbe and butter make an ointment singular good against the obstructions of the liver, experienced by some Physitions there of good account.

2 *Pinguicula sive Sanicula Eboracensis.* Butterwort or *Yorkeshire* Sanicle.

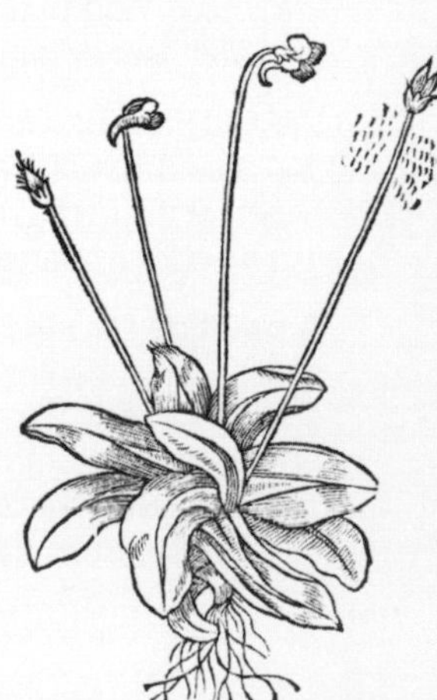

* Parkinson includes Butterwort or Yorkeshire Sanicle (*Pinguicula sive Sanicula Eboracensis*), along with other forms of Sanicle, namely Spotted Sanicle, Beares-eare Sanicle and The Shrubbe Sanicle of America.

Sanicle *Sanicula europaea*

Apiaceae (Umbelliferae)

Sanicle is a forgotten herb, which was widely used and respected until about the 1930s but has since disappeared from the European *materia medica*.

It is an easy plant to miss, as it grows in woodlands and flowers once the leaves have come out on nearby trees, but it is locally abundant where it is found. It can be grown in a shady garden, and is a plant that aroused Parkinson's curiosity – he cites botanical correspondents from Wales and other places.

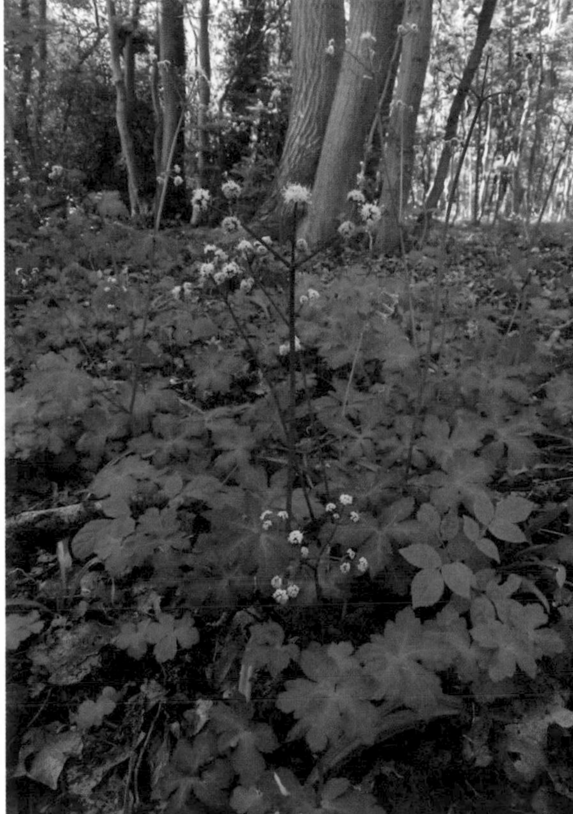

Sanicle grows in deciduous woodlands, and flowers alongside bluebells in early summer

Sanicle is bitter and astringent. Leaves are collected in the spring either before the plant flowers or while it is flowering. The root is best dug in the autumn, but can be used any time of year. The word 'sanicle' comes from the Latin 'to heal', and sanicle is one of the vulneraries ('Consounds'), with selfheal and bugle, confusingly known in English as selfheal or all-heal.

The related North American species, *S. marylandica*, was used for sore throats and fevers.

Decoction: We have made Parkinson's decoction of the leaves in water, simmered gently until the liquid is a rich golden colour and then strained and sweetened with a little honey. This can be bottled while hot, and will keep in the fridge for several weeks. The effect is at first very relaxing, then gives one the energy and clarity to get going with all manner of things one may have been putting off! It seems to work gently to make the whole body function better, but is, as Parkinson says, very good for sore throats and mouth problems. It is also beneficial for haemorrhoids and piles.

Lungs, mouth & throat: In the 1920s, English naturopath Richard Lawrence Hool wrote: 'In cases of diseases of the chest and lungs, spitting of blood, scrofula, ulcers and tumours, or internal abscesses and ulcerations, there is no plant superior to Wood Sanicle. It is useful in sore or ulcerated mouth and throat' (*Health from British Wild Herbs*, 3rd edn, Southport, 1924, p28). Given this praise, and Parkinson's, sanicle deserves another chance in treating these problems.

Bleeding: Sanicle is a good choice for stopping bleeding, either internally or externally.

Wound healing: The leaves can be crushed and applied as a poultice to injured parts. They are remarkably effective for healing and preventing bruising.

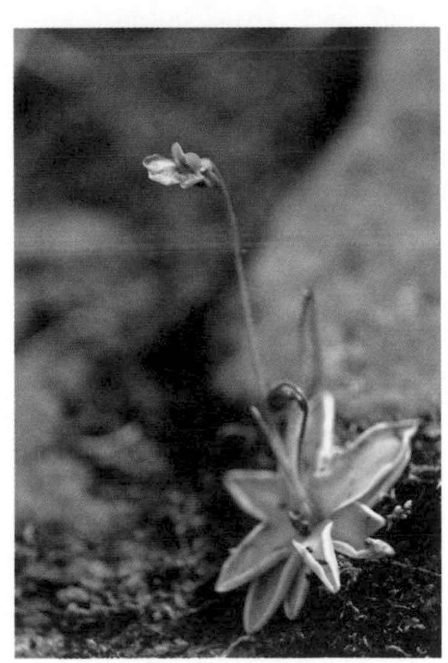

Butterwort, Pinguicula vulgaris, 'Yorkshire sanicle', is a rare insectivorous plant only found in acidic boggy conditions, and is not used by herbalists today

Sassafras or Ague Tree

Theatrum Botanicum

Tribe 17, Chapter 49, pp1606–07

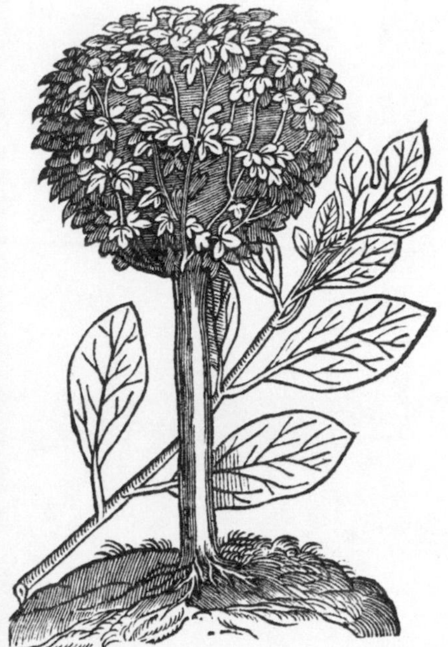

Cornel tree: dogwood
Master Iohn Tradescant: John Tradescant the Younger (1608–62), gardener and plant-hunter who travelled to Virginia
Clusius: Charles de l'Ecluse (1526–1609), French botanist
cold rheumes and defluxions: flowing of mucus
availeable: beneficial
restraineth castings: prevents vomiting
womens courses: menstruation
barrenesse: infertility
tertian and quotidian agues: malarial-type fevers
the pestilence: the plague
the French disease: syphilis

Sassaphras

[Parkinson writes in his introduction that this was a remedy for 'Agues, and swellings in their legges', taught to the French and Spanish in Florida by 'the Natives'; the origin of the name was unknown.]

… the flowers … are small and yellow made of threds very like to the Male Cornel tree as Master *Iohn Tradescant* saith … the trunke and branches are but somewhat redder [i.e. than the roots], which are most in use, being of greater force and efficacy then any other part of the tree, and taste somewhat spicelike, rellishing Fennell seede withall, but *Clusius* compareth the taste thereof unto the herbe *Tarragon*, and is hot and dry in the beginning of the third degree.

Decoction/warming & drying: The decoction whereof is familiarly given in all cold diseases and obstructions of the Liver and spleene, as also in cold rheumes and defluxions of the head, on the teeth, eyes, or lunges, warming and drying up the moisture, and strengthening the parts afterwards, and therefore is availeable in coughes, and other cold diseases of the brest, stomacke, and lungs, and restraineth castings,

Digestion: and helpeth digestion, breaketh and expelleth winde,

Urinary: the gravell and stone in the kidneyes, and provoketh urine,

Gynaecological: and womens courses, it also warmeth, heateth, and dryeth up the moisture of womens wombes, which is in most the cause of barrenesse, and causeth them to be the more apt to conceive:

Fevers/agues: it is of especiall good use in tertian and quotidian agues that come of humours, or are of long continuance: it is thought also to be good in the time of the pestilence, to weare some thereof continually about them, that the smell of it may expell the corrupt and evil vapours of the pestilence:

Venereal disease: it is generally used in all the diseases that come of cold and raw, thin, and corrupt humours, the *French* disease, and other of the like foule nature:

Wounds & sores: the Indians use the leaves being bruised to heale their wounds, and sores of whatesoever quality they be.

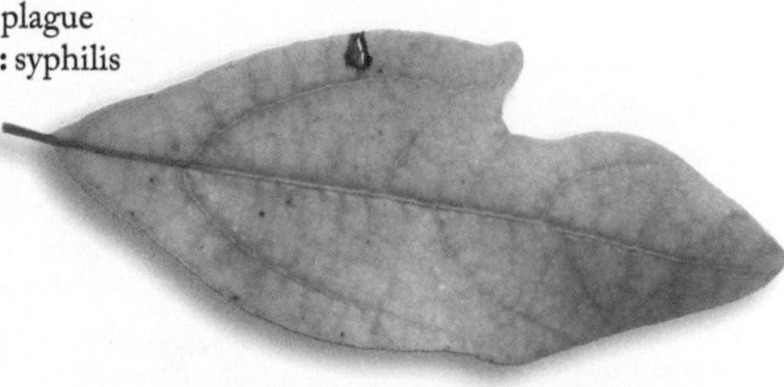

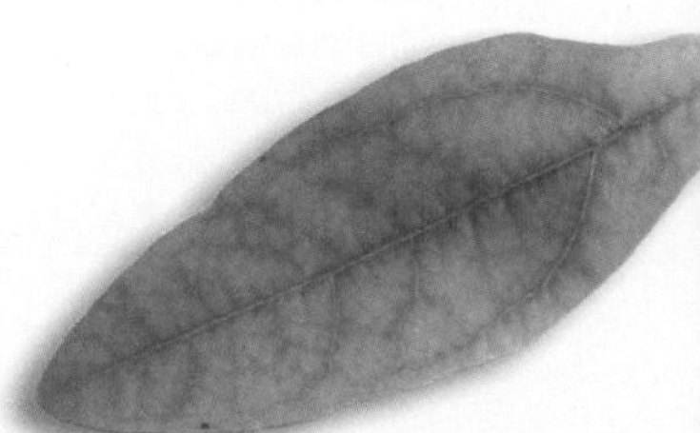

Sassafras *Sassafras albidum*

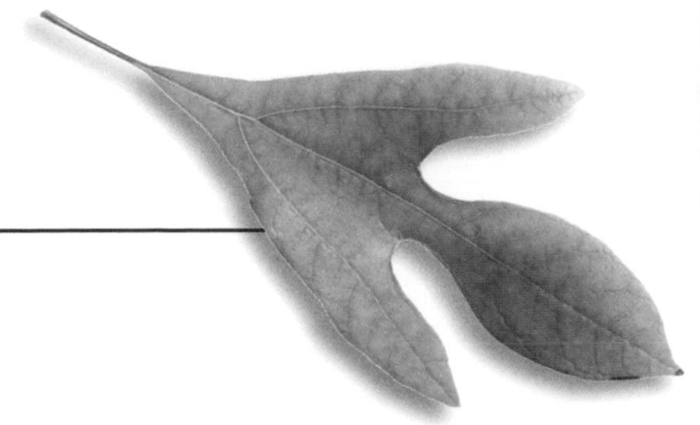

Lauraceae

Sassfras is a small tree native to eastern North America, and it grows larger in the southern part of its range. Unusually, the leaves have three shapes: an oval, a mitten shape, and a three- or even five-lobed leaf. It reached Europe in the sixteenth century, and for a while was the leading export from the Virginian colonies to England, even more valuable than tobacco.

Traditionally the roots were used to brew root beer, or boiled as a spring tonic drink. The young leaves can be dried and powdered as gumbo filé, which is used to flavour and thicken soups and stews.

Sassafras is rather neglected in herbal medicine today, but its warming tonic action remains potentially valuable.

Sassafras root and root bark were formerly widely used as a spring tonic to cleanse the blood after a winter diet. It was frequently combined with sarsaparilla root to make root beer. It is a warming and drying plant, which tones the tissues. The flowers and young leaves can be eaten in salads. As Clusius said, the taste of the leaves is similar to tarragon, but with a cinnamon overtone.

Sassafras was prized in Europe for combating fevers, and became a remedy of choice for treating venereal diseases.

Sassafras was often used to improve the flavour of other medicines. An oil contained in sassafras, safrole, is toxic in large doses and was banned by the Food & Drug Administration in the US in 1960. Sassafras is still used commercially to flavour root beer, but now in a safrole-free extract. Researcher and herbalist James Duke famously noted: 'However, the safrole in a 12-ounce can of old-fashioned root beer is not as carcinogenic as the alcohol (ethanol) in a can of beer.' The tea is low in safrole, which is not readily water-soluble, and is considered safe.

Decoction: Sassafras root decoction can be made by digging a few roots, washing them and chopping them up. Simmer gently until a good orange colour is obtained, then strain and drink. Drunk hot, it is warming and stimulating. If cooled and mixed with some mint, it is a cooling and refreshing drink.

Fevers: Sassafras probably works as well as ever in treating fevers, but fortunately fevers are not the common problem they were in past centuries.

Wounds & sores: To make a simple first aid poultice, take a few leaves of sassafras and chew them or pound them with a stone to mash them, then place over the part to be treated.

Gumbo filé or Filé powder

To make gumbo filé, dry young sassafras leaves until they are crisp. Remove stems and grind to a powder – a mortar and pestle if you feel energetic, but an electric coffee grinder or a blender also work well. Sieve to remove any large bits. Add the powder to chowder, soups and stews once they are removed from the heat, just before serving – or set a dish of the powder out for guests to serve themselves.

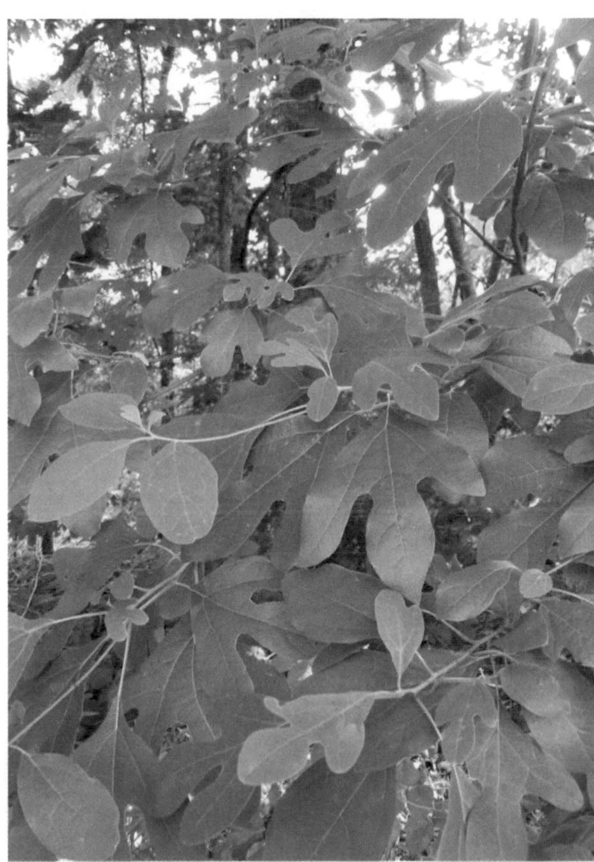

Savorie

Theatrum Botanicum
Tribe 1, Chapter 2, pp4–7

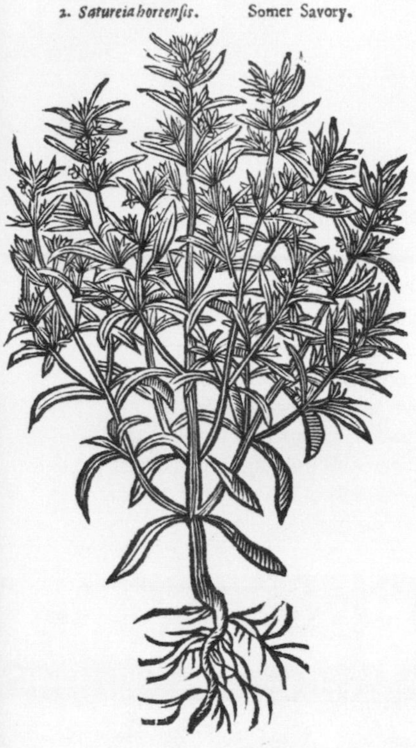

Thymbra sive Satrureia

The Vertues

Expelling wind: Our Savory of both sorts is hot and dry in the third degree, especially the summer kinde, which is both sharpe and quicke in taste, expelling winde in the stomacke and bowels, and is a present helpe for the rising of the mother procured by winde, provoketh Urine and womens courses, and is much commended for women with child to take inwardly, and to smell often thereunto:

Aphrodisiac: Some that from *Satyris* thinke *Satureia* to be derived, say it helpeth the disease called *Satyriasis* or *Pryapismus*, and to helpe dull or decayed coiture:

Appetite: others taking it to bee derived *a saturando,* say it is in familiar use with many to procure a good appetite unto meate, and to take away all manner of loathing to the same:

Expectoration: it cutteth tough flegme in the chest and lunges, and helpeth to expectorate it the more easily:

Drowsiness: it helpeth to quicken the dull spirits of the Lethargye, the juice being snuffed or cast up into the nostrills:

Eyes: the juice also is of good use to be dropped into the eyes to cleare the dull sight, if it proceede of raw thinne colde humours distilling from the braine:

Ears: the juice also heated with a little oyle of Roses, and dropped into the eares, easeth them of the noyse and singing in them, and deafenes also:

Sciatica: outwardly applyed with white flower in manner of a poultis, giveth ease to the Sciatica or hippe gowte, or paralyticall members, by heating and warming them, and taking away the paine:

Insects: it taketh away also the stinging of bees, waspes, &c.

rising of mother: upward displacement of womb
procured by winde: of a gaseous cause
courses: menstruation
Satyriasis: uncontrollable sexual desire
Pryapismus: persistent undesired erection
dull or decayed coiture: loss of libido or impotency
a saturando: relating to gluttony, appetite
cutteth tough flegme: dissolves viscous phlegm
Lethargye: torpor
snuffed: taken in nose as snuff
thinne colde humours distilling: clear watery mucus dripping down
deafenes: deafness
flower: flour
poultis: poultice
paralyticall members: paralysed limbs

Other uses: A powerful essential oil is made from both species of savory, and these are widely used today by clinical aromatherapists. The oils, which Parkinson does not mention as such, have antibacterial qualities that are used to treat candida and other fungal infections. Note that in this concentrated form they should be avoided in pregnancy.

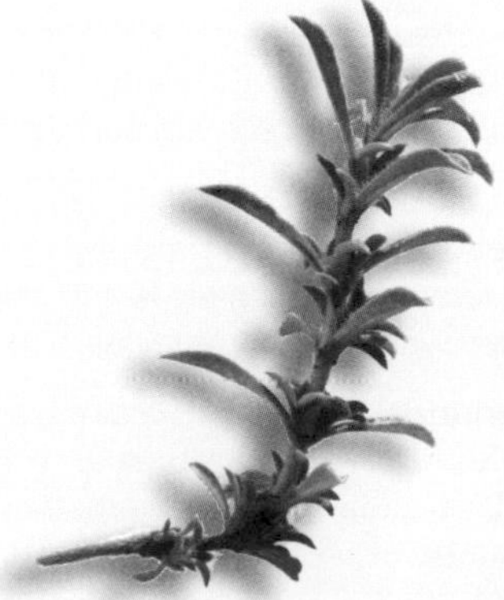

Savory *Satureja hortensis, S. montana* Lamiaceae

Savory is a small aromatic herb native to southern Europe, with two principal species used in Parkinson's time, and still today. **Summer or garden savory** (*Satureja hortensis*) is a tender annual, some 4 to 15 inches high (10–30 cm), and is softer and finer, more aromatic than its cousin. The **winter or mountain savory** (*S. montana*) (shown below) is a woody perennial, a little larger, stiffer and coarser, with bluey-white flowers and like hyssop in scent, Parkinson says. Savory was taken to the New World by early English colonists, but specific North American savories include **yerba buena or Oregon tea** (*S. douglasii*) and **Japanese peppermint** (*S. viminea*), both made into minty-tasting teas.

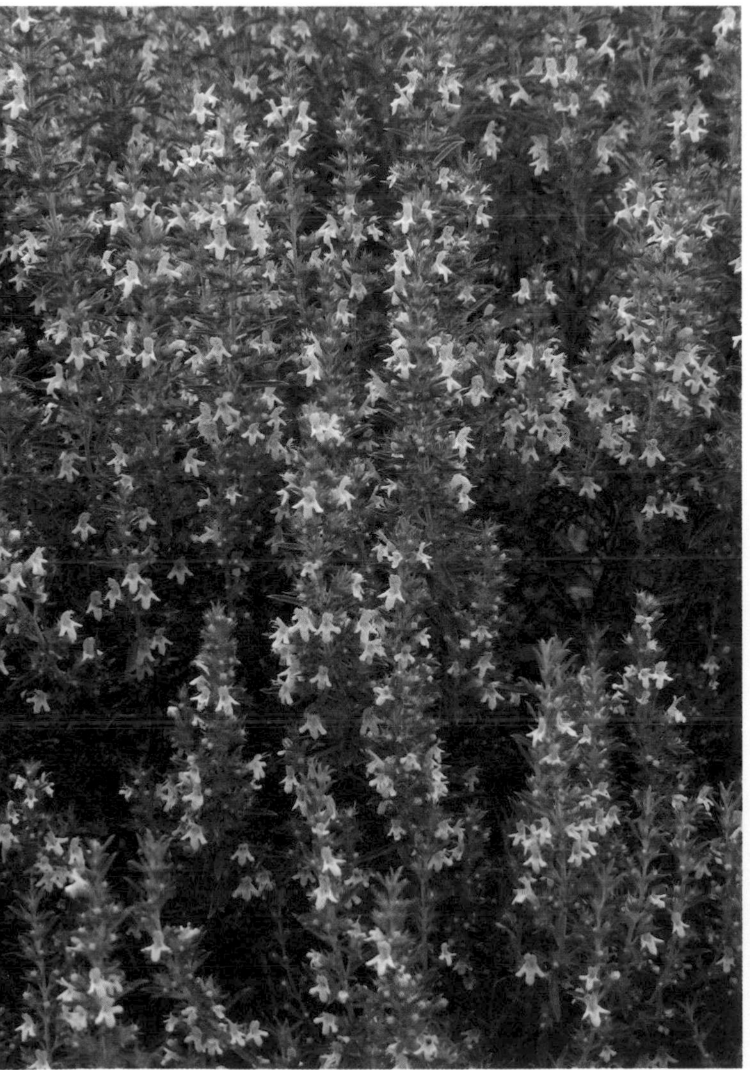

Expelling wind: Parkinson begins with the medicinal use of savory as an aromatic. He says it will expel windiness in the stomach and intestines, but also go deeper to adjust a displacement of the womb, and provoke urination and menstruation where impeded. Modern use has lost this depth, and focuses on the relief the plants can give for flatulence or colic, and stimulating the digestion.

Aphrodisiac: Savory's supposed aphrodisiac reputation is probably more a result of its provocative ancient name than its actual effects. The genus name *Satureja* is taken from *satyrus* or satyr, the drunken and lusty woodland deities, and Ovid mentions savory's amatory benefits. Parkinson isn't convinced, though concedes that it might be a sexual aid. In his time 'wind' equated to sexual desire, but he didn't include savory in his index of plants that 'provoketh unto venery'.

Appetite: Appetite in the other sense is safer ground, and summer savory especially has a peppery, stimulating taste, adding relish to vegetables, soups, meat and fish. Savory is an ingredient in the stuffing of the Thanksgiving turkey in the US, and a key herb in Turkish condiment *zatar*. German cooks know it as *Bohnenkraut*, or bean herb, for those good medieval broad beans and peas, to add flavour and counter the inevitable windiness. It is often grown with beans.

Expectoration: Cutting 'tough flegme' is an aspect of savory's warming and stimulatory action, as indeed is its wakening effects on drowsiness ('the Lethargye'); taking savory as a snuff sounds intriguing, and we will try it.

Eyes & ears: Parkinson's reported uses are probably hardly practised at all in our times, but his specificity is convincing.

Sciatica: Again, using savory as a hot poultice with white flour to ease nervous pain, gout or sciatica sounds excellent practice, but this is a forgotten remedy.

Insects: Parkinson's mention of using savory to alleviate bee or wasp stings may have its source in Virgil, who suggested growing the plant near bee hives for this purpose.

Sea wrake or Sea weede

Theatrum Botanicum

Tribe 14, Chapter 52, pp1291–95

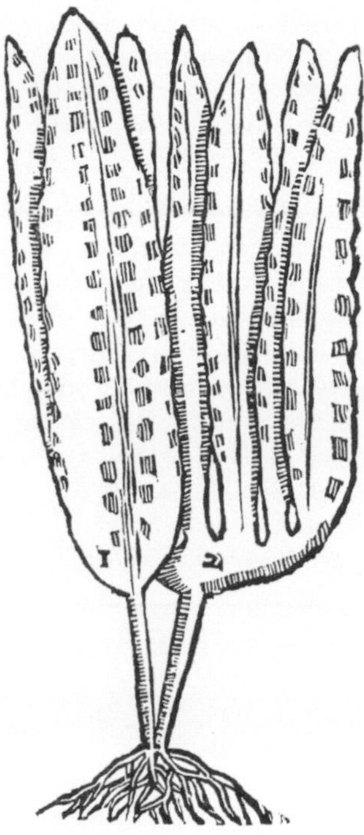

Fucus marinus sive Alga marina

The vertues

All the kindes of Wrake, saith *Dioscorides* and *Galen*, doe coole and dry, and is good to ease the Gout, and inflammations, being used fresh, but *Lacuna* correcteth the cooling word in *Galen*, and saith it doth better agree with Sea plants, to dry rather then to coole, by reason of their saltnesse, which doth binde and constraine, but not coole, *Nicander* in *Theriacis*, commendeth the red sort of *Fucus* to be good against the venome of Serpents, and other venemous creatures.

The first sort [i.e. Wrake or Sea weed] is much used by the *Venetians* instead of hay or straw, to pack up Glasses to preserve them from breaking, but at *Mompelier* and other places, they use it as a litter for their horses,

Compost: and being made into compost is excellent good manure, to refresh their barren or out eaten grounds:

As food: divers of the other sorts are eaten as sallet herbes, as the fourth [i.e. Winged Sea girdle, *F. alatas sive phosganoides*], fifth [i.e. Great Sea girdle with many Labels, *F. maximus polyschides*] and twelfth [i.e. The Sea Garland, *Opuntia marina*], the seventh [i.e. Sea weede with skinny hornes, *F. membranaceus ceranoides*] as is said, is good to represse the hurtfull longings of women with childe, and *Clusius* saith that *Cortusus* signified unto him that the commonpeople of *Corsica* did use the last, instead of *Corallina* [i.e. Hard Sea Mosse, *Muscus marinus Corallina dictus*] to kill the wormes in children.

Dioscorides: Greek-speaking Roman physician (mid-first century AD)
Galen: Claudius Galen (AD130–200), Roman physician and author
Lacuna: Andrés de Laguna (1499–1559), Spanish physician and author
sallet herbes: salad herbs
Nicander: Nicander of Colophon (2nd cent. BC), Greek physician and poet; author of a long poem, *Theriaca*
Venetians: leading traders and glassmakers in Parkinson's time
Mompelier: Montpellier was famous for its botanic garden and university in Parkinson's day
out eaten grounds: depleted soil
divers: various examples
Clusius: Charles de l'Ecluse (1526–1609), French botanist and author
Cortusus: Jacobus Antonius Cortusus (1513–1603), Italian botanist

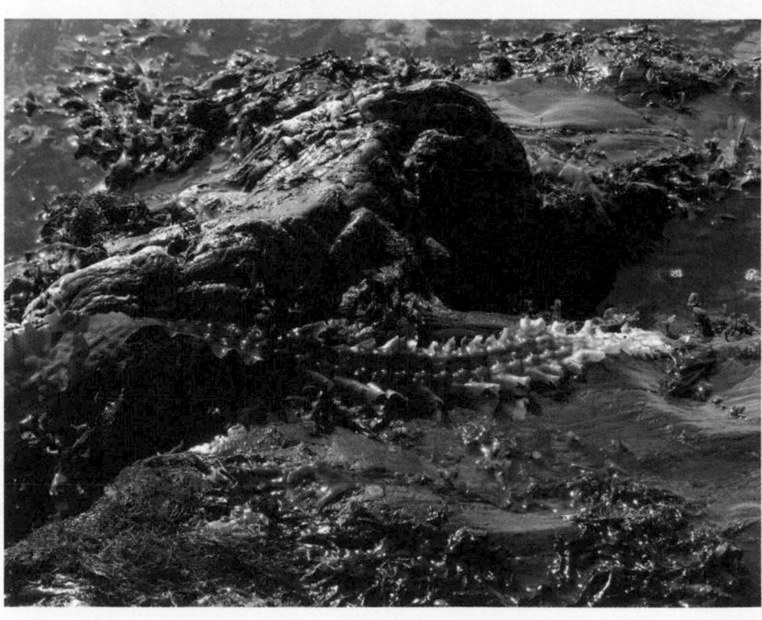

Seaweed

Parkinson describes a dozen seaweeds, wracks and kelp, but combines their virtues in one description. Seaweeds are marine algae, as he says, and are now classified as red, green or brown. They have traditionally been used as foods by coastal populations around the world, as Parkinson describes. Seaweed is still harvested for fertilizer, and it is medicinally important for its high content of minerals, notably iodine, something not known to Parkinson. Iodine is essential for thyroid function and proper metabolism, but is often deficient in inland soils/populations. The commercially traded substances agar and carageenan are extracted from seaweeds for use in the modern food industry as thickening agents and emulsifiers.

Today, as throughout history, seaweed is valued as a fertilizer, and for its minerals; we now know it as a wonderful source of iodine. Iodine is often lacking in soils away from the sea, and a deficiency causes goitre, a symptom of thyroid under-functioning. It is an essential ingredient of thyroid hormones, so seaweed can treat hypothyroidism. Bladderwrack (*Fucus*) and kelp (*Laminaria* sp. etc) are most commonly used.

Low levels of active thyroid hormone contribute to such a wide range of other health problems that seaweed supplementation can benefit most people.

The benefits are not only from the iodine content. Most seaweeds are rich in potassium and the other minerals so poorly supplied in modern diets. The mucilaginous properties are also beneficial, and algin helps eliminate heavy metals from the body.

The first written records of seaweed use are nearly 5,000 years old, in a herbal attributed to the legendary Chinese Emperor Shen Nung. Chronic pernicious iodine deficiency developed in central China after thousands of years of agriculture, and in China today kelp is grown on a large scale as a source of iodine.

Welsh laver bread (from *Porphyra* sp. and other seaweeds) can be an acquired taste. Mrs Grieve's *Modern Herbal* (1931, p112) dismissed its 'strong seaweed odour and a nauseous, saline, mucilaginous taste'. But opinions differ: many seaweeds do taste great, and are gourmet foods in Japan.

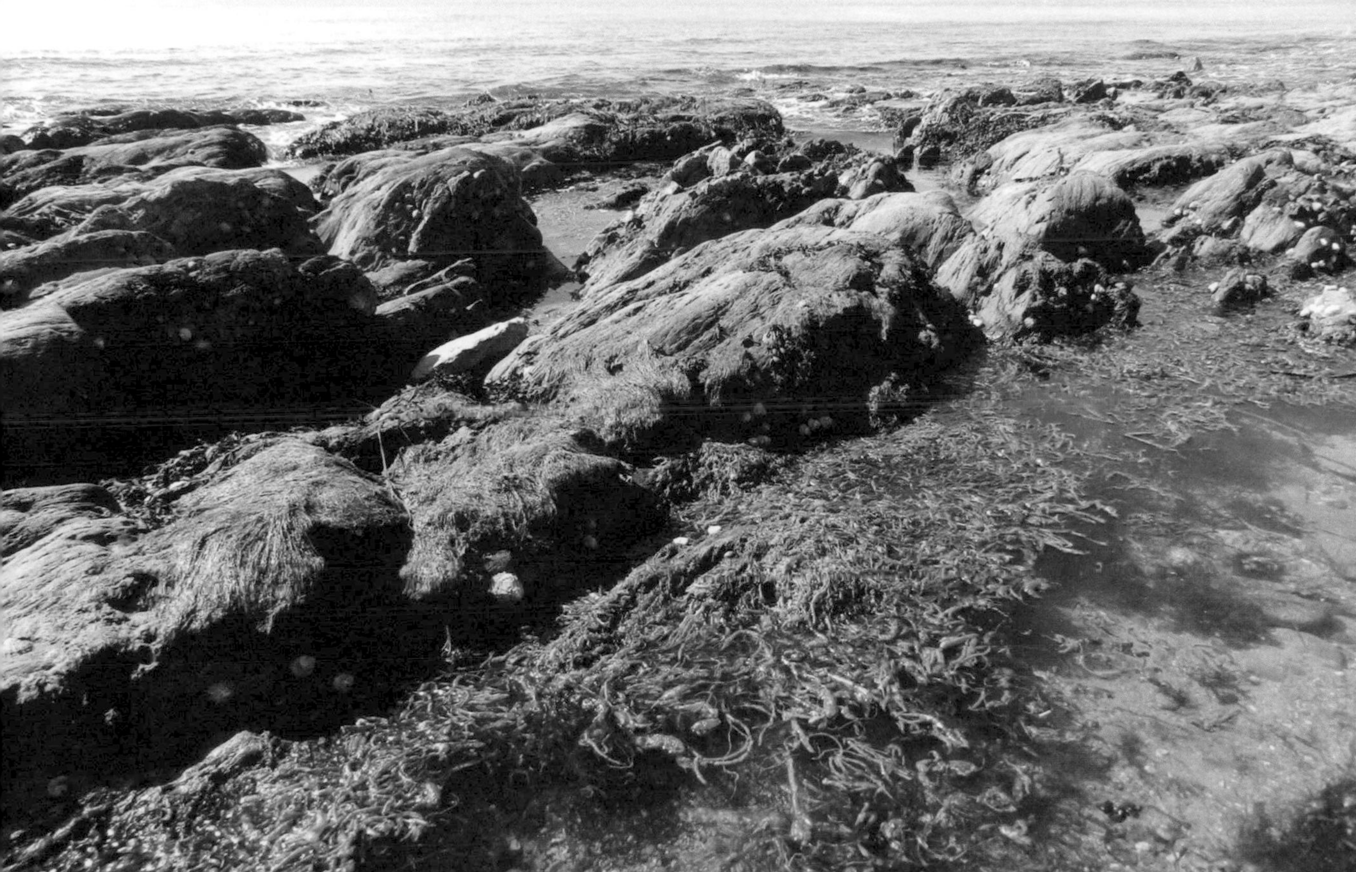

Selfeheale

Theatrum Botanicum

Tribe 5, Chapter 26, pp526–28

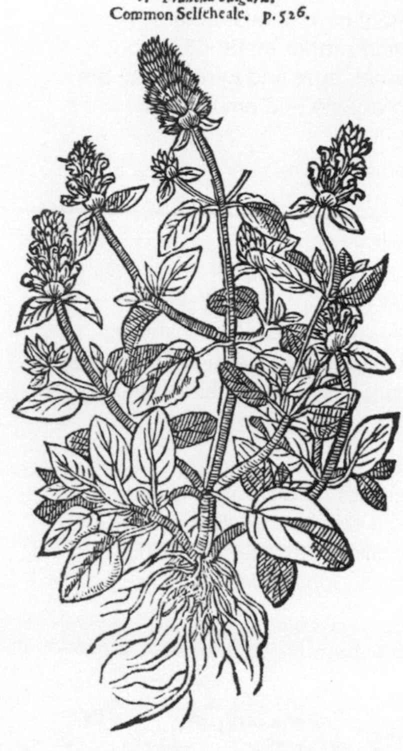

Prunella

The Vertues

The Selfeheale being so like the Bugle as I said in outward forme, is no lesse like it in the qualitie and vertues being by the bitternesse taken to be hot and drie, and yet temperate in both degrees, and by some thought to be rather more cold, in regard it is so powerfull to helpe such an hot sicknesse as the *German* disease, called *die Bruen*, which as hath bin in some part said before, commeth with inflammation and swelling both in the mouth and throate, the tongue rough and rugged or blacke, and a fierce hot continuall ague thereon, which is remedied chiefely by drinking the decoction of this herbe continually, and washing the mouth often also therewith, having some vinegar added unto it; but bloud letting must be used in the cure, and that under the tongue, without which it will not, or very hardly be effected:

Wounds & ulcers: this herbe serveth for all the purposes whereunto Bugle is applied, and with as good successe both inwardly and outwardly: for inward wounds and ulcers wheresoever within the body: for bruises and falls, and other such griefes, for if it be accompanied with Bugle, Sanicle, and other the like wound herbes it will be the more effectuall and to wash or inject into ulcers, in the parts outwardly, for where there is cause to represse the heate and sharpnesse of humours, flowing to any sore, ulcer, inflammation, swelling or the like; or to stay the fluxe of bloud in any wound or any part, this is used with good successe, as also to clense the foulnesse of all sores, and to cause them the more speedily to be healed: it is an especiall remedy for all greene wounds to soder the lippes of them, and to keepe the place from any further inconvenience:

With rose: the juyce hereof used with oyle of Roses, to annoint the temples and forehead, is very effectuall to remove the head-ach, and the same juice mixed with a little Hony of Roses, clenseth and healeth all ulcers and sores in the mouth and throate, and those also in the secret parts:

Ointment: the same ointment that is set downe in the former Chapter is made as often with this herbe instead of Bugle; if it be not at hand, or if it be, yet they are oftentimes both put together, to serve to helpe broken bones, or joints out of place:

Good health: the Proverbe of the *Germans, French*, and others, whereof is made mention in the former, is no lesse verified, as I there said then of this, that he needeth neither Physition or Chirurgion, that hath Selfeheale and Sanicle by him to helpe himselfe.

die Bruen: a mouth & throat infection, often translated as quinsy, but we think is more likely to be diphtheria
rugged: cracked
ague: fever
bloud letting: bleeding was a common medical practice
Bugle: see page 47
Sanicle: see page 189
stay the fluxe: stop the flow
greene wounds: fresh wounds
soder the lippes: join the flaps
Physition: physician
Chirurgion: surgeon

Selfheal *Prunella vulgaris*

Lamiaceae

Selfheal, also called all-heal from its reputation as a panacea (literally 'all' and 'remedy'), has a wide range of medicinal effects. It was the primary treatment for a disease of the mouth and throat known as *die Braun*, possibly a type of quinsy, and is effective against mouth ulcers.

Its other main use in Europe was for wounds and injuries of all kinds, from broken bones to bleeding cuts. In China, it is given to clear liver stagnation and congestion, and to treat and reduce swellings, especially in the neck. It is widely used for fevers, thyroid problems and infections.

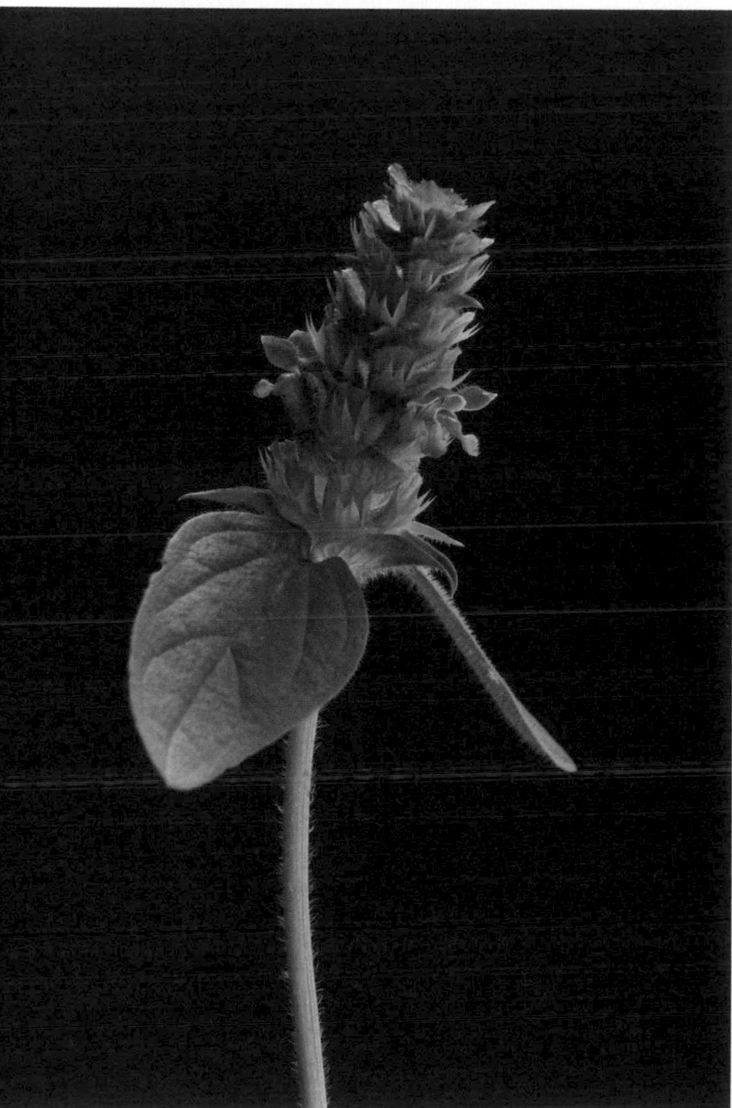

Selfheal is found across Europe, Asia and North America. It is a common wild woodland plant, and is often seen growing in lawns.

Mouth & throat problems: Selfheal is one of the foremost remedies for mouth and throat problems. It can be used for sore tongues, swollen glands, tonsillitis, mumps, goitre and laryngitis. It is helpful in promoting healing after extractions or other dental work.

Blood-letting: This is one of the very few times Parkinson mentions combining herbs with blood-letting, one of the mainstays of medicine from antiquity to the 19th century.

With rose: Parkinson suggests mixing selfheal juice with oil of roses for headaches, used externally on the forehead and temples, making a pleasant and effective treatment for many headaches. Selfheal has a relaxing effect on the nervous system, and can help reduce high blood pressure.

For mouth ulcers and genital sores, he mixes it with honey of roses. Both selfheal and rose are powerful antiviral herbs, effective against the herpes viruses that cause these problems, and the honey adds its healing properties too.

Ointment: An ointment of selfheal works well for all sorts of minor injuries. We usually make it with olive oil, infusing the herb in the sun, then straining and setting it with beeswax.

Modern uses

Selfheal is immunomodulatory, anti-inflammatory and antimutagenic. It is effective against viruses, including HIV and viral hepatitis, and has an antibiotic effect against a range of bacteria.

It has an affinity with the lymphatic system, helping clear infections and toxins, and in removal of excess uric acid from the body via the kidneys, making it useful for treating gout. A hot tea induces sweating and helps reduce fever. The cooled tea can be used as an eyewash for eye infections and inflammations.

Salomones Seale

Theatrum Botanicum

Tribe 5, Chapter 103, pp696–700

1. 3. *Polygonatum majus vulgare & majus flore majore.*
The greater ordinary *Salomons* Seale, and that with greater flowers.

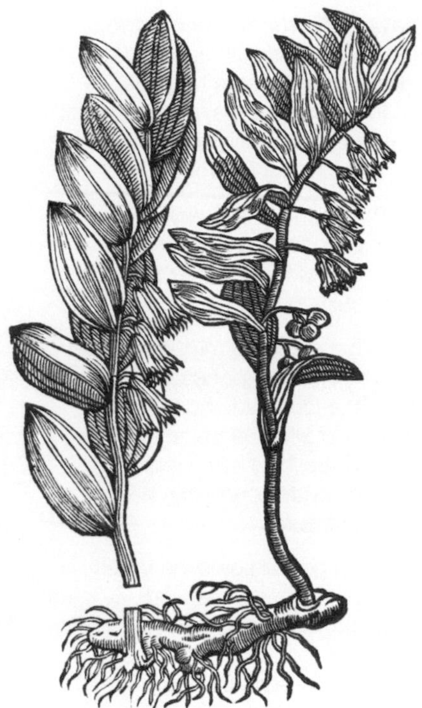

Galen: Claudius Galen (AD130–200), Roman physician and author
with us: i.e. in Britain
viscous humors: sticky mucus
rheume: thin mucus
Dioscorides: Greek-speaking Roman physician (mid-first century AD)
greene: fresh
flux of humours: irregular flows of bodily liquids
stay: stop
whits or reds: white fluids or blood
running of reines: irregular urination
late experience: recent discovery
strayned: strained
holpen: helped
divers countries: various shires
burstings: hernias
availeable: beneficial
blew: blue
morphew: skin discolouration
dames: fashionable ladies

Polygonatum sive Sigillum Salomonis

The Vertues

Root: The roote of *Salomons* Seale is of chiefest use, and hath a mixt property as *Galen* saith, having partly a binding, and partly a sharpe or biting quality, as also a kinde of loathsome bitternesse therein, hardly to be expressed, whereby it is of little use in inward medecines; which sharpenesse and loathsomenesse we hardly perceive in those that grow with us: yet some authors doe affirme that the powder of the herbe or of the seede purgeth flegme and viscous humors very forcibly, both upward and downeward; it is said also that the roote chewed in the mouth draweth downe much rheume out of the head, and put up into the nostrills causeth sneesing:

Wounds & sores: but it serveth as he and *Dioscorides* both say, and all experience doth confirme, for wounds, hurts and outward sores, to heale and close up the lippes of those that are greene and fresh made, and to helpe to dry up the moisture and restraine the flux of humors of those that are old:

Vomiting, bleeding & fluxes: it is singular good to stay vomitings and also bleedings wheresoever, as also all fluxes in man or woman, whether it be the whits or reds, or the running of the reines in men;

Broken bones & dislocations: also to knit any joynt that doth grow by weaknesse, to be often out of place, or by some cause stayeth but small time therein when it is set; as also to knit and joyne broken bones in any place of the body; the roots being bruised and applyed to the place, yea it hath by late experience beene found that the decoction of the roote in wine, or the bruised roote put in wine or other drinke, and after a nights infusion strayned hard forth and drunke, hath holpen both man and beast whose bones have beene broken by any occasion, which is the most assured refuge of helpe to the people in divers countries of this Land, that they can have:

Ruptures & bruises: it is no lesse effectuall to helpe ruptures and burstings, to be both inwardly taken, the decoction in wine, or the powder in broth or drinke, and outwardly applyed to the place: the same also is availeable for inward or outward bruises, falls or beatings, both to dispell the congealed blood, and to take away both the paines and the blacke and blew markes that abide after the hurt:

Skin: the same also or the distilled water of the whole plant used to the face or other part of the skinne, clenseth it from morphew, freckles, spots or markes whatsoever, leaving the place fresh, faire and lovely, which the *Italian* dames as it is said doe much use.

Solomon's seal *Polygonatum multiflorum* Liliaceae

Parkinson describes 12 kinds of *Polygonatum*, and illustrates two in the woodcut opposite. The medicinal properties of the species are comparable, with *P. odoratum* and *P. biflorum* used most frequently today; the latter is found mainly in deciduous woods of the eastern and central states of the US. The False solomon's seal (*Maianthemum racemosum*) looks similar, inhabits the same North American habitats and even has similar uses; it has terminal flowers in a raceme and red berries, as against pendulous two-by-two flowers in the 'true' seal, and blue berries. Parkinson's account indicates a remarkable and forgotten plant.

Solomon's seal has often attracted champions who rescue it from neglect, though, as Parkinson notes, Galen had few good words to say for inward use of the roots. John Gerard contradicts Galen (and Dioscorides), writing in his *Herball* (1597) of the positive experience of 'the vulgar sort of people from Hampshire' who gather the root to add to ale for treating their musculo-skeletal woes. Gerard recommends the plant unreservedly, while Parkinson confirms it is 'the most assured refuge of helpe to the people' – to man or beast alike.

But after all his good words, Gerard blots his copybook when his misogynist side emerges: he says solomon's seal will heal bruises 'gotten by fals or women's wilfulness in stumbling on their hastie husband's fists'. Parkinson is more discreet: it 'is availeable for inward or outward bruises, falls or beatings'.

Contemporary American herbalists Matthew Wood and Jim McDonald make strong cases for restoring the plant to the top table. The root of solomon's seal in wine (Parkinson) or tincture (modern preference) is a major, if largely ignored, remedy for lubricating and knitting bones, cartilage and tendons. McDonald says the root has 'the remarkable ability to restore the proper tension to ligaments', while acting as a connective tissue anti-inflammatory. McDonald suggests a key indication for using the plant is inflammation alongside dryness.

It has only slightly less spectacular success with wounds, bleeding, ruptures and bruises, as Parkinson explains and modern practice confirms.

Interestingly, in both McDonald and Wood's practice small drop doses prove effective.

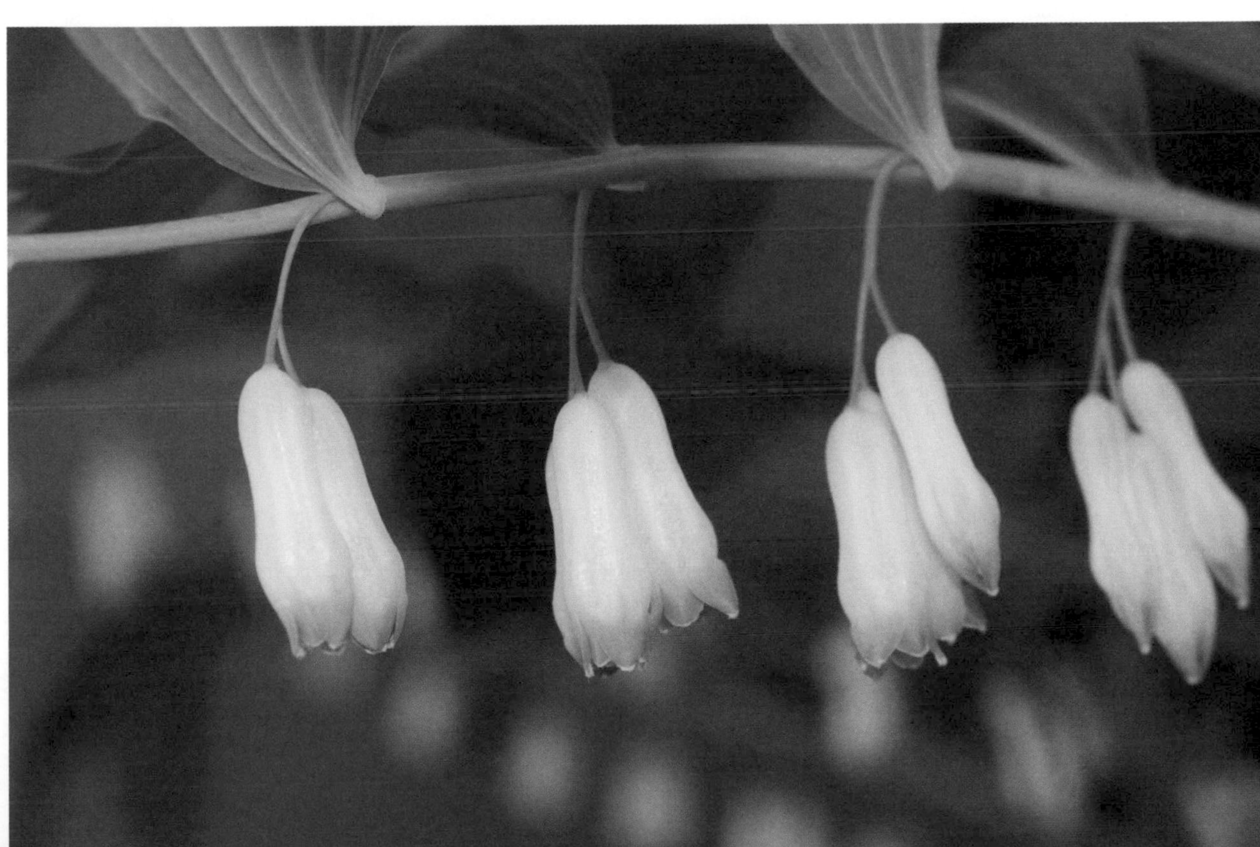

Sorrell or Soure Dock

Theatrum Botanicum

Tribe 6, Chapter 10, pp742–45

Acetosa

The Vertues

Sorrell is cooling and drying in the second degree, and is prevalent in all hot diseases to coole any inflammation and heate of bloud in agues pestilentiall or chollericke or other sicknesses and fainting, rising from heate, and to refresh the overspent spirits with the violence of furious or fiery fits of agues, &c, to quench thirst, and to procure an appetite in fainting or decaied stomackes; for it resisteth the purtrefaction of the bloud, killeth wormes,and is as a cordiall to the heart which the seede doth more effectually, being more drying and binding, and thereby also stayeth the hot fluxes of the menstrues, or of humours in the bloudy flixe, or fluxe of the stomacke:

agues pestillentiall: infectious fevers
cholericke: bilious
decaid stomackes: weak digestion
bloud: blood
cordiall: tonic
menstrues: menstruation
bloudy flixe: bloody dysentery
fluxe of the stomache: vomiting
jaundise: jaundice
raines: kidneys
blacke jaundise: leptospirosis
Fumiterrie: fumitory, *Fumaria officinalis*
soveraine helpe: effective remedy
frettings: sores
gallings: rubbed places
tetters: ringworm or eczema
discusse: disperse
scrophules or kernells: scrophula or swollen glands
Colewort: *Brassica oleracea*, wild cabbage or a cultivar
empostume: purulent abscess or swelling
botch: blemish
bile: boil

Roots: the rootes also in a decoction or in powder, is effectuall for the said purposes: both rootes and seede, as well as the herbe is held powerfull to resist the poison of the Scorpion, so that he that shall eate thereof shall feele no paine being stung: the decoction of the rootes is taken to helpe the jaundise, and to expell gravell, and the stone in the raines or kidneyes:

Decoction: the decoction of the flowers made with wine and drunke helpeth the blacke jaundise, as also the inward ulcers of the body or bowells.

Syrup: A Syrupe made with the juyce of Sorrell and Fumiterrie is a soveraine helpe to kill the sorce of those sharpe humours that cause the itch:

Juice: the juyce thereof with a little Vinegar, serveth well to use outwardly for the same cause, and is also profitable for frettings and gallings of the skin in any part, and for tetters, ringwormes, &c. it helpeth also to discusse the scrophules or kernells in the throate, and the juyce gargled in the mouth helpeth the sores therein: the leaves wrapped up in a Colewort leafe, and roasted under the embers, and applied to an hard empostume, botch, bile, or plague sore, both ripeneth and breaketh it:

Juice: the juyce of Sorrell dropped into the eares of such as are hard of hearing helpeth oftentimes: the distilled water of the herbe is of much good use for all the purposes aforesaid.

The lesser wilde Sorrell, and so all the other are of the same qualitie, and are no lesse effectuall in all the diseases before spoken of.

Acetosa vulgaris.
Our ordinary Sorrell.

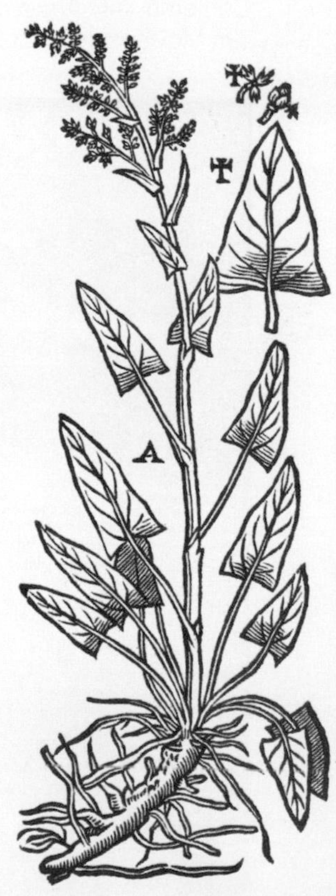

Sorrel *Rumex acetosa, R. acetosella, etc*

Polygonaceae

Sorrel is more used in cooking than in medicine today, but we can take inspiration from Parkinson's description of its many virtues and from its use around the world. It is rich in vitamin C, and is a cooling remedy for all sorts of hot conditions.

Parkinson's name of sour dock is accurate, in that sorrels are now classified as *Rumex* species, the same as the docks, and they are certainly sour. In Parkinson's time, lemons and other citrus were not always readily available, and sorrel was often used instead to give a lemony tang to dishes both sweet and savoury. He mentions 15 different kinds of sorrel, including the British buckler-leaved sorrel (*R. scutatus*) and sheep's sorrel (*R. acetosella*), and a large leaved sorrel of Germany, which is the kind most people grow in their gardens today.

John Evelyn, in his 1699 salad book *Acetaria* (pp42–3), describes sorrel as 'imparting so grateful a quickness to the rest, as supplies the want of *Orange*, *Limon* and other *Ompachia*, and therefore never to be excluded'. Wild sorrel is certainly one of our favourite and regular salad ingredients.

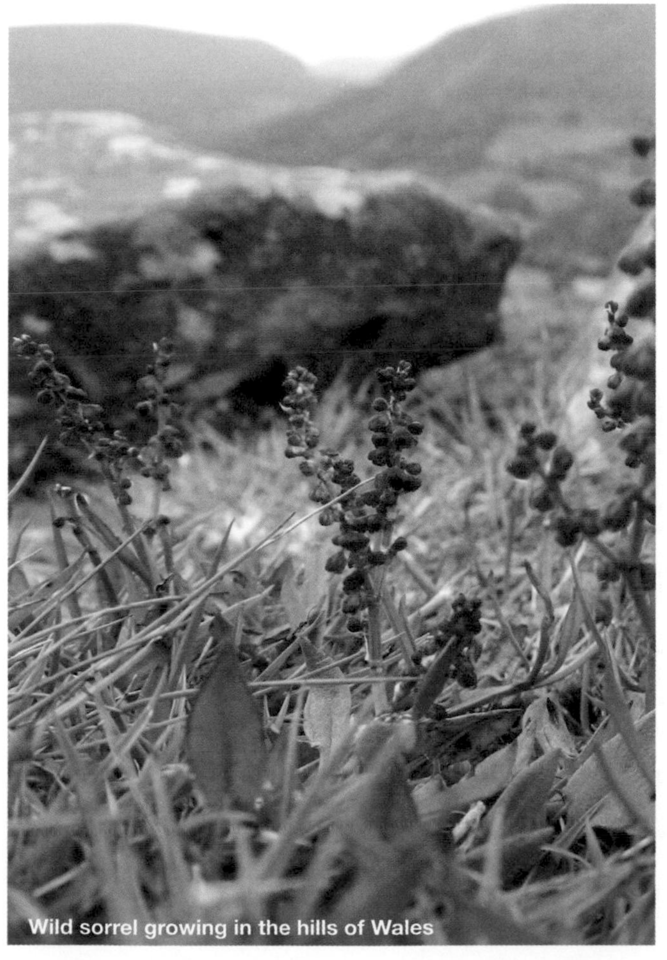

Wild sorrel growing in the hills of Wales

The lemony tang of sorrel is from oxalic acid, so the theoretical advice is to avoid eating large quantities if you have kidney stones, and yet sorrel has a traditon of use for kidney stones and other kidney and bladder complaints – another example of a whole plant differing in its action from isolated constituents. Parkinson suggests the decoction of the roots to expel gravel and stone from the urinary tract. It is also diuretic in its effect.

Inflammation: Parkinson recommends the cooling action of sorrel for fevers, inflammation and other hot conditions. A poultice of the roast leaves is used to soften and draw boils and swellings.

Thirst: Sorrel can be made into a kind of lemonade to quench the thirst.

Appetite: Sorrel sharpens the appetite, especially useful after a fever or long illness that has left the digestion weak.

Skin complaints: The juice, especially mixed with vinegar, is an effective folk treatment for ringworm, a fungal skin infection. It is also a good mouthwash to gargle for sore throats.

Sorrel is high in vitamin C and has been used successfully to treat scurvy. It is considered an alterative, or herb that gently returns one to normal health.

Maurice Mességué, a French herbalist writing in the 1970s, used sorrel for all the things Parkinson mentions, and found it good for blockages in the stomach or intestines.

Sheep's sorrel, *R. acetosella*, is an ingredient of the famous Essiac formula.

St John's Wort

Theatrum Botanicum

Tribe 5, Chapter 50, pp572–74

1. *Hypericum vulgare.*
Ordinary S. *Iohns* wort.

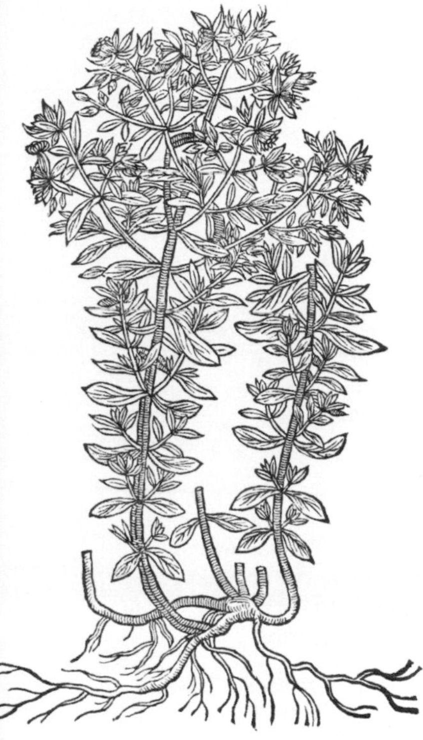

subtill: subtle
soder: hold together
Knotgrasse: *Polygonum* species
womens courses: menstruation
pouder: powder
mesentery veines: veins that drain blood from the intestines
fits of agues: fever or shivering
tertians: occurring every second day
quartaines: occurring every four days
Falling sicknesse: epilepsy
Palsie: paralysis and tremors
greene wounds: fresh wounds
oyle Ollive: olive oil
Balneo: kettle, double boiler

Hypericum

The Vertues

S. *Iohns* wort is as singular a wound herbe as any other whatsoever, eyther for inward wounds, hurts or bruises, to be boyled in wine and drunke, or prepared into oyle or oyntment, bathe or lotion outwardly, for being of an hot and drying quality, with subtill parts, it hath power to open obstructions, to dissolve tumours, to consolidate or soder the lips of wounds, and to strengthen the parts that are weake and feeble;

Injuries: the decoction of the herbe and flowers, but of the seed especially in wine, being drunke, or the seed made into pouder and drunk with the juice of Knotgrasse, helpeth all manner of spitting and vomiting of blood, bee it by any veine broken inwardly, by bruises, falls or howsoever: the same also helpeth all those that are bitten or stunge by any venemous creature:

Urinary & gynaecological: And is good for those that are troubled with the stone in their kidneys, or cannot make water, and being applyed provoketh womens courses:

Seed & leaves: two drams of the seede made into pouder, and drunk in a little broth, doth gently expell choller, or congealed blood in the stomack, and mesentery veines; the decoction of the leaves and seeds being drunk somewhat warme before the fits of agues, whether they be *tertians* or *quartaines,* doth helpe to alter the fits, and by often using taketh them quite away; the seede is much commended being drunke for 40. dayes together, to helpe the Sciatica or Hippe Goute, Falling sicknesse and Palsie also.

Distilled wine: The herbe, that is, both the leaves, flowers and seede, steeped in wine for 12. houres, and then distilled in an ordinary Still, the water hereof being drunke with a little Sugar therein, is accounted as effectuall as any decoction or other preparation, and killeth the wormes in the belly or stomacke.

Oil: The oyle of S. *Iohns* wort, eyther simple or compound, but the compound is more effectuall, is singular good both for all greene wounds, and old sores & ulcers, in the legs or else where, that are hard to be cured, and is effectuall also for crampes and aches in the joynts, and paines in the veines and sinewes, and is also good for all burnings by fire, to be presently used, or the juice of the green leaves applyed;

Powder: the hearbe dryed and made into pouder, is as effectuall for wounds and sores to be strowed thereon, as the oyle or juice.

An infused oil: The simple oyle is made of foure ounces of the flowers infused in a pint of oyle Ollive, called Sallet oyle, and three ounces of white wine, for 10. or 12. dayes to bee set in the Sunne, and afterwards boyled in a *Balneo* or Kettle of seething water, strayned forth, and refreshed with new flowers, so set in the Sunne, and in the same manner boyled, strained forth and renewed the third time

St John's wort *Hypericum perforatum* Hypericaceae

Today, most people think of St John's wort primarily as a herb for depression, but it is so much more than that. It is a wonderful liver herb, and was valued for thousands of years as a premier wound herb. Parkinson calls it 'as singular a wounde herbe as any other whatsoever'. St John's wort is also nervine, pain-relieving and antiviral.

Parkinson's first few lines summarize the uses of St John's wort as a hot, drying, opening and strengthening herb.

Injuries & wounds: St John's wort is used today to treat puncture wounds, cuts and bruises, and has the additional benefit of speeding up the healing of surgical scars. This is referred to by Parkinson as 'to consolidate or soder the lippes of wounds'.

Seed: From medieval times into Parkinson's era, the seed of St John's wort – rarely considered today – was used to treat a wide range of ailments. St John's wort seeds have been found in archaeological digs at Soutra Aisle, Scotland's largest medieval hospital. From Parkinson's account, it appears that the effects of the seed are stronger than that of the flowers and leaves, as one would expect.

Urinary & gynaecological: Parkinson says the plant is powerful enough to dissolve stones and indeed tumours, and is stimulant enough to restart the menstrual cycle.

Bites & stings: St John's wort is still used for animal bites. Through its action on the liver, it helps eliminate poisons from the body.

Distilled wine: We made Parkinson's distilled St John's wort wine, and certainly have not suffered from worms in the belly since!

Infused oil: St John's wort oil, infused in the sun, is still a major herbal remedy. It is great for achey muscles, backache, painful joints, neuropathy, neuralgia, arthritis, scars, bruises and sprains. Parkinson's triple method is 'singular good' but calls for considerable patience in the medicine-maker. Gerard's method is still painstaking but takes less time, while the mixed compound oil (with earthworms) sounds a potent preparation.

As Parkinson says, the oil can be used for burns, and also for soothing sunburn. While taking St John's wort internally can make people more sensitive to sunlight, applying the oil externally provides some protection against the sun's rays.

The oil is also one of the best external remedies for shingles, being pain-relieving and specifically helping the healing of nerve endings; we now know it also brings antiviral benefits into its healing pattern.

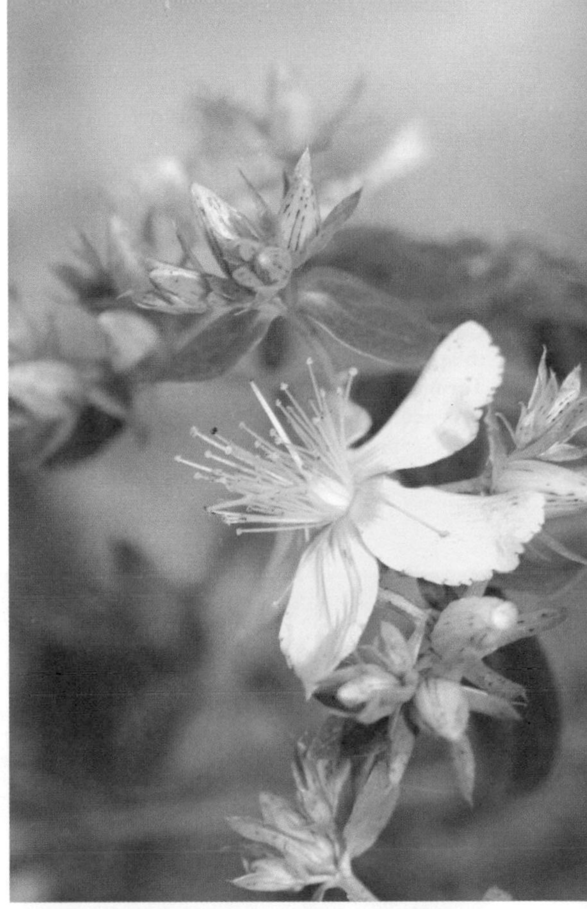

Modern uses of St John's wort

Depression: St John's wort has been the subject of much research, and is recognized as an effective treatment for mild to moderate depression. It is also helpful for the winter blues and SAD (Seasonal Affective Disorder).

Homeopathy: As Hypericum it is the best homeopathic first aid remedy for nerve pain. It was used in the Second World War for gunshot wounds and is prescribed for puncture wounds.

Other: St John's wort is used for post-operative pain and neuralgia, and can help protect against radiation.

turpentine: oleoresin from terebinth tree, *Pistacia terebinthus*, or from pine trees
Gerard: John Gerard (1545–1612) barber-surgeon, gardener and author
Sallet oyle: olive oil
oyle of Turpentine: distilled turpentine resin
Dittanie of Candy: dittany of Crete, *Origanum dictamnus*
Gentian or Felwort: *Gentianella amarella*
Cardus Benedictus or Blessed thistle: *Centaurea benedicta*
Tormentill: *Potentilla erecta*
strayned: strained
close stopped: sealed

with fresh flowers, which after they have lastly stood in the Sunne a fortnight or more, are to be boyled in the sayd *Balneo* or Kettle of seething water, strayned forth, and the oyle, having some fine turpentine dissolved in it whiles it is hot, and so kept, is singular good for the purposes aforesayd.

Gerard's oil: Like hereunto *Gerard* hath set downe a way, which is, with Sallet oyle two parts, white wine and oyle of Turpentine one part, set in the Sunne, with the leaves, flowers and seedes of S. *Iohns* wort, for 8. or 10. dayes, and boyled and renewed the third time, in the manner aforesayd.

Compound oil with earthworms: But the compound oyle is made of the simple oyle, after the last infusion being strained forth, there is added, *Dittanie* of Candy, *Gentian* or Felwort, *Cardus Benedictus*, or Blessed thistle, and *Tormentill* of each a small quantitie, and some earth wormes washed and slit, and all of them infused in the sayd oyle, and set in the Sunne, and after boyled, strayned forth, and Turpentine and oyle of Wormewood put thereto, which then is to bee reserved in some pot, or glasse close stopped, to be used as occasion doth require.

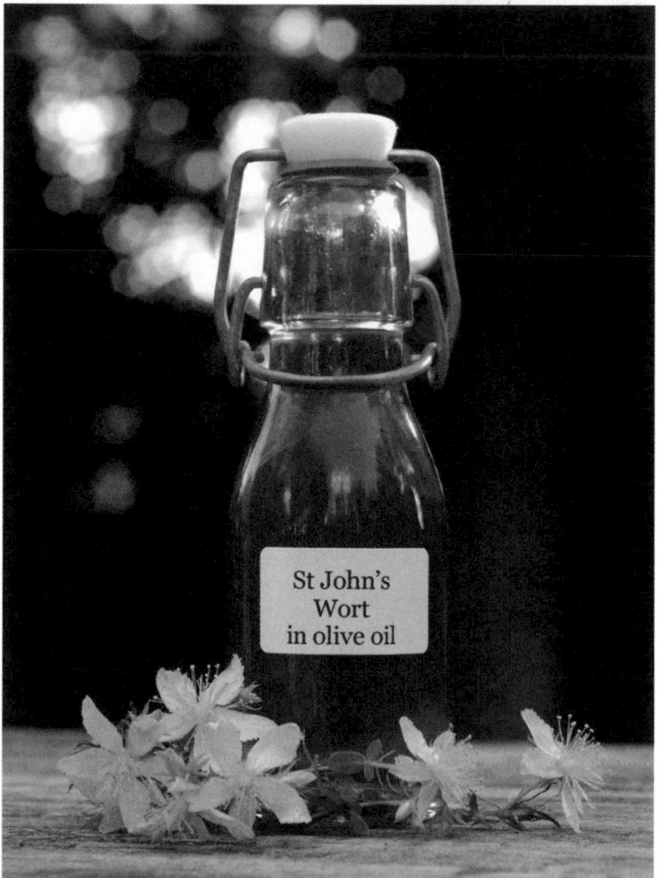

Earthworms: This is the only recipe in all of Parkinson's 'vertues' we have read so far that uses earthworms, but they were a popular ingredient in medicines of his time.

Culpeper's *Pharmacopoeia Londinensis*, his 1649 English translation of the official Latin list of medicines prescribed by doctors and made up by apothecaries, specifies living creatures, their parts and excrements, that were recognized and approved medicines. Examples include sparrow's brain, crab's eyes, duck's liver, elk's claws, frog's liver, man's skull and unicorn's horn. Earthworms were in good company.

A recipe by Dr Richard Mead (Physician to St Thomas's Hospital, London) for snail water appeared in *Pharmacopoeia Pauperum* in 1718. This is a distillation of earthworms, snails, and nine different herbs and spices in water and wine. An interesting source of further earthworm herbal lore is the Old Operating Theatre and Herb Garret, St Thomas's Hospital, London.

Caution: St John's wort can weaken the effects of many prescription medicines, and should not be taken if you are already using antidepressants. It can cause sensitivity to sunlight, in cattle as well as humans.

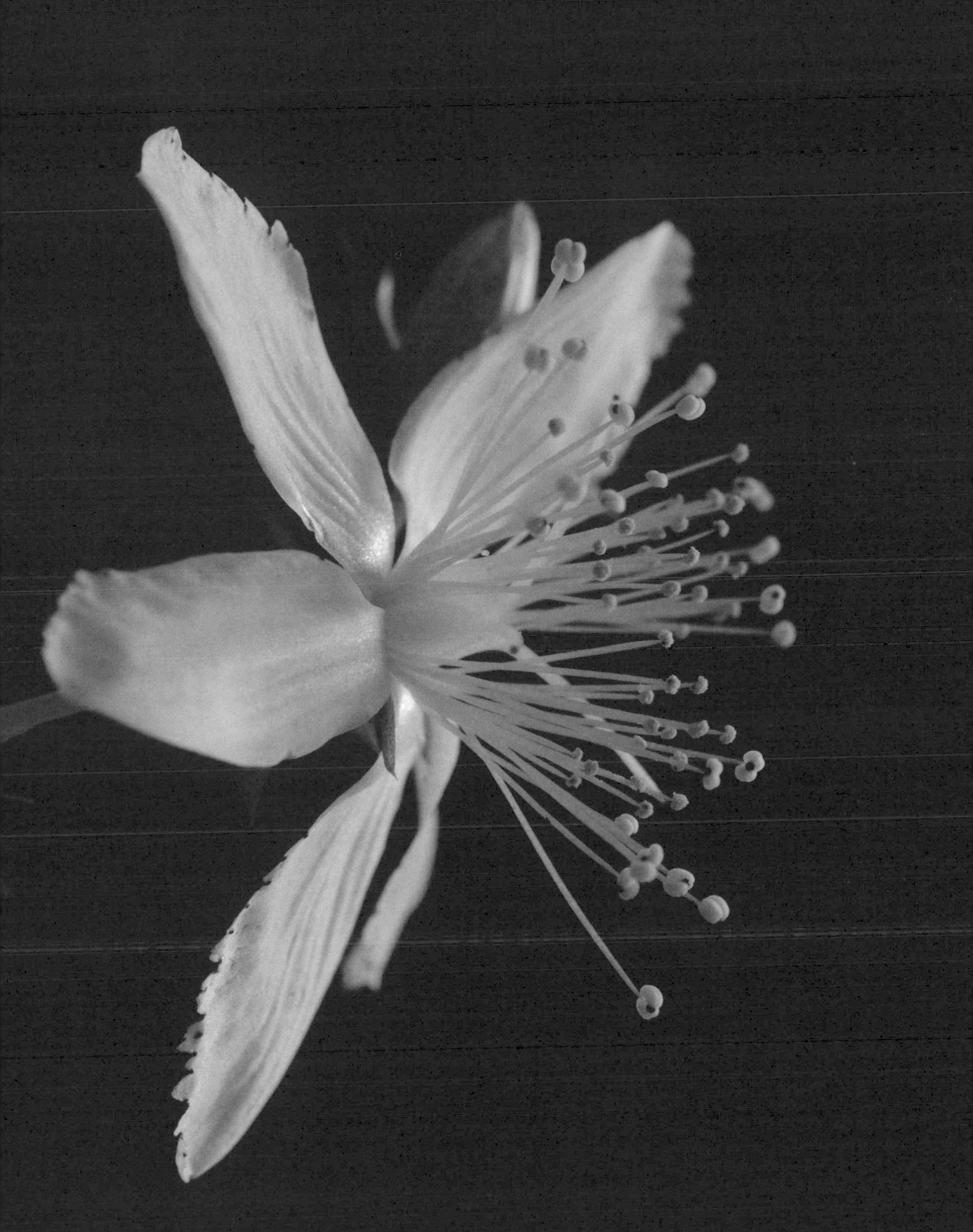

Strawberries

Theatrum Botanicum

Tribe 6, Chapter 16, pp757–59

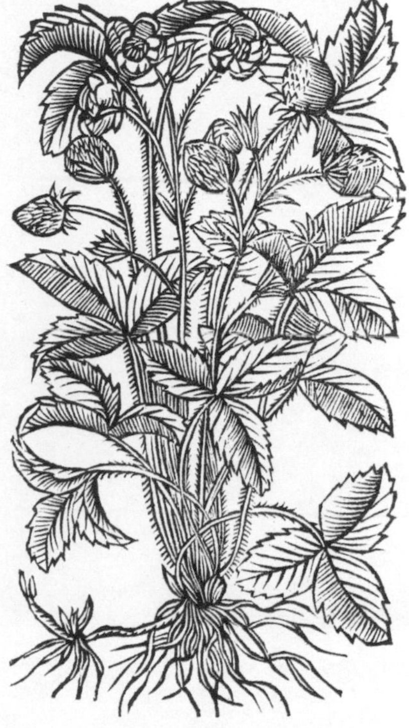

Fragaria

The Vertues

These Strawberries that are here set forth and fit to be eaten, are of the same qualitie with the other garden kinds expressed in my former Booke, the leaves of them all being cooling in the first degree, and yet some say hot and drying in the second, the roote is more drying and binding, the berries while they are greene are cold and drie, but when they are ripe they are cold and moist:

Berries: the berries are excellent good to coole the liver, the bloud and spleene, or an hot chollericke stomacke to refresh and comfort the fainting spirits, and to quench thirst: they are good also for other inflammations, yet it behoveth one to be cautelous, or rather to restraine them in a fever, least by their putrefying in the stomacke, they encrease the fits and cause them to be the more fierce:

Leaves & roots: the leaves and rootes boiled in wine and water and drunke, doe likewise coole the liver and bloud, and asswage all inflammations in the raines and bladder, provoketh urine, and allaieth the heate and sharpenesse thereof: the same also being drunke staeith the bloudy flixe and womens courses, and helpeth the swellings of the the spleene:

Distilled water & juice: the water of the berries carefully distilled, is a soveraigne remedy and cordiall in the palpitations of the heart, that is, the panting and beating of the heart, and is good for the overflowing of the gall, the yellow jaundise; the juyce dropped into foule ulcers, or they washed therewith or with the decoction of the herbe and roote, doth wonderfully clense them and helpe to cure them.

Leaves & roots again: All lotions and gargles that are made for sore mouthes or ulcers therein, or in the privie parts, or else where are made with the leaves and rootes hereof, which is good also to fasten loose teeth, and to heale spungie foule gummes: the same also helpeth to stay catarrhes or defluxions of rheume into the mouth, throate, teeth or eyes: the juyce or water is singuler good for hot and inflamed eyes, if some thereof be dropped into them, or they bathed therewith, the said juyce or water is also of excellent propertie for all pushes, wheales, and other eruptions of hot and sharpe humours into the face or hands, or other parts of the body to bath them therewith, and helpeth to take away any rednesse in the face, and spots or other deformities of the skinne, and to make the skin cleare and smooth: some use thereof to make a water for hot inflammations in the eyes, and to take away any filme or skin that beginneth to grow over them, or other defects in them that any outward medicine can helpe in this manner:

Recipe: Take what quantitie of Strawberries you please, and put them

former Booke: i.e. the *Paradisi* (1629)
drying and binding: astringent
hot chollericke: overheated
behoveth one to be cautelous: it is wise to be cautious
fits: chills of a fever
asswage: moderate
raines: kidneys
allaieth: cools
staeith the bloudy flixe: stops bloody diarrhoea
courses: menses
soveraigne: superior
cordiall: medicinal for the heart
defluxions of rheume: dripping of mucus
pushes, weales: skin eruptions
hot and sharpe humours: thin, hot phlegm

Strawberry *Fragaria vesca, F. spp.*

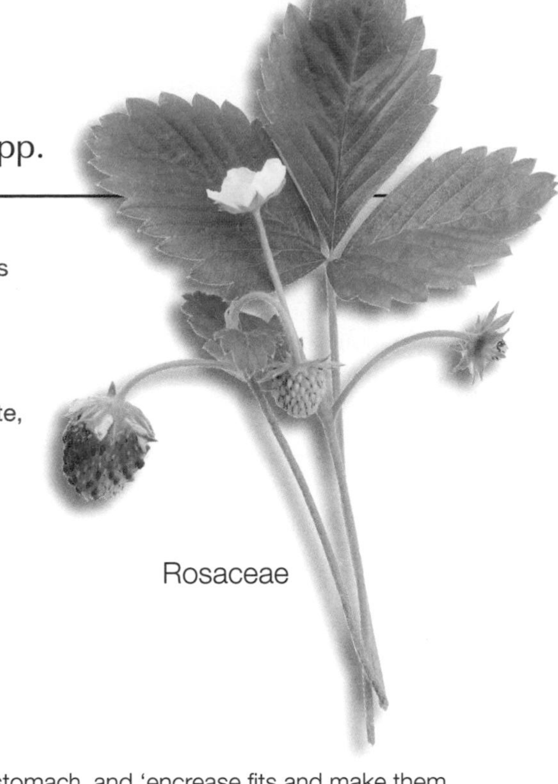

Rosaceae

Strawberries as we know them did not exist in Parkinson's time, when wild woodland strawberries were transplanted into gardens to grow. Modern strawberries are a cross made in Europe in the mid-1750s between two New World strawberries, *Fragaria chiloensis* and *F. virginiana*, to create our 'strawberry', *F. x ananassa*. The European wild or woodland strawberry, *F. vesca*, might be small, but the flavour and aroma of the fruit are exquisite, and repay the effort in gathering.

It is worth repeating that Parkinson is describing the wild strawberry, and would have been unhappy to see what we commonly call strawberry now. But we can still find and transplant wild strawberries into our gardens, as he did, and use them herbally – it surely is the most welcome weed of all. Buying the organic fruit is the next best option, and even if it sounds counter-intuitive, you will need some supply of strawberry leaves for your herbal medicine-making.

The fruit: For all that Parkinson wishes to say about the medicinal benefits of strawberry, he starts with those that 'are fit to be eaten'.

He writes in the *Paradisi* in 1629 that the berries, as he terms the fruit, are eaten at table, 'whereunto claret wine, creame or milke is added with sugar, as every one liketh'. They make 'a good cooling and pleasant dish in the hot Summer season' (p528).

This is not quite the enthusiasm for strawberries expressed by Dr William Butler (1535–1618), royal physician to James I and a contemporary Parkinson must have known. Butler is reported as saying: 'Doubtless God may have made a better berry, but doubtless God never did.'

But Parkinson in the *Theatrum* is eager to get to the medicinal value of the berries, which he says are cold and dry when green but cold and moist when ripe. It is this cooling quality he picks up on, describing the fruit as 'excellent good' to cool the liver, blood and spleen or a hot, choleric stomach and to quench the thirst.

In modern terms, strawberry is diuretic, laxative, detoxicant and nutritive. Its core area of action is the digestive and urinary systems, where it is both nutritive as well as potentially laxative. As a diuretic, it has been used to good effect to settle gout and arthritis. The great Linnaeus, for example, undertook strawberry fasts for his gout and started a trend in the second half of the 18th century.

It is also true that overeating the fruit can lead to constipation and discomfort for some, though the danger Parkinson mentions that in a fever an excess of the fruit will putrefy in the stomach, and 'encrease fits and make them more fierce', is less likely today.

The juice: Strawberry juice was used more herbally in Parkinson's time than currently, and his suggestion of the juice or distilled water to treat or wash 'foule ulcers', and for hot, inflamed eyes, could repay further investigation. Its use for a 'filme or skin that beginneth to grow over them' and more serious eye conditions is untested.

On the other hand, using the juice externally for treating sunburn, skin blemishes and for removing tartar from teeth were and remain good home remedies. Strawberry juice has been a handy cosmetic rouge for many fair-skinned ladies at various times in northern Europe. Note, though, that some people develop an allergic reaction, such as urticaria, when using strawberry juice on the skin.

The juice can also be made into strawberry wine or cordial, the favourite drink of the adventurer Sir Walter Raleigh, and many of the early settlers travelling across North America. The French *grande dame*, Madame Tallien (1773–1835), went further: she was said to have 10 kg (22 lb) a time of fresh strawberry juice in her bath, though we are told she did not bathe daily. More prosaically, the juice is the basis of a delicious fruit leather.

into a brasse vessell, and with a little salt cast upon them, which being covered, set into a wine cellar for eight dayes, in which time the berries will be dissolved into a greene water, which being cleared from the rest, keepe in a glasse close stopped to use when you neede: a droppe or two put into the eyes serveth for the purpose aforesaid:

greene water: greenish fluid
cleared from the rest: separated
close stopped: sealed
morphew: discoloration of skin
leprey: a form of leprosy
large destillatory or body of glasse: large still or similar glass arrangement

Another recipe: some in misliking both salt and brasse for the eyes, make a water both for the eyes and for the deformities in the skinne, be it morphew, leprey, or the like in this manner: Into a large destillatory or body of glasse, they put so many Strawberries as they thinke meete for their use, if a few, the lesser glasse body will serve, which being well closed, let it be set in a bed of hot horse dung for twelve or fourteene dayes, and after distilled carefully and the water kept for your use.

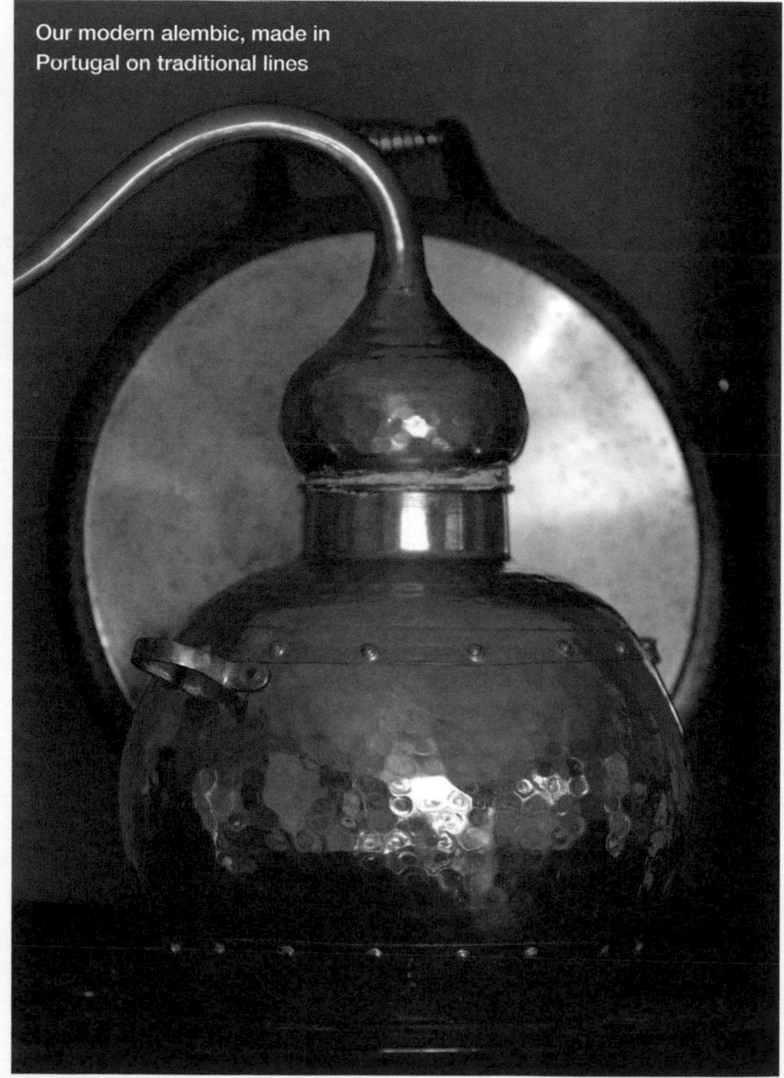

Our modern alembic, made in Portugal on traditional lines

Wild v cultivated: no contest

For a true believer sounding off on this unequal comparison, look no further than French herbalist Maurice Mességué: 'Now I am not going to talk about the cultivated strawberry, selected, sterilised, manipulated, de-natured, stuffed up with chemical fertilisers and insecticides, that comes to us from the Cape in the winter months and that has no flavour to it except a vague sort of sweetness.' The wild strawberry, by contrast, he says, is 'sweet and delicious'; it is 'a blood-red jewel in the enchanted woodlands of the lovely month of May'. *The Health Secrets of Plants and Herbs* (London, 1979), p268

The leaves: Strawberry leaves are the most used herbal form, often as a tea. The qualities are similar to those of other parts of the plant and to those of raspberry or blackberry leaves. The slight astringency makes the tea an excellent remedy for diarrhoea, and the bitterness acts as a tonic and appetiser.

Parkinson recommends the leaves and roots cooked in wine or water to cool the liver and blood, assuage inflammations of the kidneys and bladder, and provoke urine, as well as stop dysentery or undue menstruation. In his terms he is describing the range of diuretic action strawberry tea can offer. A modern insight would be that strawberry is strongly alkaline and reduces the over-acidity that can lead to stones and tartar build-up, and urinary tract inflammation.

Michael Moore, the American herbalist, writes in *Medicinal Plants of the Mountain West* (Santa Fe, 1979, p150) about using the leaves for sore gums: 'I met a Scottish gentleman on one occasion who placed the fresh leaves under his dentures whenever his gums were inflamed and sore.'

The roots: Parkinson notes that the root is more drying and binding than other parts of the plant. It makes a stronger diarrhoea and dysentery treatment when this is necessary, and it helps to settle internal bleeding. Parkinson mixed it with the leaves for lotions and gargles to bind loose teeth and to dry up catarrh and 'defluxions of rheume'. These uses might be revisited as home remedies, though few may initially think of growing and harvesting strawberry for its roots.

Distilled water: Parkinson specifies this as the best remedy for palpitations and jaundice. We have not had occasion to test this on ourselves or others, but we did two distillations of strawberries, using large modern ones as we couldn't collect enough wild strawberries. One was a straight water distillation of fresh berries, and for the other we adapted Parkinson's second recipe. Instead of hot horse dung we went for the modern equivalent of an airing or warming cupboard to keep the crushed berries warm and fermenting for a week. Both distillates had and retain a wonderful aroma of fresh strawberries, but did not differ much in quality.

We should admit that one of the waters went mouldy, because the glass vessel we used was not perfectly sterile. Learn from our mistake, and check your equipment carefully. You don't have the alcohol of a tincture here to cover up your mistakes!

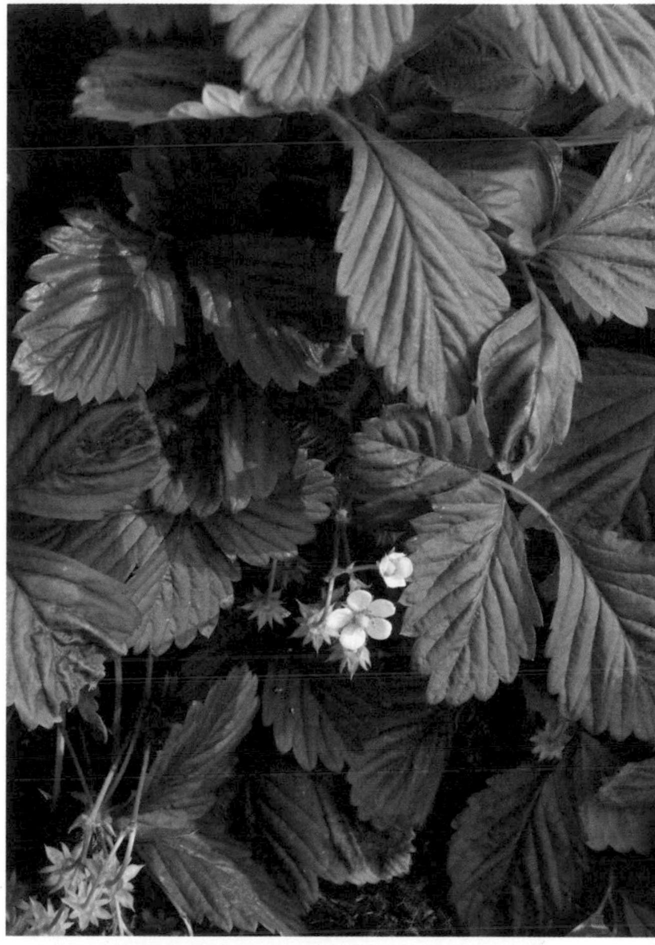

A gardener who earned Parkinson's praise

Parkinson, as a compulsive gardener, was highly competitive, but, like the best gardeners, he would recognize a fellow grower's success. In the *Paradisi* (p528) he talks of the Bohemia strawberry, which he names *Fraga Bohemia maxima*, as 'the goodliest and greatest' variety. Some of its berries 'have beene measured to bee neere five inches about'. He writes how the 'industrious' Flemish immigrant 'Master Vincent Sion', who 'dwelt on the Banke' side, had been given some roots, and in 18 months planted half an acre with 'the increase from them, besides those he gave away to his friends'. Parkinson saw this for himself. He also obtained one of his beloved double daffodils from Sion, but for all its promise the Bohemia strawberry disappeared.

Tyme

Theatrum Botanicum

Tribe 1, Chapter 3, pp6–9

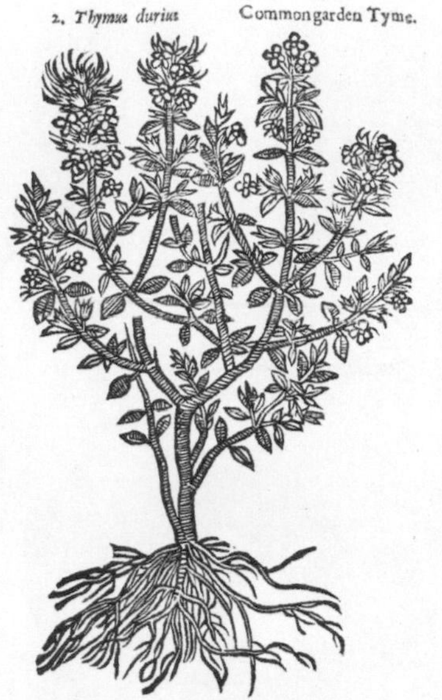

Thymum & Serpillum

Vertues

Phlegm & breath: The true Tyme, or in the want thereof our garden Tyme, (as nearest thereunto, although not altogether so effectuall) doth helpe somewhat to purge flegme, if as *Dioscorides* saith, it be taken with hony salt and vinegar: the decoction thereof is good for those, that are troubled with shortnes or straightnesse of breath:

Menstruation & birth: it killeth the wormes in the belly, procureth the monethly courses of women, expelleth the secondine or afterbirth, after it hath holpen the delivery of the child, & causeth easie expectorations of tough flegme, being taken with hony in an Electuary;

Tumours & warts: it dissolveth tumours or swellings when they are fresh; the juyce thereof being annoynted or bathed on the place with some vinegar, taketh away loose or hanging warts:

Sciatica, eyesight & wind: it helpeth those that have the Sciatica, applyed with wine and meale: it helpeth those that are dull sighted, and is of good use in meates and brothes, to warme and comfort the stomacke, and to helpe to breake winde as well for the sicke as the sound. *Galen* saith the same things almost.

Gout & swellings: It is found by experience saith *Ætius,* that if 4. dragmes of dried Tyme in powther, be given in Oxymel fasting, to them that have the gowte it helpeth them, for it purgeth choller and other sharpe humours, and that if one dragme thereof bee given fasting with meade, it dissolveth the hard swellings of the belly:

Other swellings: It is profitable for those that have swellings in their sides, and paines in their loynes and hippes: it is likewise given fasting to those that have great paines in their eyes, and are bleare-eyed: it is with wine applyed to the cods that are swollen.

Mother of thyme: Wild Tyme or Mother of Tyme if it be boyled and drunke, moveth urine, and the monethly courses, helpeth such as have griping paines in the belly, or that have cramps, or are bursten bellied, or are troubled with inflamation of the liver:

For the head: being taken inwardly, or applyed outwardly with Rosemary and vinegar to the head, it ceaseth the paines thereof, and is very helpefull to those, that are troubled with either Frensye or Lethargy: four dragmes of the juyce drunke with a little vinegar, is very availeable to those that spitt or vomit blood: taken with hony, licoris and aniseede in wine, it helpeth a dry cough, and is comfortable both to the head, stomacke and reines, and helpeth to expell winde:

For the head again: the distilled water therof applyed with vinegar of Roses to the forehead, easeth the rage of Frensye, & expelleth Vertigo that is the swimming or turning of the braine, & helpeth to breake the stone in the bladder.

Dioscorides: Greek-speaking Roman physician (mid-first century AD)
shortnes or straightnesse: shortness of breath, tightness of chest
procureth the monethly courses: restarts menstruation
holpen: assists in
Electuary: herb powder in honey
annoynted: rubbed
meale: coarse-ground grain
Galen: Claudius Galen (AD130–200), Roman physician and author
Ætius: Aetius of Antioch, 4th century theologian and doctor
four dragmes: four drams, ½ ounce
Oxymel fasting: powder, taken in honey and vinegar, while not eating
meade: mead, honey drink
profitable: effective
loynes, hippes: thighs, hips
cods: male genitalia
Mother of tyme: wild or creeping thyme, *Thymus serpyllum*
bursten bellied: hernia of stomach
Frensye: over-activity
Lethargy: under-activity
availeable: absorbed easily
comfortable: acceptable
reines: kidneys

Thyme *Thymus polytrichus* Lamiaceae

Parkinson's text expresses an understanding of thyme that has been almost lost: the fact that it is such a powerful remedy, 'deeply dredging the system, opening it up so that heat and toxins can be removed and thinning phlegm' (the words of contemporary American herbalist Matthew Wood, In *The Earthwise Herbal*, Berkeley, 2008, p483). While thymol or oil of thyme is often preferred today for treating 'deep' issues, Parkinson can be read to remind us how effective the plant itself is for infections and inflammations of the respiratory and digestive tracts, and much more.

Thymes are notorious for their many chemotypes and for promiscuous hybridization, meaning that the chemistry of the plant and its oil can vary markedly. It is indicative that Parkinson in *Paradisi* describes a garden wild thyme! For the present let us generalize that the more 'wild' and 'Mediterranean' the thyme, the more aromatic, heating and powerful it will be; conversely, the more hybridized, cultivated and cool the origin (as in *T. vulgaris*, garden thyme, or *T. x citridorus*, lemon thyme) the less pronounced the effects.

The old Greek name for thyme was *thumon*, meaning either (or both) courage or cleansing, depending on translation. The cleansing aspect is found in the use of thyme in ancient Egyptian and Etruscan mummification, in medieval plague remedies and for its **antiseptic properties**. In ancient Greece dried thyme was burned as a fumigant smoke, to keep away insects, and later was an inhalation for sinusitis.

Thyme's antiseptic role was confirmed in 19th century research showing it boosted immunity to infections like anthrax, typhoid and diphtheria. A syrup from dried thyme is a soothing gargle, and cooled thyme tea helps diseased gums.

Thyme is best known, perhaps, as a **respiratory** herb, which improves expectoration ('purges phlegm') and relieves coughs, especially dry ones. It was a specific antispasmodic for whooping-cough, after Parkinson's time, but he knew the decoction as helpful for asthmatic-type breathing issues.

It is equally a **digestive** herb, which warms and dries the gastrointestinal tract, soothing colic, indigestion and irritable bowel; it is good for children's diarrhoea. It is also a herb for **nervous relaxation**, and the tea or syrup are excellent remedies for stress, headaches, depression and poor sleep.

Another area of its action is **uterine**, regularizing menstruation, and, as Parkinson explained, even helping expel the afterbirth. In Ayurveda, the ancient herbal tradition of India, thyme is an important aphrodisiac. As an **anti-inflammatory**, thyme reduces various swellings, as Parkinson explains.

Finally, in an area unidentified in Parkinson's era, thyme is an **immune-supporting** herb, with known affinity with the lymphatic system, spleen and thymus gland.

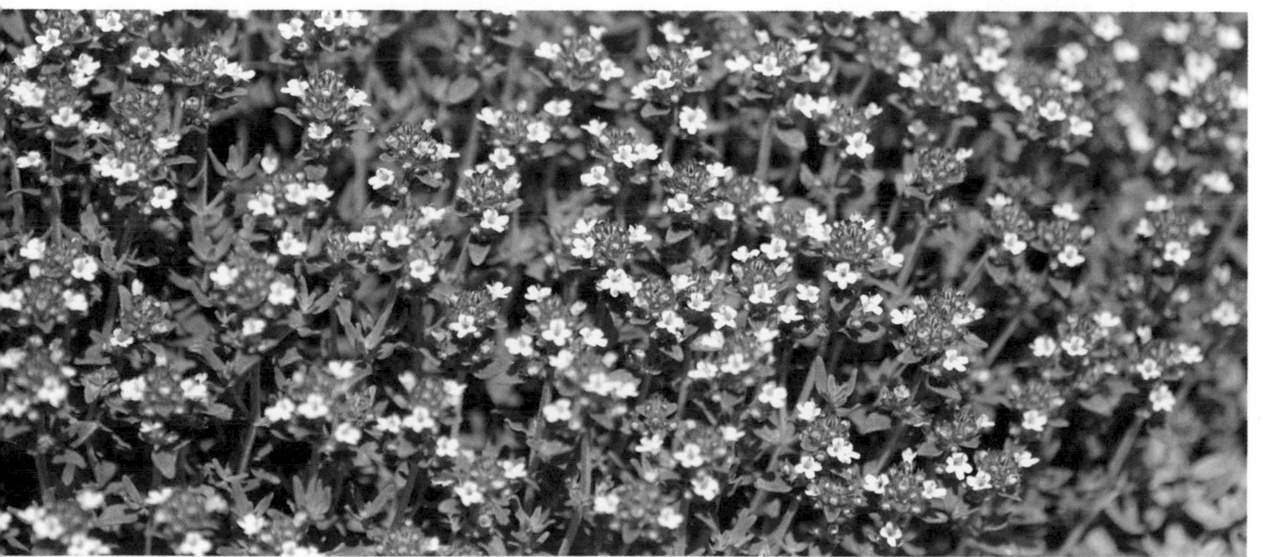

English Tobacco

Theatrum Botanicum

Tribe 5, Chapter 109, pp711–12

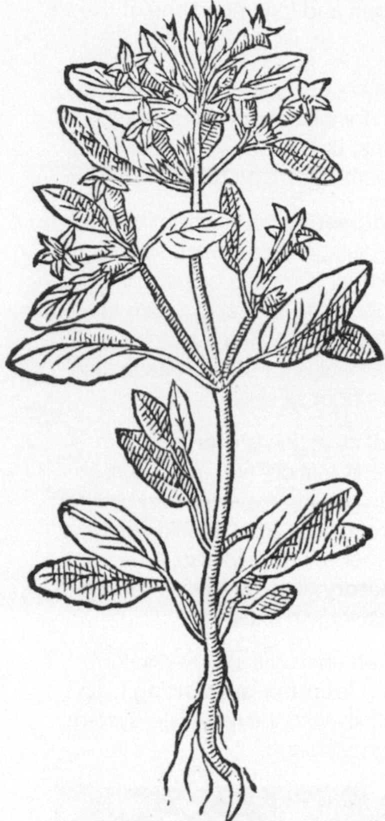

Tabacco Anglicum

The Vertues

This kind of Tabacco although it be not thought so strong, or sweete for such as take it by the pipe, (and yet I have knowne Sr. *Walter Raleigh*, when he was prisoner in the Tower, make choice of this sort to make good Tobacco of, which he knew so rightly to cure as they call it, that it was held almost as good as that which came from the *Indies*, and fully as good as any other made in *England*:) nor yet so effectuall for inward diseases, because it is not so much used as the other,

yet it is availeable by good experience for to expecterate tough flegme out of the stomacke, chest and lungs, that doth offend them: the juice thereof being made into a Syrupe, or the distilled water of the herbe drunke with some Sugar, or without as one will, or else the smoake taken by a pipe as is usuall, but fasting. The same also helpeth to expell wormes in the stomacke and belly, as also to apply a leafe to the belly, and to ease the paines of the head, or the Megrime, and the griping paines in the bowells, although to some it may seeme, to bring or cause more trouble in the stomacke and bowells for a time:

Kidney stone: it is also profitable for those that are troubled with the stone in the kidneyes, both to ease paines, and by provoking urine to expell gravell and the stone engendred therein, of that viscous matter, and to heale the parts;

Uterus: and hath beene found very effectuall to suppresse the malignitie and expell the windy and other offensive matters, which cause the strangling of the mother:

Mouth: the seede hereof is much more effectuall to ease the paines of the toothach, then any Henbane seede, and the ashes of the burnt herbe to clense the gummes and teeth and make them white:

Contra-indications: it hath beene thought not to have beene safe for weake bodies and constitutions, nor for old men, but of both sorts I have seene the experience that it hath bin profitable being taken in a due manner, that is fasting, and to bed ward and before meate. *Thevet* saith that the Women in *America* forbeare the taking of Tobacco, because that they have beene taught that it will hinder conception and bodily lust:

Scrofula & dropsie: the herbe bruised and applyed to the place of the Kings Evill, helpeth it in nine or ten dayes effectually: it is said also to bee effectuall to cure the dropsie, by taking foure or five ounces of the juice fasting, which will strongly purge the body both upwards and downewards.

Sr. Walter Raleigh: the adventurer, courtier and spy (1552–1618); Parkinson had visited him in prison
availeable: beneficial
expecterate tough flegme: cough up thick, sticky phlegm
offend: distress
megrime: migraine
gravell: small calcified crystals
strangling of the mother: constriction of the womb
Henbane: *Hyoscyamus niger*
Thevet: André de Thevet (1516–90), French priest, explorer and writer
Kings Evill: scrofula
dropsie: oedema

Tobacco *Nicotiana rustica*

Solanaceae

This species of tobacco is often referred to as wild tobacco, and is still used by native Americans as a sacred and medicinal herb. Today, most cigars and cigarettes are made from the large-leaved *Nicotiana tabacum*, but in India and Indonesia *N. rustica* is still used for cigarettes. *N. rustica* generally has much higher levels of the alkaloid nicotine, though the chemistry of the plant varies with growing conditions. It is a soft fuzzy annual, with smaller leaves than commercial tobacco. It is easy to grow, as we have found, and, following Parkinson's recommendations, it is now our favourite plant for speedily healing minor wounds.

Tobacco has had a chequered history, from its origins in the Americas, where it was used by shamans and healers as a sacred plant, to today's huge tobacco industry and all the health problems caused by regular smoking or chewing. Tobacco was cultivated in Peru more than 4,000 years ago, and is thought to have been traded north, appearing in North American archaeological sites much later.

In his first book (1629, p364) Parkinson writes shrewdly about the two sides of tobacco: 'The herbe is, out of question, an excellent helpe and remedy for divers diseases, if it were rightly ordered and applyed, but the continuall abuse thereof in so many, doth almost abolish all good use in any.'

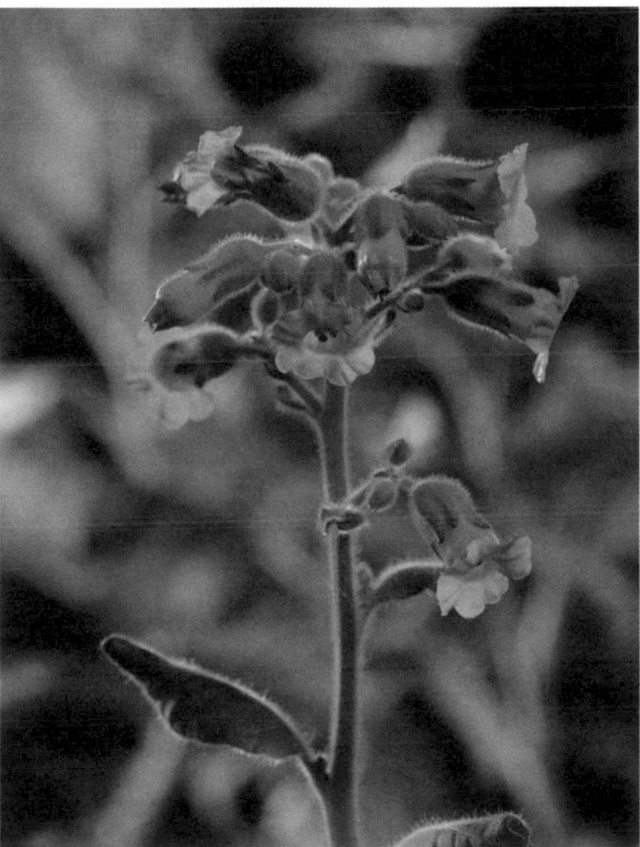

The medicinal properties of tobacco were quickly embraced when the plants reached Europe, as were its recreational uses. Some of this may have arisen from its exotic nature, but there is no doubt that tobaccos are plants with a powerful and addictive chemistry.

Monardes, a doctor from Seville, wrote a pioneering book (1574) on the medicinal properties of plants from the 'West Indies', listing 36 maladies that tobacco could help. An English translation appeared in 1577, and in 1595 Anthony Chute praised the plant in *Tabaco: The distinct and severall opinions of the late and best Phisitions that have written of the divers natures and qualities thereof*.

It was *Nicotiana rustica*, which grew wild in eastern North America, that first arrived in England. Sir Francis Drake was an early tobacco user, but it was Sir Walter Raleigh, the Queen's favourite courtier, who first made smoking fashionable in Elizabethan England, and he even encouraged the Queen to try it.

Overall, tobacco had a mixed reception. In 1604 King James I published his famous booklet *A Counterblaste to Tobacco*, writing that smoking is a 'filthie custome', 'lothsome to the eye, hatefull to the nose, harmefull to the braine, daungerous to the Lungs', and did his best to discourage the habit. This same year he introduced an import tax of 4,000% on tobacco. But tobacco remained popular with many, and soon the king was making so much money from the tobacco tax that by 1620 he gave up trying to discourage its use.

Tobacco really took off after John Rolfe planted seeds of a West Indian variety of tobacco, which produced larger plants and a stronger, sweeter tobacco than that previously grown in Virginia. This new crop, *Nicotiana tabacum*, became the major cash

Monardus: Nicolás Monardes (1493–1588), Spanish physician and botanist; an advocate of tobacco to cure almost everything
Alexipharmacum: antidote
the fit of an Ague: chills brought on by a fever
faeces of the herbe: residue of the leaves
fimo calido: hot dung
sellar: cellar
running vlcers: open weeping sore
greefes: ailments
greene: fresh
salve: ointment, unguent
streine: filter
rosen: rosin, distilled oil of turpentine
sheepes tallow: sheep fat
deares suet: deer fat
turpentine: resin of a coniferous tree
Aristolochia rotunda: round-leaved birthwort, now known to contain toxic compounds
olibanum: *Boswellia*, frankincense
imposthumes: purulent swellings

Bites: *Monardus* saith it is an *Alexipharmacum* or Counterpoison, for the biting of any venemous creature, and to apply the herbe also outwardly to the hurt place.

Distillation of tobacco: The distilled water is often given with some Sugar before the fit of an Ague, both to lessen the fits and to alter them and take them quite away in three or foure times using; which water above many other will taste of the sharpnesse of the herbe it selfe, but will yeeld no oyle or unctuous substance, as most other herbes will doe, although divers have boasted to make an oyle thereof; if the distilled *fæces* of the herbe having beene bruised before the distillation, and not distilled dry bee set in *fimo calido*, to digest for 14. dayes, and afterwards hung up in a bagge in a wine Sellar, that liquor that distilleth therefrom is singular good to use for Cramps, Aches, the Gout and Sciatica, and to heale itches, scabbes and running Ulcers, Cankers, and foule sores whatsoever:

Juice & salve: the juice also is good for all the said greefes, and likewise to kill lice in childrens heads: the greene herbe bruised and applyed to any greene wound is commonly knowne to country folkes, to cure any fresh wound or cut whatsoever: and the juice put into old sores both clenseth and healeth them, for which purpose many doe make a singular good salve hereof in this manner.

Parkinson's tobacco salve: Take of the greene herbe three or foure handfulls, bruise it and put it into a quart of good oyle of Olives, boile them on a gentle fire untill the herbe grow dry and the oyle will bubble no longer, then streine it forth hard and set it on the fire againe, adding thereto Wax, Rosen and Sheepes Tallow, or Deares Suet which you will, of each a quarter of a pound, of Turpentine two ounces, which being melted put it up for your use: Some will adde hereunto of the powder of *Aristolochia rotunda*, round Birthwort, and of *Olibanum*, that is, white Frankinsence of each halfe an ounce, or six drams, which are to bee put in when it is nigh cold, and well stirred together: this salve likewise will helpe imposthumes, hard tumors, and other swellings by blowes or falls.

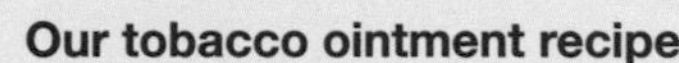

Our tobacco ointment recipe

15 to 20 wild tobacco leaves
250 ml olive oil
10 g beeswax

Put the leaves and oil in a small saucepan, and simmer gently until the leaves are crisp – just as Parkinson says, it stops bubbling when all the moisture has gone. Strain through a fine sieve, then return the oil to the pan. Add the beeswax and stir until it has melted. Pour into clean jars and allow to set.

crop in Jamestown and the Virginian colonies, and was even legal currency in Maryland and Virginia for a time. In 1620 a trade agreement between the Crown and the Virginia Company banned commercial tobacco growing in England, in return for a lower duty on Virginia tobacco.

The herbalist Nicholas Culpeper was an early tobacco addict, and smoking contributed to his death in 1654; this was not long after Parkinson, but Culpeper was only 37.

In his book *Nicotiana* (1832) Henry James Meller wrote about *Nicotiana rustica*: 'This is commonly called English tobacco, from its having been first introduced here, and being much more hardy than the other sorts, insomuch that it has become a weed in many places.' Today, it can still be found occasionally in parts of England, as an alien on rubbish heaps, and it grows wild in several southern US states.

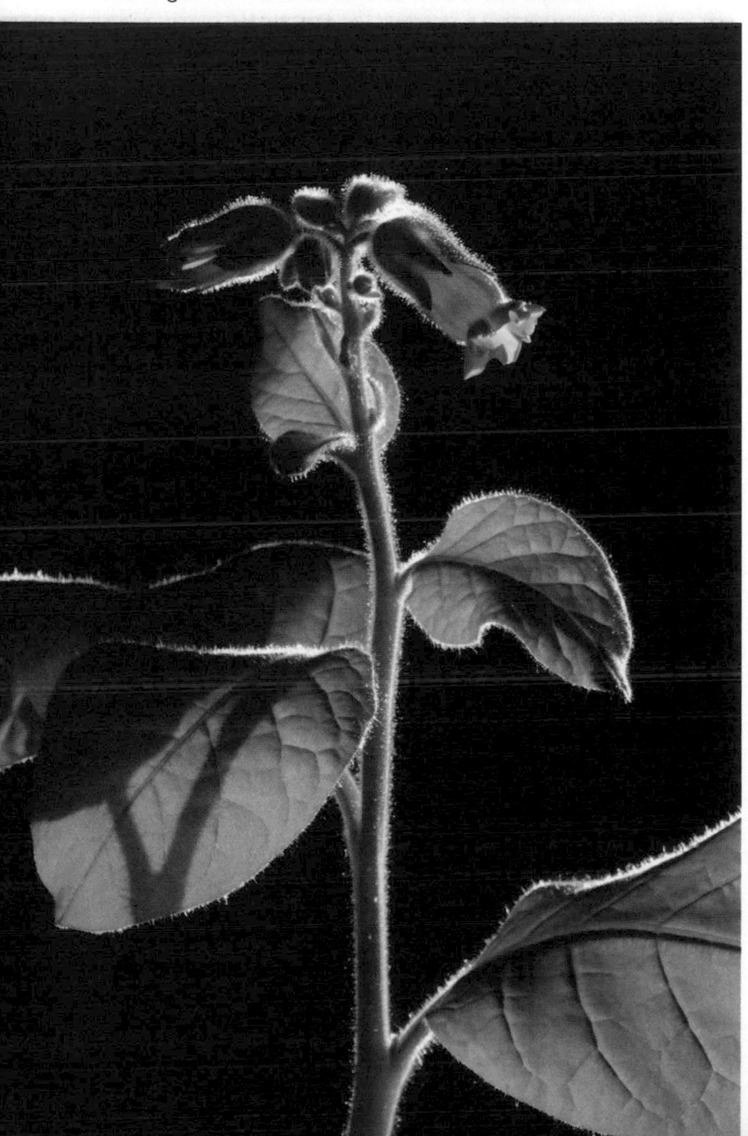

Tobacco is still used as the homeopathic remedy tabacum, which treats a symptom picture including dizziness, motion sickness, diarrhoea and dry cough – the symptoms that tobacco causes in a first-time user.

Mouth: Tobacco is made into a powder to clean and whiten the teeth in India, and is even used there in commercial toothpastes.

In our own experience, chewing a leaf of the fresh plant relieves toothache, but the narcotic properties render it a less than perfect remedy unless you want pain relief with a buzz!

Bites: Venomous creatures are luckily less of a problem for most of us than they were for Monardes, but the fresh leaf, bruised and rubbed on flea and other insect bites, brings quick relief for itching and burning. The young leaves are soft and very juicy. We've found that they are effective for several hours before another application is needed.

If you don't happen to have wild tobacco growing, the chewed-up tobacco from an ordinary cigarette will work, as Parkinson would say, for the aforesaid purpose.

Insectcide: Tobacco is still used to make an insectcide for use on garden plants, so it makes sense that it would work for lice.

Wounds: We have found the juice of fresh wild tobacco leaves to be excellent in speeding up the healing of wounds. It stings at first if the skin is broken, but the pain soon stops and healing is rapid. We've used it for broken blisters, scratches from thorns, splinters and for all sorts of cuts and grazes.

Nicotine: The main alkaloid in tobacco has been the subject of copious research. Nicotine patches were introduced as a way to help smokers quit, by giving them a small amount of the addictive chemical without the inhalation of other harmful chemicals. Nicotine has been found to improve cognitive function in older people, including those with Alzheimer's disease. Because of its effect on brain chemistry and neurotransmitters, it also has possibilities for helping with depression and other neurological conditions.

Love Apples

Theatrum Botanicum

Tribe 3, Chapter 9, pp352–54

Poma amoris majora media & minora

The Vertues

Madde apples are eaten being first boyled in fat broth, with vinegar or salt, oyle and pepper, as a continuall juncket with the Genveses and others, as *Scaliger* saith, and neither breed frensyes nor any other harme, and therefore he saith, *minus sano judicio insana dicuntur*.

Yet *Avicen lib.* 2, *cap.* 455. condemneth them, saying that those that are old are very noisome and hurtfull, although the fresh ones be better: for by their bitternesse and acrimony it is gathered, that they are hot and dry in the second degree, and that therefore they engender Melancholly, the Leprosie, Cancers, the Piles, Imposthumes, the Headache, and a stincking breath, breed obstructions in the Liver and Spleene, and change the complection into a foule blacke and yellow colour, unlesse they be boyled in Vinegar; so that it is to be admired, that *Averrhoes* should commend them, being drest in some fashion.

Fuschius saith that there is a superaboundant coldnesse, and moisture, in the Madde apples, as there is in Cowcumbers and Mushroomes: yet the beauty of the fruite worketh in some, and the insatiable desire of delight to the palate in others, and the inciting to Venery in the most, (which these are thought to procure) doe so farre transport a great many, that in *Italy* and other hot countries, where they come to their full maturity, and proper rellish, they doe eate them with more desire and pleasure than we doe Cowcumbers, or the like, and therefore prepare and dresse them in divers manners;

as some doe eate them raw, as Cowcumbers, some doe roast them under the Embers, and others doe first boyle them, pare them and slice them: and having strowed flower over them, doe frye them with oyle or butter, and with a little pepper and salt, serve them to the table. Some also doe keepe them in pickle, to serve for to spend in the Winter and Spring:

but it is certainely found true, that they doe hardly digest in the stomacke, whereby they breed much windinesse, and thereby peradventure bodily lust; that they engender bad blood and Melancholicke humours, and give little nourishment at all unto the body, and that not good:

the Apples of *Ethiopia*, are of the same quality, although of a firmer substance, not yeelding any good nourishment, but rather offensive to the body, for these two are *congeneres* in forme, and therefore most likely in quality.

The golden apples or apples of love, are cold and moist, more then any of the former, and therefore lesse offensive, these are eaten with great delight and pleasure in the hotter Countries, but not in ours, because their moisture is flashy and insipide, for want of the sufficient heate of the Sunne in their ripening.

5. *Pomum amoris majus,*
The greater love Apples.

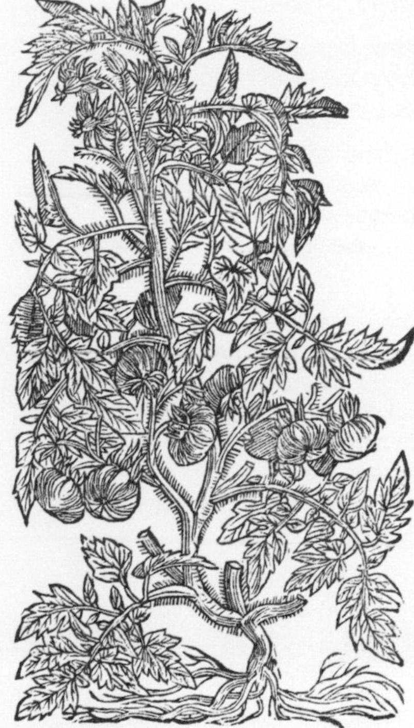

fat broth: rich soup
juncket: sweet concoction
Genveses: inhabitants of Geneva
Scaliger: Joseph Justus Scaliger (1540–1609), Dutch preacher and historian
minus sano judicio insana dicuntur: it is not right to say mad apples drive you mad
frensyes: delirium
Avicen: Avicenna, Ibn Sina (980–1037), Persian scholar and physician
noisome: noxious
acrimony: pungency
piles: haemorrhoids
imposthumes: large, deep abscesses
Averrhoes: Averroes, Ibn Rusd (1126–98), Moroccan scholar and philosopher
Fuschius: Leonhart Fuchs (1501–66), German botanist and author
cowcumbers: cucumbers
inciting to venery: provoking lust
strowed flower: sprinkled flour
offensive: unpleasant
congeneres: in same genus, resembling

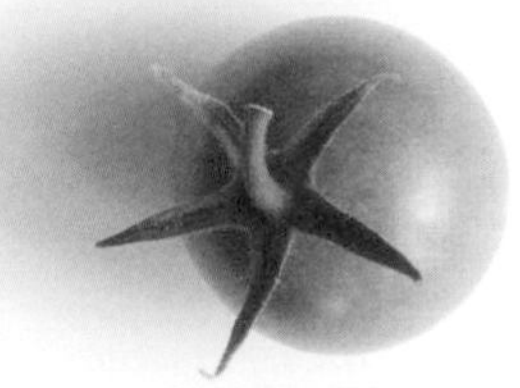

Tomato *Solanum lycopersicum* Solanaceae

We thought it would be interesting to see what Parkinson wrote about some of the recently introduced plants of the New World, which feature in the golden age of botanical exploration that he lived through and recorded in his books. Our entries on chilis, coca, corn, sassafras and tobacco come into this category, and here we examine tomato, known to Parkinson as apples of love or love apple.

Parkinson's chapter on *Solana pomifera*, his Applebearing Nightshades, covers six species, with the following English names: Lobel's red berried Nightshade, the Winter Cherry Tree, Madde Apples of Syria, Madde Apples of Ethiopia, Madde Apples of Europe, and Apples of Love, of a greater, lesser, and middle size.

He devotes most space in his virtues to madde apples – kinds of eggplant (*Mala insana)* – with only one sentence on love apples. He questions the name madde apples ('but many doe much marveile, why they should be so called, seeing none have beene knowne to receive any harme by the eating of them', TB, p354). At least one of his madde apples is still recognized: the *Solanum aethiopium* or Ethiopian eggplant.

The madde apples, he says, are prepared for the rather obscure 'continuall junckct with the Genveses', but give no trouble (neither 'breed frensyes nor any other harme'). His discussion of Avicenna probably relates to some other more toxic Solanum-type plant of the Middle East, whose mature fruits are hot and dry, and cause various severe reactions.

The actual date of the tomato arriving in Europe is a tangled terrain. Some have argued for Columbus in the 1490s and others for Cortéz in the 1520s; no doubt it was introduced at various times before making an impact. Such history is hard to recover, but the generally agreed first book reference is in Matthiolus, who in 1544 described *pomo d'oro*, the golden apple; in a later edition of 1554, he adds the red tomato.

By that time the evocative Latin name *Lycopersicum* or wolf peach (which is still used today) was being applied to the plant in Germany. Here is the echo of older werewolf legends; perhaps such legends – also hinted at in 'nightshade' itself – were a social protective valve to caution people about the dangers of eating and using potentially toxic plants? Certainly tomato was considered poisonous or dangerous for most of its first two and even three hundred years in Europe. It is curious why tobacco was accepted so readily while tomatoes were not.

Parkinson does not use 'tomato', the closest he comes being in citing Guilandinus (German botanist, 1520–89), who 'saith it is called *Tumatle* by the Americans [i.e. the Aztecs]'. Parkinson mentions Fuchs in his comparison of madde apples and cucumbers and mushrooms. All are cold and moist (the love apples more so), and despite their relish, their incomplete digestion, both agree, leads to windiness and 'thereby peradventure bodily lust'.

Parkinson writes of tomato, somewhat plaintively in both his books, as a curiosity plant that has limited chance of fully ripening in the English climate, but you get the impression he will keep on trying. Ask any English gardener today: growing the plants outside from seed is still problematic without glasshouses. But Parkinson didn't say that 'the whole plant is of a ranke and stinking savour'. These words in Gerard's *Herball* (1597) are said to have set tomato-growing in England back by decades.

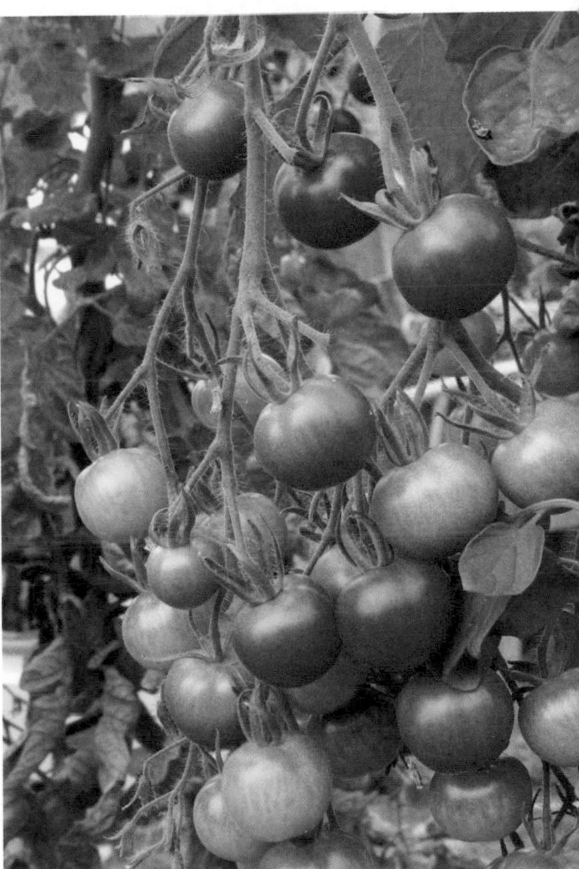

Land Caltrops

Theatrum Botanicum

Tribe 11, Chapter 26, pp1097–98

Tribulus terrestris

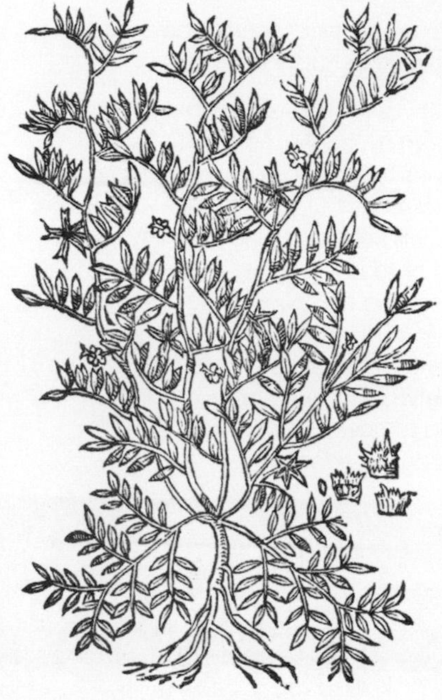
Tribulus terrestris. Land Caltrops.

The Vertues

The Land Caltrops are of an earthly cold qualitie and thereby astringent and hindering of the breeding of inflammations and Imposthumes, and against the flux of humors:

Kidney stones: moreover being of thinne parts it doth much helpe to breake and waste the Stone in the Kidneyes:

Mouth & throat: a Lotion made therewith healeth all sores and Ulcers in the mouth, and all corruptions that breede in the gummes and throate:

Eyes: the juice doth clense the inflammations and other hot rheumes in the eyes:

Poisons: it likewise cureth the venome of the Viper and other poysons, if a dram thereof bee taken in wine.

Pliny & Galen: The *Thracians* saith *Pliny* and *Galen* that dwell neare the River *Strimon* did feede their Horses with the greene herbe, and lived themselves of the fruit or kernells, making them into a sweete bread which bound the belly;

Pliny addeth that the roote being gathered by a caste persons doth consume Nodes and Kernells:

Swellings: the seede bound to the swollen veines in the Legs, or other parts of the body taketh the swellings away, and easeth the paines.

Imposthumes: purulent abscesses or swellings
corruptions: infections
hot rheumes: watery, hot secretions
Pliny: Pliny the Elder (AD 23–79), Roman naturalist
Galen: Claudius Galen (AD130–200), Roman physician and author
kernells: the burs
a caste persons: [unknown]
Nodes and Kernells: swollen glands and cysts

Caltrops and chestnuts: further explanations

'Caltrops' refers to a passive weapon made up of metal spines so arranged that one of them always points upward, designed to effectively disable soldiers and animals. The idea for metal caltrops probably came from burs such as tribulus, which do this naturally.

Parkinson calls tribulus 'land caltrops' to differentiate it from the water caltrops, *Trapa natans*, the name for water chestnut, which has seeds of a similar shape. Water chestnut's starchy seeds were an important European food until the late twentieth century, but the wild plants are quite rare now except in Turkey and the Balkans. Water chestnuts grow in parts of Africa and across Asia, and are an invasive species in parts of Australia and the US.

What we know as 'water chestnut' in Chinese restaurant menus in Europe is another plant, *Eleocharis dulcis*, a grass-like sedge grown for its edible corms.

Tribulus *Tribulus terrestris*

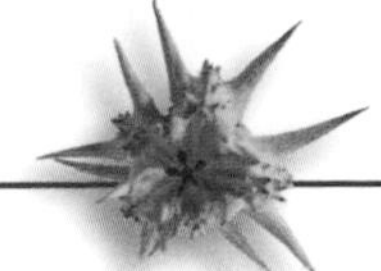

Zygophyllaceae

This herb has been largely forgotten in Western European herbalism until recently, but it has had a long history of continued use in Eastern Europe, the Middle East, India and China. It was found as a British wild flower in Parkinson's time: 'wee finde it many times in our owne Land', he wrote.

Tribulus is a small creeping plant with pinnate green leaves, pretty yellow flowers and vicious spiny burs. It is found today growing all around the world in subtropical waste ground: we have seen it next to African waterholes, on Peruvian highway verges and Australian footpaths.

Kidney stones & urinary tract: The burs are still used to treat kidney stones, helping break down gravel and stone in the kidneys and bladder. They are also valuable for prostate problems, urinary infections, renal colic, urinary retention, obstructed urine flow, blood in the urine and cloudy urine.

Mouth & throat: The astringency of the herb adds to its usefulness for weak gums, mouth ulcers and throat lesions. Make a strong tea of the seeds or whole plant, and let it cool before using as a mouthwash. The tincture can also be taken, diluted with water.

Eyes: In Chinese medicine, tribulus is used to brighten the eyes and treat itchy, swollen or painful eyes.

Swellings: This treatment is no longer current, but tribulus' astringency would make sense of this use.

Other current uses of tribulus

Reproductive: The aerial parts and burs increase virility, fertility, lactation and sperm production. In Ayurveda, the plant is used to rejuvenate the reproductive system in both sexes. Tribulus is sold online as an aphrodisiac and performance enhancer.

Nervous system: Tribulus contains harmaline, an alkaloid that has a MAO (monoamine oxidase)-inhibiting action, making it useful for treating depression and other nervous system imbalances.

Skin: Tribulus is used in both Ayurveda and modern Chinese medicine (TCM) to treat itchy skin, eczema and psoriasis.

Athletic performance: Tribulus products to enhance athletic performance are widely available. Bulgarian weightlifters owe much of their competitive prowess to tribulus supplements. Indeed, research shows that only the Eastern European tribulus species contains significant levels of protodioscin, which increases levels of usable testosterone in the body.

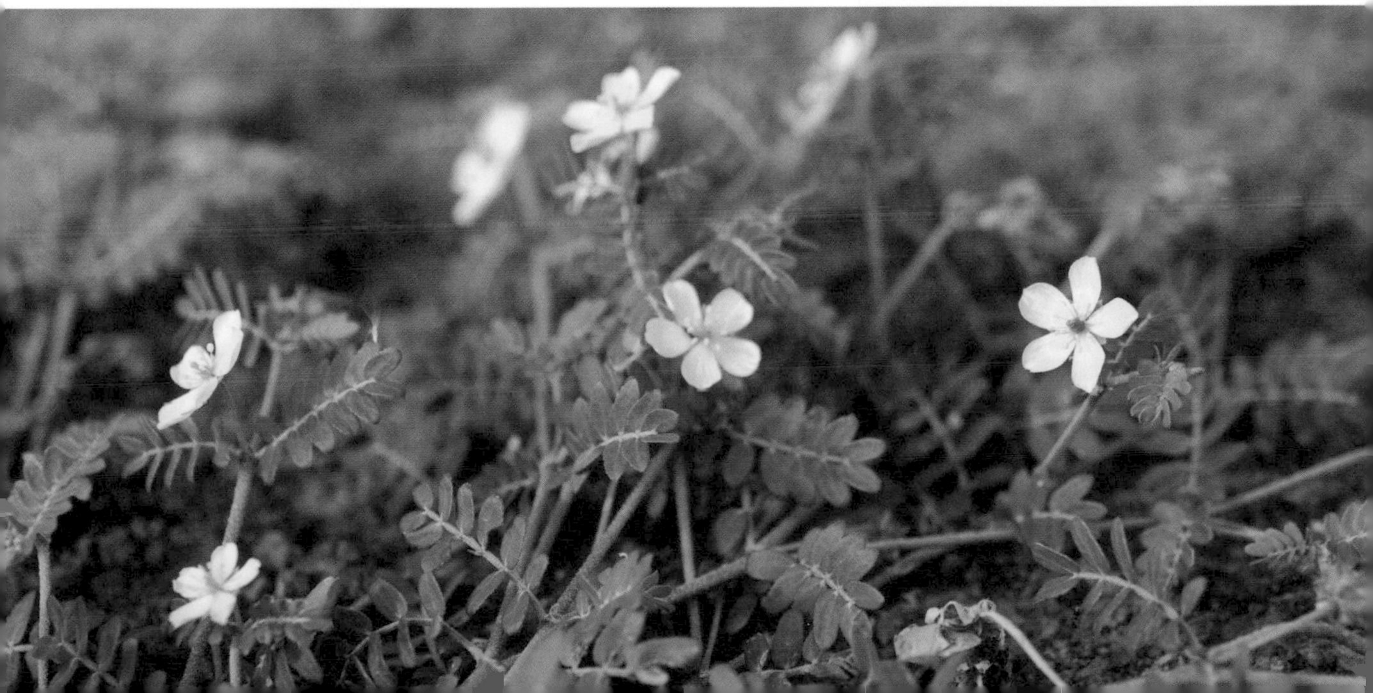

Vervaine

Theatrum Botanicum

Tribe 5, Chapter 92, pp674–76

1. Verbena vulgaris.
Common Vervaine.

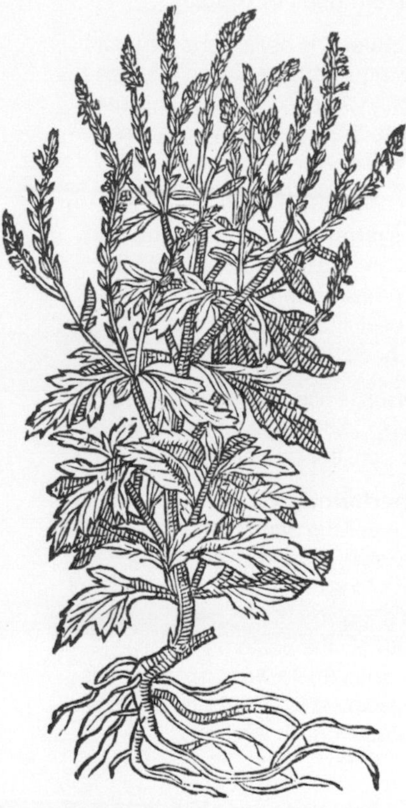

Jaundies: jaundice
Dropsie: oedema
Reines: kidneys
tertian Ague: two-day fever
quartaine Ague: four-day fever
Piony: peony
ingendreth: gives rise to
Fistulaes: hollow channels
Hogs grease: pig lard
inveterate paines: chronic painsß
frensy: extreme mental agitation
morphew: discoloration of skin
pustulaes: pus-filled growths
greene wounds: fresh wounds

Verbena

The Vertues

Vervaine is hot and dry, bitter and binding, and is an opener of obstructions, clenseth and healeth: for it helpeth the yellow Jaundies, the Dropsie and the Goute, as also the defects of the Reines and Lungs, and generally all the inward paines and torments of the body:

the leaves being boyled and drunke, the same is held to be good against the bitings of Serpents and venemous beasts, and the Plague or Pestilence, against both *tertian* and *quartaine* Agues, killeth and expelleth the Wormes in the belly, and causeth a good colour in the face and body, strengthneth as well as correcteth the diseases of the Liver and Spleene, is very effectuall in all the diseases of the Stomacke and Lungs, as Coughs, shortnesse of breath and wheesings,

and is singular good against the Dropsie, to be drunke with some Piony seedes, bruised and put thereto, and is no lesse prevalent for the defects of the Reines and Bladder, to clense them of that viscous and slimy humour which ingendreth the stone, and helpeth to breake it being confirmed, and to expell the gravell:

Wounds, ulcers & haemorrhoids: it consolidateth and healeth also all wounds, both inward or outward, and stayeth bleedings, and used with some honey, healeth all old Ulcers, and Fistulaes in the legs or other parts of the body, as also those Ulcers that happen in the mouth, or used with old Hogs grease, it helpeth the swellings and paines of the secret parts of man or woman, as also for the piles or hemorrhoides:

Headache: applyed with some oyle of Roses and Vinegar unto the forehead and temples, it helpeth to ease the inveterate paines and ache of the head, and is good also for those that are fallen into a frensy:

Skin: the leaves bruised or the juice of them mixed with some Vinegar, doth wonderfully clense the skinne, and taketh away all morphew, freckles, pustulaes, or other such like inflammations, and deformities of the skinne in any part of the body:

Distilled water: The distilled water of the herbe when it is in his full strength, dropped into the eyes, clenseth them from filmes, clouds or mist that darken the sight, and wonderfully comforteth the opticke veines. The said water is very powerfull in all the diseases aforesayd, eyther inward or outward, whether they bee old corroding sores, or greene wounds. The female Vervaine is held to be the more powerfull for all the purposes being spoken of;

Vervain *Verbena officinalis* Verbenaceae

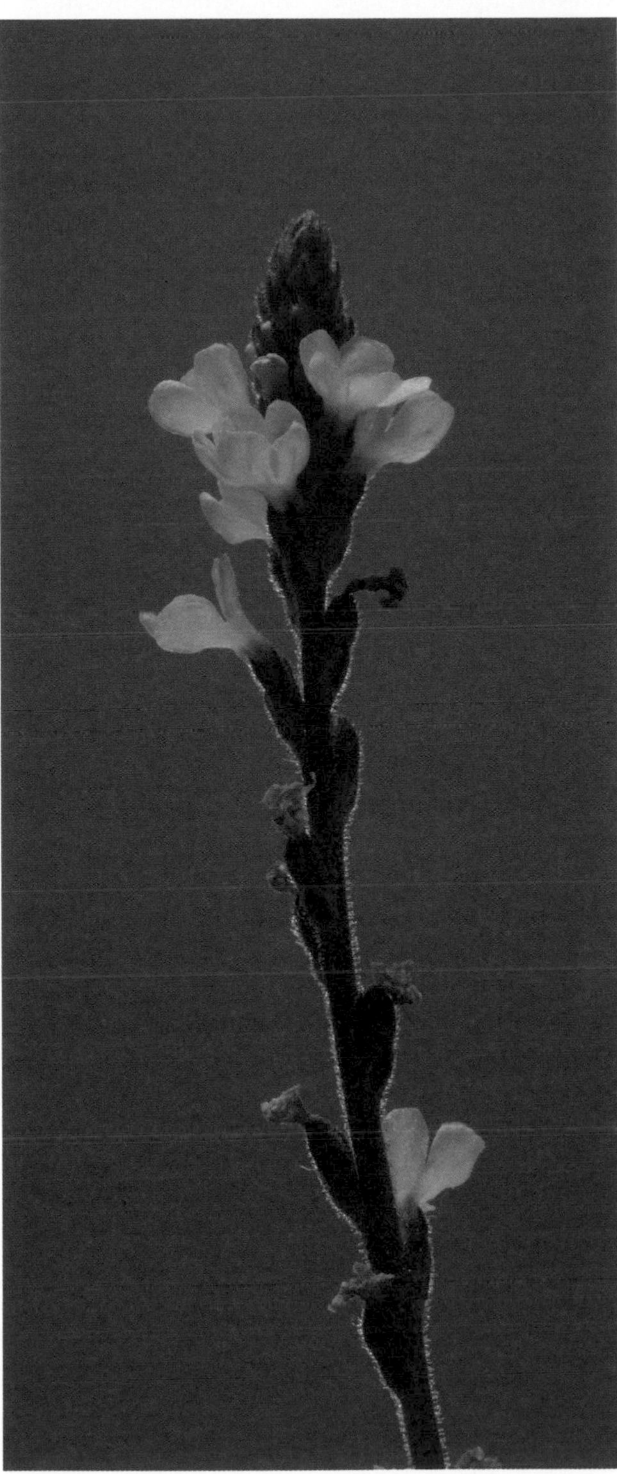

Vervain is a wonderful restorative, protective tonic to the nervous system. It helps invigorate appetite and digestion, is used for liver and gallbladder problems, and helps clear the kidneys and bladder.

It calms anxiety, relieves stress, alleviates headaches and eases restlessness. Externally, it is effective for cuts, scratches, insect bites and a range of skin problems.

Vervain gives us another example of a bitter herb that Parkinson classifies as hot and which most modern herbalists classify as cooling.

V. officinalis is native to Europe, Asia and north Africa and is naturalized in other areas. The North American blue vervain, *V. hastata*, is used very similarly.

Vervain has a gentle and widespread action, making it effective for a range of different problems. As Parkinson says, it is good for 'generally all the inward paines and torments of the body'. It is a relaxing nerve tonic, a bitter digestive with an affinity for the liver, gallbladder and spleen. Vervain also works on the lungs, kidneys and urinary system.

It is pain-relieving, reduces inflammation, stops bleeding and heals wounds. It is used to expel worms, treat headaches, heal ulcers and balance hormones.

Vervain is still used for 'the frensy' just as in 1640, in calming an overactive nervous system. Herbalists think of it for restlessness and irritability. It has been a popular treatment for madness through much of its history.

It is useful as a cooling herb for menopausal hot flushes, and for fevers, and is considered antimalarial. It increases sweating, promotes lactation and stimulates the uterus.

Vervain can help ensure good sleep, but may need to be taken for a while before it takes effect. It is a great restorative after periods of stress or nervous exhaustion.

The uses in Chinese medicine are very similar to those in Western herbalism.

Monardus: Nicholás Monardes, physician of Seville (1493–1588)
West Indies: generic term for Spanish South America
divers Physitians: various physicians
avoided, avoyding: vomited up
roules: rolls

Peruvian vervain: but that of *Peru* goeth farre beyond them both, for *Monardus* reporteth divers very admirable cures which that herbe hath performed in the *West Indies*; as of a certaine noble woman, who having used the helpe of divers Physitians in vaine, an *Indian* Physitian very skilfull in herbes, gave her the juice of that Vervaine to drinke with some Sugar mixed therewith, for to allay somewhat of the bitternesse thereof, by whose use shee avoided in a few dayes a thicke long worme (which shee called a snake) being hairy, of a foot in length, and double forked at the taile, after which shee grew well; the same noble woman commended the same medicine to another noble woman in *Peru*, who had not beene well of a long time, who having taken it in the same manner for certaine dayes, avoided many small and long wormes, and among the rest, one very long, like unto a long white girdle, after which time shee became well againe. Which medecine was by advice given to many others that complained of Wormes, and they were all soone holpen by avoyding wormes, either more or lesse, and some also roules or balls of haire, and other things:

it is held also to bee no lesse effectuall against all poyson, and the venome of dangerous beasts and serpents, as also against bewitched drinkes or the like. Many other examples of cures *Monardus* setteth downe which are too long here to recite, seeing these are sufficient to shew how prevalent that herbe is for many diseases.

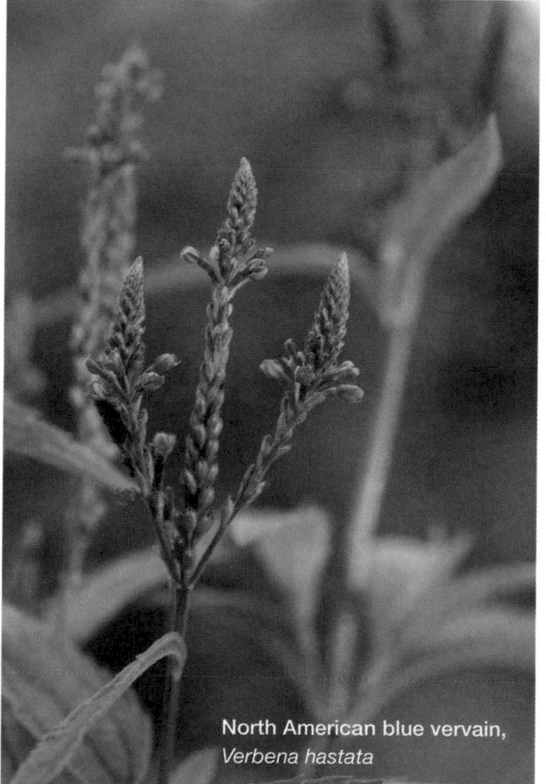
North American blue vervain, *Verbena hastata*

There are around 250 species of vervain, *Verbena* spp., mostly native to South America.

It is hard to know which species is being referred to by Monardes, who says (p187): 'Moreover the gentleman wrote unto me from the Peru that in the rivers of the mounteins of that country neere unto them, ther groweth a great quantity of Vervaine, like unto those of Spaine, [from] which the Indians doo profite themselves in their cures, for many infirmities, and in especially against all kind of poyson.'

The tall upright vervain (right) was photographed in a river valley leading down to the Sacred Valley in the mountains of Peru, and certainly fits the description of being similar to European vervain.

Monardes was a physician from Seville, who published several books, including *Historia medicinal de las cosas que se traen de nuestras Indias Occidentales* (completed 1574). This was translated into Latin by Charles de l'Ecluse and then into English by John Frampton (1577) with the title *Joyfull newes out of the newe founde worlde*. Parkinson used this book and was certainly impressed by the reports from Monardes.

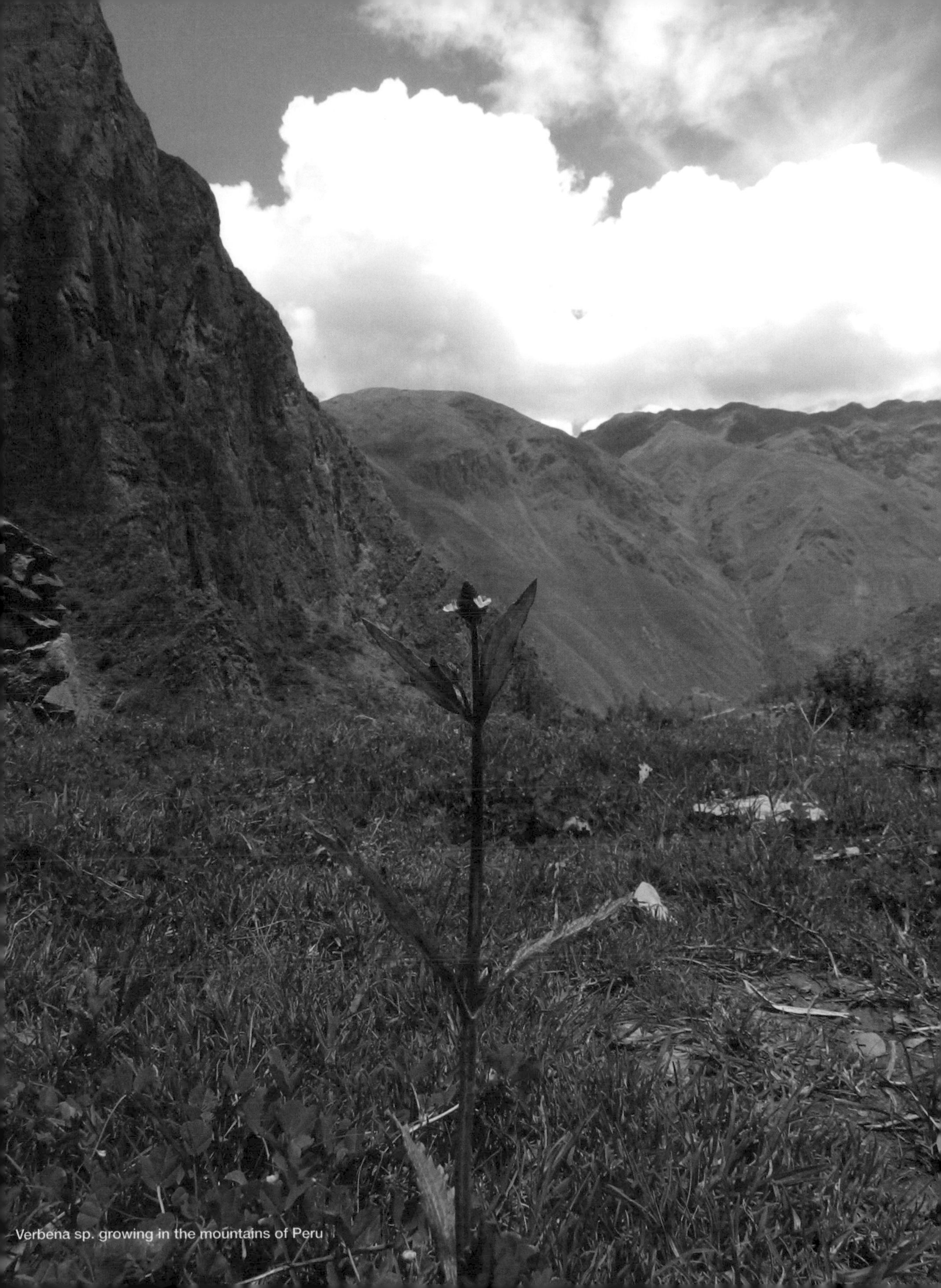

Verbena sp. growing in the mountains of Peru

Violets

Theatrum Botanicum

Tribe 6, Chapter 15, pp755–57

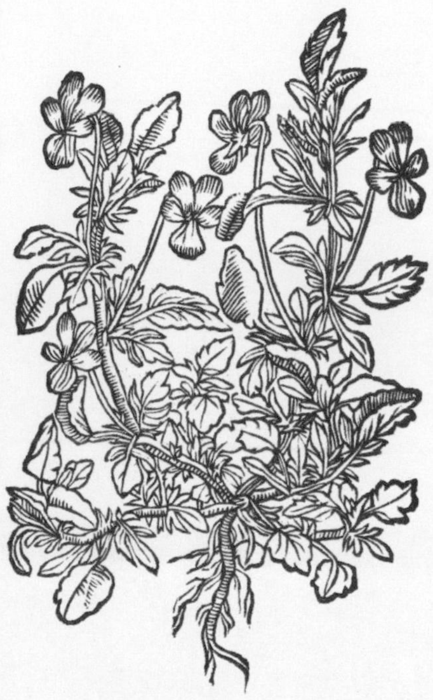

distemperature: erratic temperature
mother: womb
fundament: anus or buttocks
fallen downe: prolapsed
Imposthumes: abscesses
poultis wise: like a poultice
dram: apothecary weight, ⅛th oz
chollerick humors: hot, dry and fiery conditions
Quinsie: throat inflammation
Falling sicknesse: epilepsy
Plurisie: pleurisy
lenifie: moderate
rheumes: watery discharge
reynes: kidneys or kidney area in back
Iaundies: jaundice
agues: fevers

Viola

The Vertues

Cooling & anti-inflammatory: The Garden Violets and so likewise the wilde kindes are cold and moist while they are fresh and greene, and are used to coole any heate or distemperature of the body, eyther inwardly or outwardly, the inflammations in the eyes in the mother or in the fundament when they are fallen downe & are full of paine, Imposthumes also and hot swellings, to drinke the decoction of the leaves or flowers made with water or wine, or to apply them poultis wise to the grieved place,

Head: it likewise easeth paines in the head, which are caused through want of sleepe, or in any other place arising of heate applyed in the like manner, or with oyle of Roses:

Dried violets: a dram weight of the dryed leaves of the flowers of Violets, (but the leaves more strongly) doth purge the body of chollerick humors, and asswageth the heate being taken in a draught of wine or any other drinke:

Purple violets: the powder of the purple leaves of the flowers onely pickt and dryed, and drunke in powder with water is said to helpe the Quinsie and the Falling sicknesse in children, especially in the beginning of the disease:

White violets: the flowers of the white Violets ripeneth and dissolveth swellings: the seede being taken resisteth the force of the Scorpion: the herbe or flowers while they are fresh, or the flowers when they are dry are effectuall in the Plurisie and all other diseases of the Lungs, to lenifie the sharpenesse of hot rheumes and the hoarsenesse of the throate, the heate also and sharpenesse of urine, and all paines of the backe or reynes and the bladder: it is good also for the Liver and the Iaundies, and in all hot Agues helping to coole the heate, and quench thirst:

Syrup of violets: but the Syrupe of Violets is of most use and of better effect being taken in some convenient liquor, and if a little of the juice or Syrupe of Lemons bee put to it or a few drops of the oyle of Vitrioll, it is made thereby the more powerfull to coole the heate and to quench the thirst, and besides the effect giveth to the drinke a Claret wine colour and a fine tart rellish pleasing to the taste.

With honey or sugar: Violets taken or made up with hony doth more clense then coole, and with Sugar contrariwise: the dryed flowers of Violets are accounted among the Cordiall flowers and are used in cordialls, drinkes powders and other medicines, especially where cooling cordialls, as Roses and Saunders are used:

Violets & heartsease

Violaceae

The Viola genus has some 500 species worldwide, but for our purposes can be divided into two broad groups: the **violets**, which have three upper petals and two below, and the **violas and pansies**, with four above and one below. The violets are usually perennial, with heart-shaped leaves, side petals and tend to be single-coloured; they include sweet and dog violet. The viola/pansy group are annual or perennial, with irregular leaves, a flat 'face' of flowers and are often multicoloured; they include pansies and heartsease. The medicinal uses are similar, with some significant variation, as Parkinson explains.

Cooling, anti-inflammatory: Parkinson characterizes garden and wild violets as cold and moist. He explains by humoural theory their capacity to cool any inward and outward 'distemperature', including inflammations of the eyes, hot abscesses and other swellings, and the pain of prolapse of the womb. He recommends drinking a decoction of the leaves or flowers, or applying as a poultice on the 'grieved place'.

This generic use of violets for inflammation was supplemented by a more specific application in the chest area, with violet classified as a pectoral and demulcent herb. This included its use to treat colds and bronchitis, whooping cough and as an effective expectorant. Parkinson goes on to discuss the use of white violets for respiratory problems.

Head: The engaging account of French folk medicine by Jean Palaiseul, *Grandmother's Secrets* (1973), p306, quotes the 19th century naturopath Abbé Kneipp as saying that a violet decoction is good for headaches and 'great overheatings of the head'. This usage is at least as old as classical Greece, with Hippocrates (c.460–c.370BC) suggesting violets for headaches and hangovers, and Roman times, when violet leaf wreaths and flowers were worn after alcoholic binges.

Doctors of the Salerno school in the 13th century agreed, with this recipe from the *Liber*

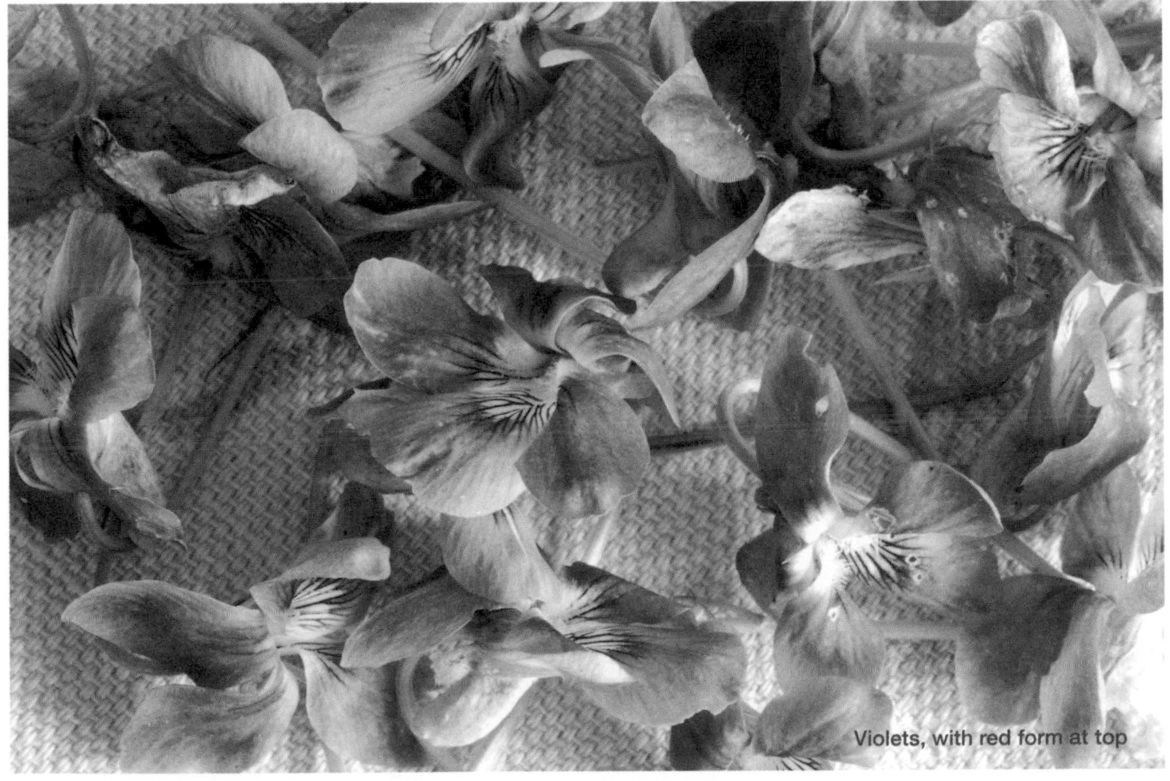

Violets, with red form at top

Viola tricolor major & vulgaris.
Greater and leſſer Panſyes or Hearts eaſe.

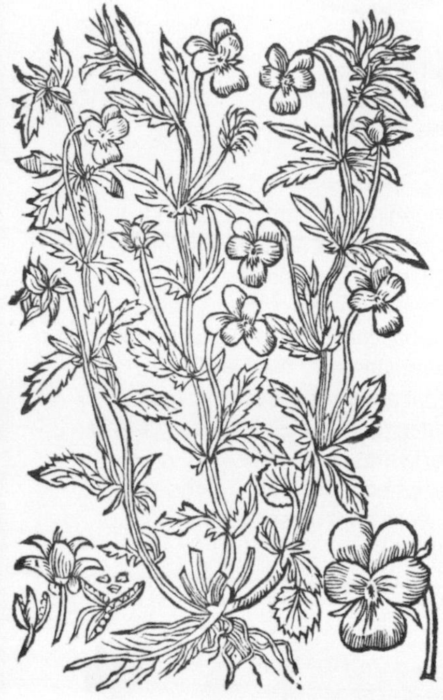

Poultices: the greene leaves are alway3s used with other herbes to make Cataplasmes and Poultises for inflammations or swellings, and to ease paines wheresoever arising of heate and for the piles also being fryed with Yolkes of Egges and applyed thereto.

Pansies or heartsease: Pansyes or Hearts ease is like unto Violets in all the parts thereof, but somewhat hotter and dryer, yet very temperate, and by the viscous or glutinous juice therein doth somewhat mollifie, yet lesse then Mallowes:

it is conducing in like manner as Violets to the hot diseases of the lungs and chests, for agues, for convulsions, and the falling sicknesse in children: the places also troubled with the itch or scabs being bathed with the decoction of them doth helpe much: it is said also to soder greene wounds, and to helpe old sores to use the juyce or the distilled water:

French violets: *Lugdunensis* setteth it downe that many sacks full of the flowers and herbes are transported from *Marseilles* in *France* unto *Alexandria*; and other parts of *Egypt* where they use them boyled in water, which onely by their religion they are enjoyned to drinke, not onely thereby to make it the more wholesome to be drunke: but they are perswaded also that it helpeth the diseases of the lungs and chest, and the falling sicknesses.

oyle of Vitrioll: sulphuric acid
Cordiall: comforting, stimulating
Saunders: sandalwood (*Santalum album*)
Cataplasmes: poultices with herbs
piles: haemorrhoids
mollifie: soften
Mallowes: *Malva sylvestris*
soder greene wounds: join fresh wounds
Lugdunensis: the *Historia Plantarum Lugdunensis* (1586), a noted French botanical text, published anonymously; elsewhere Parkinson identifies the author as Jacques D'Aléchamps (1513–88)
their religion: i.e. Islam

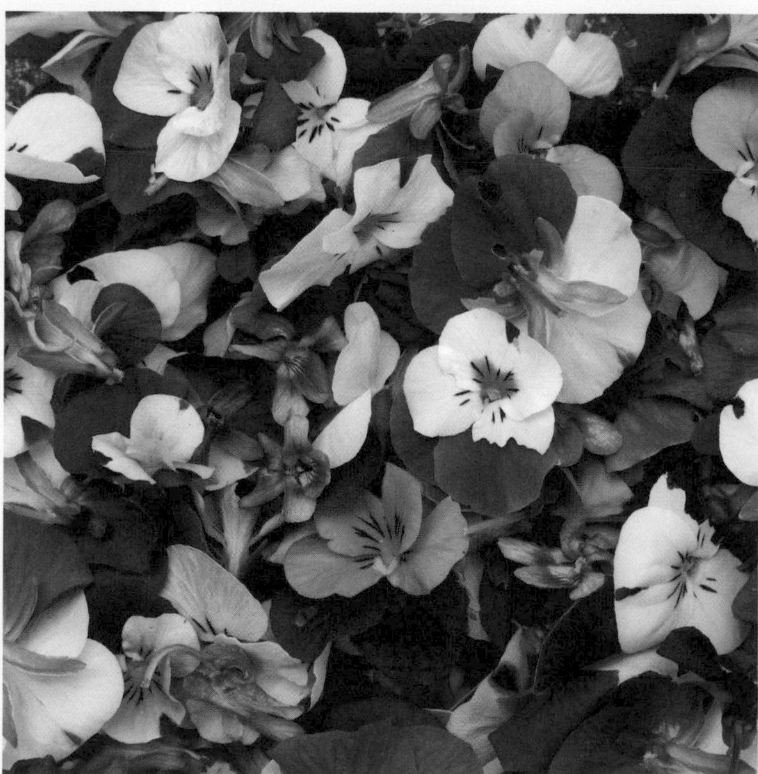

Heartsease, violets and violas from our garden

de Simplici Medicina, rendered in English verse as: 'To dispel drunkenness and repel migraine / The violet is sovereign; / From heavy head it takes the pain, / And from feverish cold delivers the brain.' Parkinson adds sleeplessness to his list of 'paines in the head'.

Dried violets: There is also a tradition that violets are mildly laxative and purgative, the leaves more than the flowers and the roots more so again. This supports another old, probably medieval, belief in *Viola odorata* treating some forms of cancer, especially of the lungs, stomach and chest.

In this connection *Bartram's Encyclopedia of Herbal Medicine* (1995), p444, gives an interesting example. When Catherine, the wife of General Booth, founder of the Salvation Army, was dying of cancer in 1890 the one drink that gave her relief from pain was violet leaf tea. Sweet violets were gathered from railway embankments by concerned members of the Army.

There is ongoing medical research into the use of large and continuous doses of violets following breast or stomach cancer, the goal being to prevent growth of further tumours.

Purple violets: Parkinson reports ('is said to') use of a violet powder drunk in water to treat the onset of throat inflammations and epilepsy in children. Epilepsy would not be treated at home today, but this seems a powerful preparation.

White violets: There is no continuing tradition that white-flowered violets are stronger in effect – sufficient to counter scorpion bite, he believes. On the other hand the use of violets in general, fresh or dried, for treating respiratory ailments, including pleurisy, is of long duration. Both sweet violet and heartsease are 'official' in the *British Herbal Pharmacopoeia* (1996) as expectorants, which not only assist in removing mucus but soothe the throat and respiratory tract.

Parkinson also mentions treatment of urinary tract infections, related back pain in the kidney area, jaundice and fevers; he repeats that violets cool excess heat, and also quench thirst.

Syrup of violets: Such applications are more efficacious, he suggests, with syrup of violets, added to 'some convenient liquor'. He now proposes adding syrup of lemons or a few drops of sulphuric acid. How many people today would find using the acid an appealing idea, even if the violets look like a claret or add a 'fine tart rellish pleasing to the taste'?

With honey or sugar: He finds violets with honey more cleansing than cooling, which suggests more purgative, while with sugar the reverse is true. This subtlety has been lost, but syrup of violets was until recent times a treatment of choice for children's coughs and chest colds. Parkinson notes the cordial nature of violet preparations, while adding roses and sandalwood sounds wonderful, with a little astringency from the roses adding depth to the violets' sweetness.

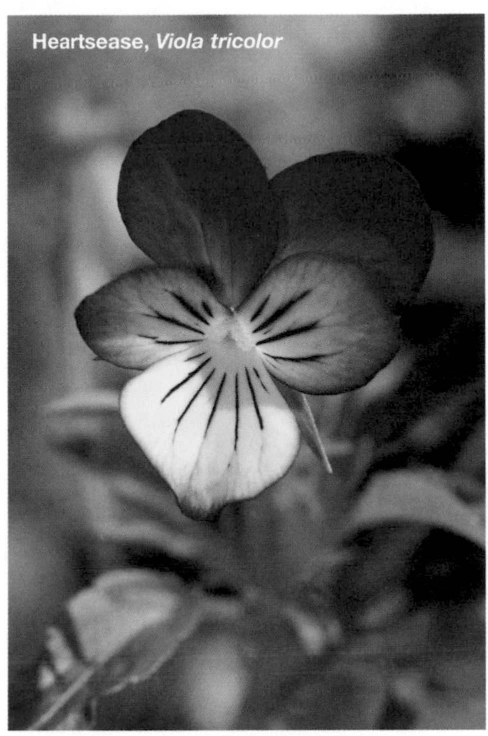
Heartsease, *Viola tricolor*

Poultices: Again violet leaves in poultices or cataplasms are soothing and cooling, he says, and mixed with egg yolk can ease piles.

Pansies or heartsease: Parkinson has drawn the balance well: sweet violets (*V. odorata*) and pansies/heartsease (*V. tricolor*) are broadly similar but their differences add to the versatility of the group as a whole. He finds pansies marginally hotter and drier, yet still temperate, and equally effective in cooling hot diseaes of the chest and lungs, and for fevers and epileptic conditions of children.

He describes pansies as more used for treating itch and scab problems, which would include eczema; indeed, this use is still 'official' in Britain. The Chinese violet, *Viola yezoensis*, has also been researched for treating childhood eczema.

French violets: In a diversion, he now describes the French violet industry of some time before his. This is not the French perfume industry, as might be expected, but the sale of violets from Marseilles to Egypt for a non-alcoholic violet drink, taken for pleasure and for medicine.

Water Cresses

Theatrum Botanicum

Tribe 14, Chapter 19, pp1238–40

Nasturtium aquaticum

3. *Nasturtium aquaticum amarum.* Bitter water Cresses.

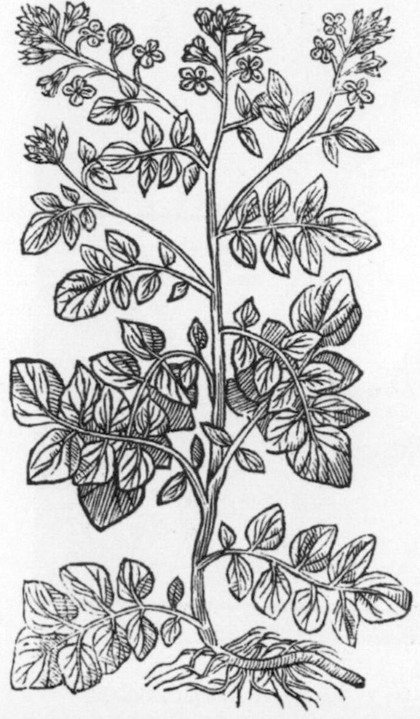

The Vertues

The Water Cresses are hotter in taste then Brookelime, and more powerfull against the Scurvy, and to clense the blood and humours, and for all the other uses whereunto Brookelime is before said to be availeable, as to break the stone, to provoke urine and womens courses: the decoction thereof is said to be good to wash foule and filthy Ulcers, thereby to clense them and make them the fitter to heale:

The leaves or the juice is good to be applyed to the face or other parts troubled with freckles, pimples, spots or the like at night, and taken away or washed away in the morning, the juice mixed with vinegar, and the forepart of the head bathed therewith is very good for those that are dull and drowsie, or have the Lethargy.

Brookelime: *Veronica beccabunga*, a blue-flowered plant of damp places
availeable: beneficial
breake the stone: dissolve or weaken internal crystalline concretions
women's courses: menstruation
the Lethargy: extreme tiredness, possibly a form of chronic fatigue

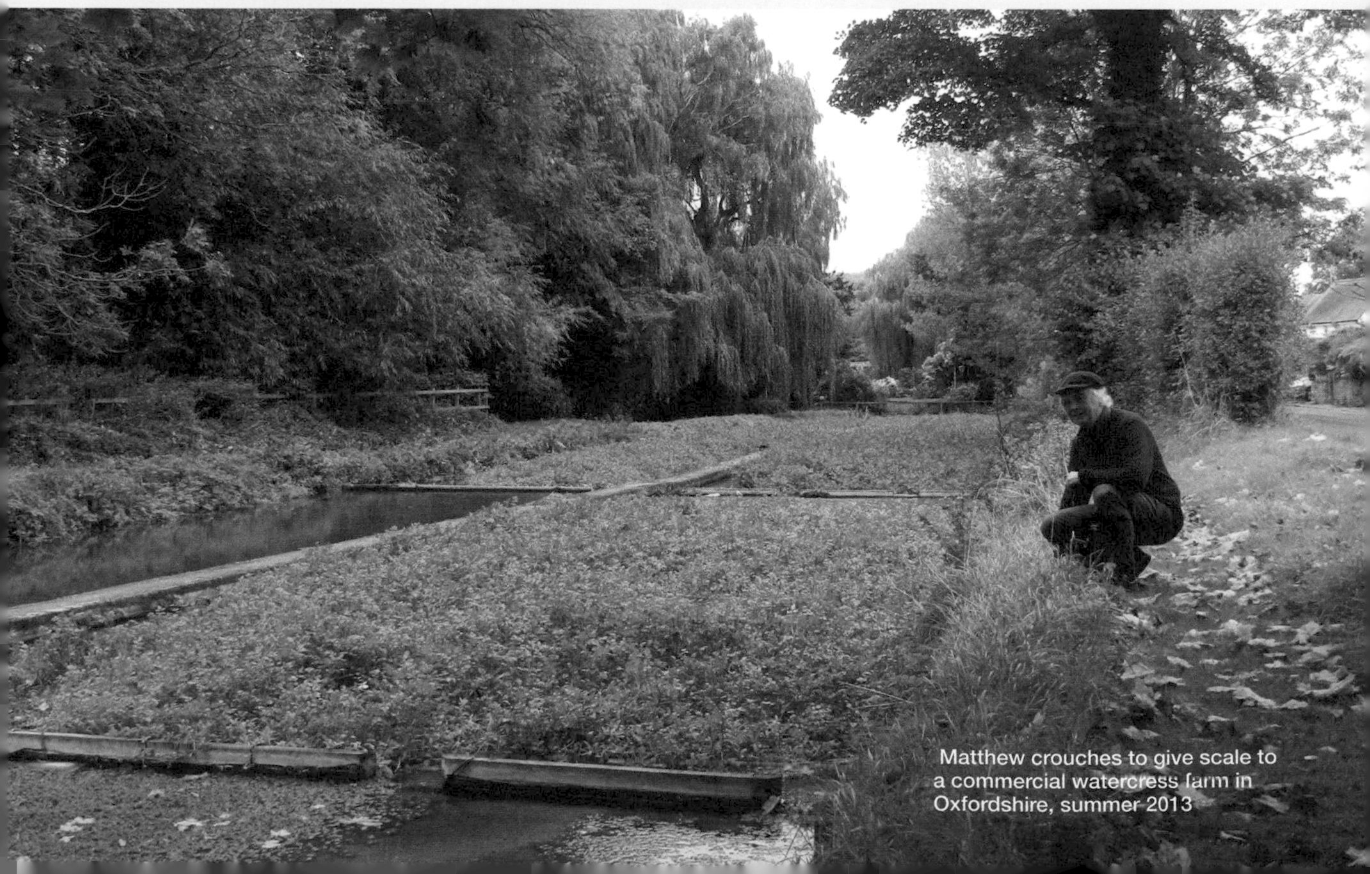

Matthew crouches to give scale to a commercial watercress farm in Oxfordshire, summer 2013

Watercress *Rorippa nasturtium-aquaticum* Brassicaceae

Parkinson does not specify eating watercress for pleasure, but using it in salads or soups today is a tasty way to take in mild bitters and leafy vitamins. His wild watercress was probably more peppery than the commercial varieties we buy in the shops, and accordingly had a more powerful range of uses. He compares watercress to the wonderfully named *Veronica beccabunga* or brooklime, which is now hardly used at all herbally.

Untypically, Parkinson does not go into the naming or history of this plant. Both are interesting.

Watercress was a popular food and medicine for the Greeks, with the general and historian Xenophon (431–355BC) describing how he gave leaves to his troops as a battle tonic. Hippocrates called it a stimulant, and Dioscorides an aphrodisiac. Its juice was used by Romans and Anglo-Saxons to treat baldness. Watercress, or stime, was one of the nine sacred herbs of the Anglo-Saxons; other evocative old English names for it were tang-tongues and tongue-grass (from its peppery taste), rib, creese and kerse.

The official names are also colourful. The plant was until recently known as *Nasturtium officinale* in the Cruciferae, but is now classified as *Rorippa* in the Brassicaceae or cabbages. Some authorities, going back to Pliny, believe *nasturtium* to derive from *nasi-tortium*, or nose-twisting (again a reference to the hot taste), but others prefer a Greek origin as *mnastorgion*, translated as 'which longs for wet soil'.

The golden age of watercress growing in England (and the US) was from the 19th to the mid-20th centuries, during which it was the main cultivated green salad plant. It could be gathered wild but was increasingly farmed. It grew readily in clear running water, often on chalk-fed streams (as recognized in the name of its close relative brooklime), with many crops a year, including mid-winter. It was an ideal small-scale but productive crop for countrymen to supply to nearby big cities or to sell in local markets.

Demand was insatiable. In his *Cyclopaedia of Botany* in 1824 Richard Brook wrote of London: 'Every morning throughout the year, although there are something like two million of inhabitants they have all Water-cresses within call, and can have them to breakfast if they choose.' Fresh watercress, with its still unknown vitamin content (the word was first used in 1912), saved many urban lives in Victorian England.

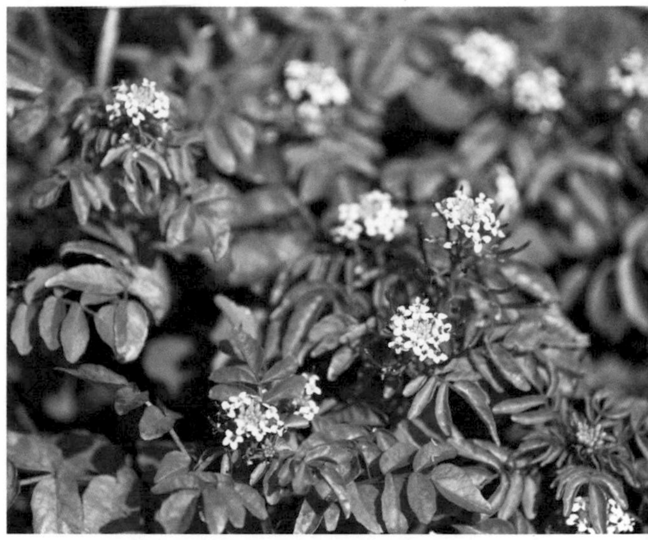

Parkinson, interestingly, knew how good watercress was for treating scurvy (the first book reference to this specific use had been in 1617). His other internal uses, in provoking urination and menstruation, cleansing the blood and clearing ulcers would be given other names today, but their validity remains. Watercress is a blood-builder, with an impressive palette of vitamins, minerals and trace elements; it detoxifies and regulates the metabolism, and nourishes the endocrine, nervous and immune systems – deficiencies in the last of which Parkinson may be referring to as 'Lethargy'.

Externally, watercress juice as a wash for the complexion, freckles, pimples and spots has been a popular folk remedy wherever watercress grows. Similarly, Parkinson's mixture of the juice with vinegar (or honey) to bathe the head was well known both before and after he wrote.

There are modern downsides he could not have known about. The most serious is the possibility of the plants carrying the parasitic liver fluke (*Fasciola hepatica*), which affects livestock and potentially humans. There is not normally a problem with purchased watercress but care is needed with wild-gathered plants. Cooking the leaves kills the flukes, and picking from fast-flowing streams is safest.

The mustard-like glycosides of watercress give it its pungent flavour, but for some people large amounts or long use irritate their gastric mucosa or bladder.

Welde

Theatrum Botanicum

Tribe 5, Chapter 64, pp602–04

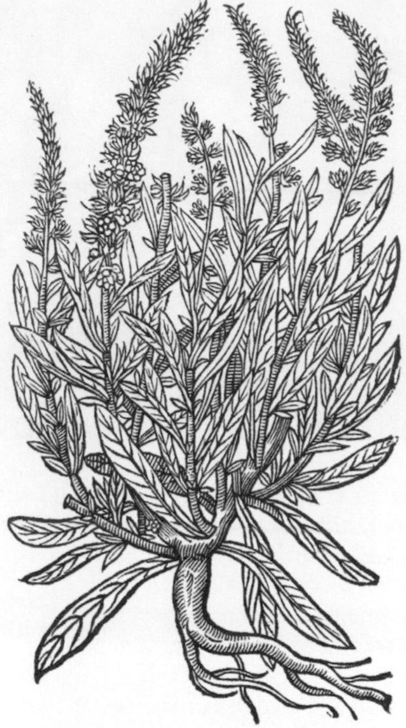

Luteola vulgaris

The Vertues

Root: *Matthiolus* saith, that the roote hereof, is hot and dry in the third degree, and that it cutteth tough flegme, it maketh grosse humours thinne, it doth resolve hard tumours, it digesteth raw flegme, and openeth obstructions.

Venom & pestilence: Some doe not onely commend it, against the bitings of any venemous creatures, to be applyed as well outwardly to the wound or hurt place, as to be taken inwardly, to expell the poyson therhence: but also much commended it to be used against the Plague or Pestilence:

Wounds: the people in some Countries of this Land, doe use to bruise the herbe, and lay it to the cuts or wounds, they chance to make in their hands, or legges, &c.

Dye: the chiefest use otherwise they have thereof, is to dye cloth, either wollen or linnen, or silke, raw or woven into a yellow colour, and also to give a greene colour to those clothes or silkes, have first been dyed with Woade, into a blue colour, which *Vitruvius* it seemeth was not ignorant of in his time, for he speaketh thereof in the aforesayd place, both booke and chapter, that a yellow colour upon a blue, is changed into greene, and for these uses, there is great store of this herbe spent in all Countries, and thereof many fields sowen for the purpose.

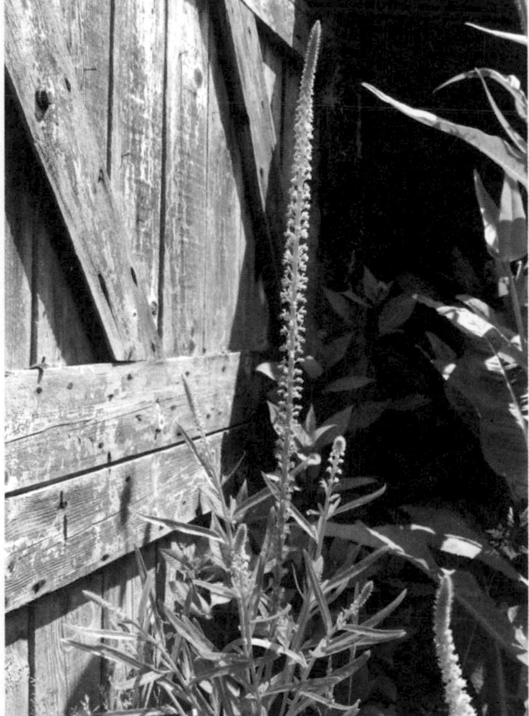

Matthiolus: Pierandrea Mattioli (1501–77), physician and author
cutteth tough flegme: breaks up thick sticky phlegm
grosse humours thinne: dilutes and thins mucus
resolve hard tumours: reduce solid tumours without pus forming
digesteth raw flegme: dissolves or dilutes thick phlegm
openeth obstructions: clears internal passages
Woade: *Isatis tinctoria*, the well-known blue dye plant
Vitruvius: Marcus Vitruvius Pollio (c.80–c.15BC), Roman military engineer and author of a ten-volume work, *De Architectura*; in his Names coverage of weld Parkinson quotes from book 7, chapter 14
sowen: sown

Weld *Reseda luteola* Resedaceae

Weld is a tall, wild perennial member of the Mignonette family with graceful arching spikes of yellow-green flowers. A native of Eurasia and introduced to North America, it is best known as a yellow dye plant, as suggested in its common names of dyer's rocket, dyer's weed, yellow and yellow rocket. Parkinson also uses the old name 'would'. Weld is related to wild mignonette, *Reseda lutea*, and the garden mignonette, *R. odorata*.

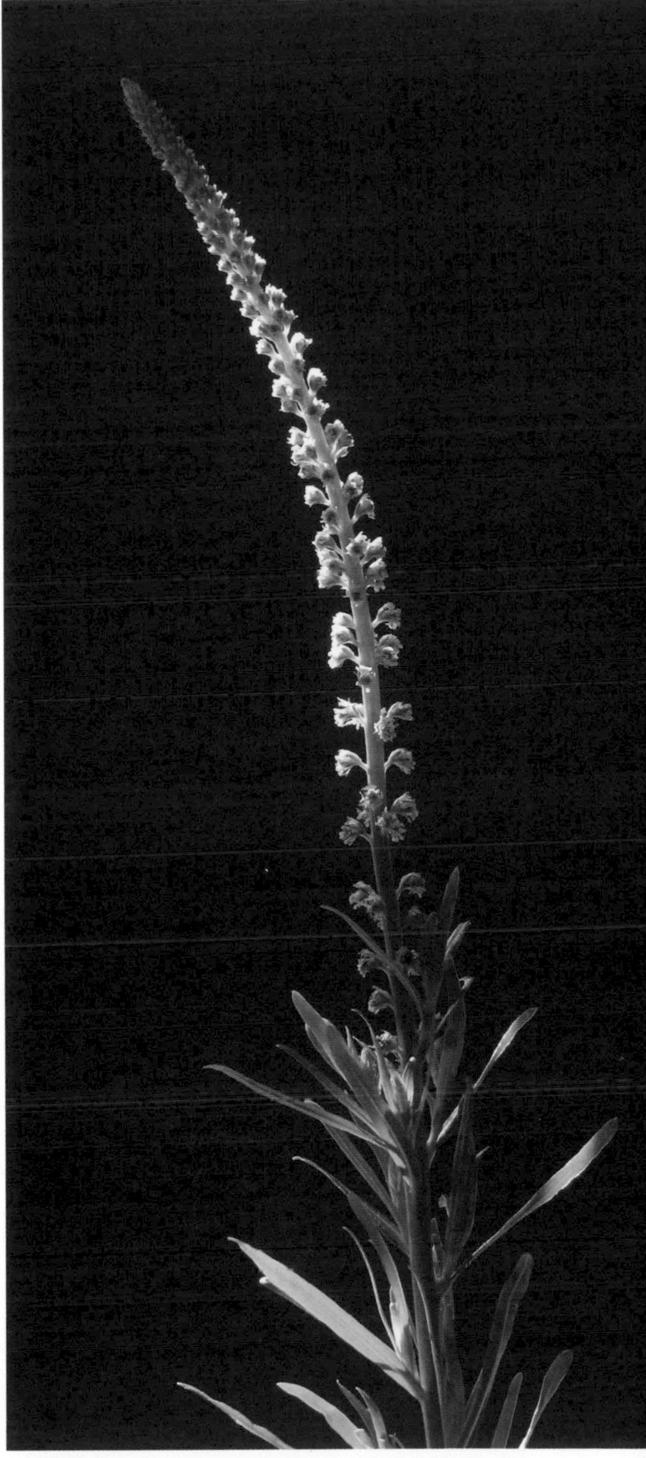

Root: Parkinson quotes Matthiolus as saying the root of weld is hot and dry in the third degree. As such it has a cleansing, clearing effect on 'tough' and 'gross' humours, opening internal obstructions and reducing hard tumours without suppuration. Parkinson reports that it was considered powerful enough to treat plague and pestilence.

Venom & pestilence: When Parkinson says 'some' commend weld to treat 'bitings of any venemous creatures' he is probably referring to Pliny, who seemed mildly obsessed by this misfortune.

Wounds: The outward use of the plant, 'bruised' to lay on wounds, poultice-style, also reflects old Roman practice.

What is new is that recent research (2010) on luteolin extract, the yellow flavonoid in weld flowers, shows 'antiproliferative and 'pro-apoptotic' activity, i.e. controls tumour growth. If this finding is repeated, it would support what Parkinson and others said so long ago.

Other research suggests that luteolin may protect the skin from UV rays and reduce 'photoaging'.

Dye: In terms of weld as a dye plant, Parkinson confirms that it gives a superior yellow finish to various fabrics and that when applied to cloth already made blue by woad it yields a strong green. This is often called Lincoln Green. The mordant (fixative) was often alum (potassium aluminium sulfate), a use that goes back at least to ancient Egypt, if not the Neolithic.

Weld was held in 'great store' until the synthetic dyes of Victorian times. The botanic writer Anne Pratt noted the decline in 1866: 'even in recent times it [weld] was planted on chalk or limestone where little else would grow, and was gathered in July, bound up in bundles and hung up to dry for the dyer's use' (*Haunts of the Wild Flowers*, p198).

Woodroofe

Theatrum Botanicum

Tribe 5, Chapter 44, pp562–63

1. *Aſperula aut Aſpergula odorata.* Common Woodroofe.

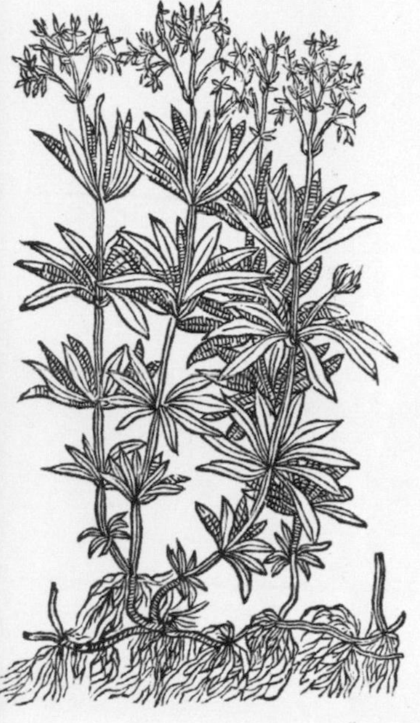

familiarly: frequently
Burnet: *Sanguisorba officinalis*
melancholly passions: bouts of depression and misery
stomacke dejected: loss of appetite
oppressed and obstructed: blocked and poorly functioning
noisome: offensive
imposthumes: cysts or abscesses
greene wound: fresh wound
effectuall: beneficial

Asperula

The Vertues

WINE: The *Germanes* doe account very highly of this Woodroofe, using it very familiarly in wine, like as we doe Burnet to take away melancholy passions, to make the heart merry;

STOMACH & LIVER: and to helpe the stomacke dejected, unto a good appetite, and the Liver being oppressed and obstructed:

INFECTIONS: it is held also to be good against the Plague, both to defend the heart, and vitall spirits from infection, and to expell the noysome vapours that are received:

CYSTS & CUTS: it helpeth also to dissolve hard imposthumes, being bruised and applyed, and in the same manner many Country people use it, for any fresh or greene wound, or cut in the flesh any where:

DISTILLED WATER: the distilled water of the herbe is no less effectuall, for the purposes aforesayd, either inwardly or outwardly.

A look behind the 'Names'

Let us take a moment to look at Parkinson's 'Names section' for woodruff as an example of the thoroughness of his scholarship. He cites the following authorities: Gesner, Pliny, Galen, Brunselsius, Tragus, Thalius, Dodoneus, Lobel, Lugudensis, Clusius, Pena, Cordus, Dioscorides, Tabermontanus, Camerarius, Turner, Bauhinus and Columna. This is 18 scholars, ancient and modern, whose work he has examined, and for only a little plant, of no particularly great merit (to judge by the small size of his 'Vertues' section).

Parkinson has been criticized for drawing on the encylopaedic *Pinax Theatri Botanici* (1623) by the French botanist Gaspard Bauhin (Bauhinus in Parkinson's list). The *Pinax*, a work of forty years' labour – Parkinson's took fifty – described briefly and classified some 6,000 plants, nearly 2,500 more than Parkinson did in his book. Intriguingly, Bauhin, a contemporary of Parkinson's (1560–1624), was planning another huge work, to be called *Theatrum Botanicum*, in twelve parts; only one was published (in 1658), and long after the author's death.

In Parkinson's defence, the *Pinax* was the outstanding classificatory work of the time, an heroic attempt to marry Greek and Roman botany with all known modern sources. This was Parkinson's grand aim too, so what better practice than refer often to Bauhin? Parkinson brought selected findings into English from Bauhin's Latin, a service in itself; he did not copy everything or choose uncritically, but, as with all his source material, he engages with previous authors, however eminent, as an equal, often rejecting them as insufficient.

Woodruff *Galium odoratum* Rubiaceae

In looking at woodruff, Geoffrey Grigson's invaluable book *The Englishman's Flora* (1958), p365, records the Old English name 'wudurofe', saying it suggested a woodland plant that spreads. The dean of British woodland studies, Oliver Rackham, uses the presence of woodruff as a leading indicator of ancient woodland.

Grigson explains how the plant in full flower was woven into 'wodrove' garlands to be hung up in churches, and the loose plant strewn on St Barnabas' Day, 11 June – it was an unplanned coincidence that Julie took her woodruff photos in our garden on this exact date. Grigson also records the delightful historic regional names kiss-me-quick, new-mown hay, scented hairhof and musk-in-the-woods, hinting at an aphrodisiac past as well as a sweet-scented one.

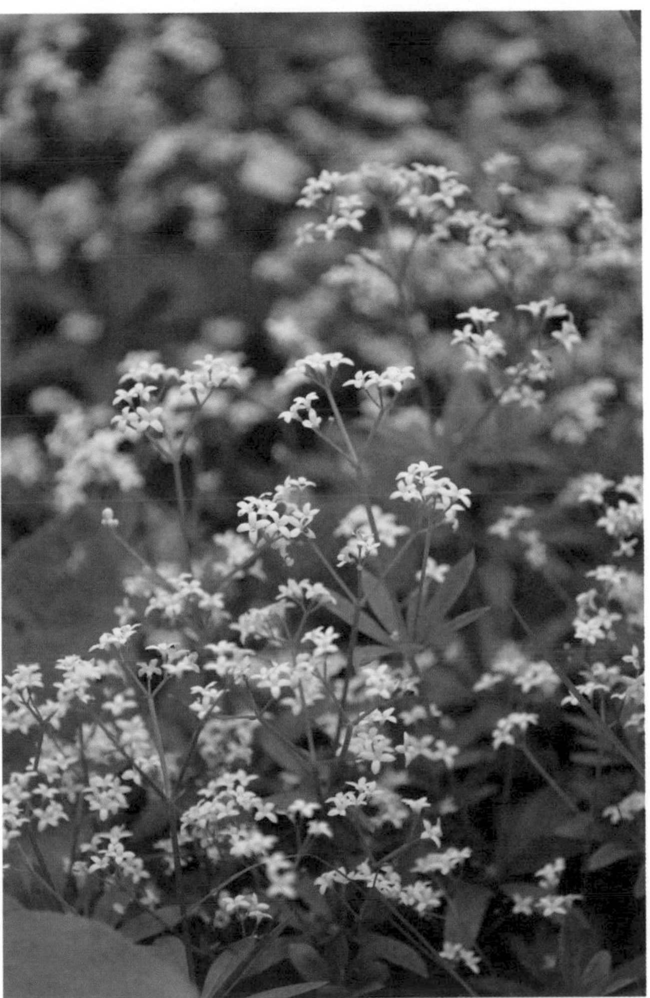

Woodruff had an ancient and medieval reputation, and was already disappearing from herbal use in Parkinson's time. British herbalist Julian Barker thinks it has all gone too far: '… [woodruff] does not deserve to have become so neglected. In reasonable doses, it is safe and pleasant to take' (*Medicinal Flora*, West Wickham, 2001, p335).

Woodruff is a healing *Galium*, alongside other white bedstraws like cleavers and the yellow lady's bedstraw. Another common name, 'sweet woodruff', and the Latin *odoratum*, highlight its pleasing fresh hay scent on drying. Mrs Grieve in her 1931 *Modern Herbal* already knew the reason: organic chemical coumarins emerging as the plant dried out.

As a scented and widely available wild plant, woodruff was in demand for strewing on floors, filling mattresses and layering with linen in drawers, much as we use lavender today, to keep clothes fresh and repel moths.

Wine: Parkinson writes of a German wine from woodruff; this was the famous *Maibowle*, drunk on May Day, but again less so now than formerly. The wine, or a woodruff cordial with apple juice, were celebratory and meant to dispel headaches and melancholy. Grigson says, 'in a full sense it is a herb of cordiality'.

Stomach & liver: A woodruff tea is delicious: make it with very hot rather than boiling water, respecting the plant's delicacy, and allow a long infusion, say 20 minutes. This tea brings out the plant's stomachic and sedative qualities, promotes appetite and decongests the liver. It was once a significant liver herb, clearing obstructions in the bile duct, including gallstones, and in treating jaundice.

Infections: Using woodruff against the plague was fanciful, although it gave a degree of protection from mild infection.

Cysts & cuts: Parkinson reports on 'Country' usage of the bruised leaf externally for alleviating cysts, cuts and much else too.

Distilled water: We have not yet made this, but can imagine how fresh, summery and cheering it must be.

Yarrow

Theatrum Botanicum

Tribe 5, Chapter 102, pp693–96

1. *Millefolium vulgare album vel rubrum.*
Common Yarrow or Millfoile, with white or red flowers.

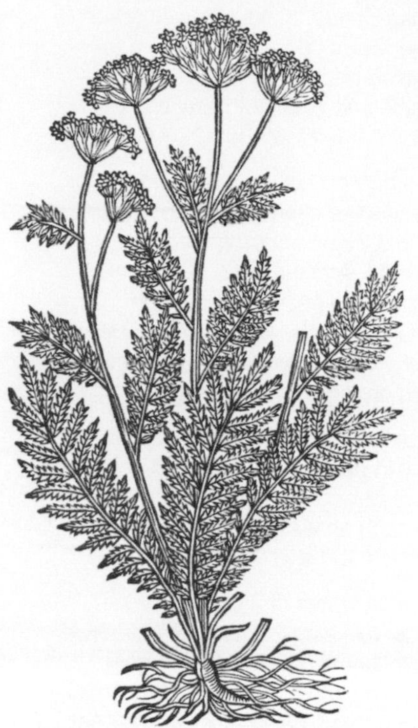

Dioscorides: Greek-speaking Roman physician (mid-first century AD)
Galen: Claudius Galen (AD130–200), Roman physician and author
sodereth: fuses
stayeth: stops
flux of blood: menstrual bleeding
sit over: i.e. a steam bath
greene wounds: fresh wounds
Fistulaes: channels or passageways
Comfrey: *Symphytum officinale*
Plantaine: *Plantago* spp.
quartaine Ague: four-day fever
fits: episodes of high fever
running of the reines: continuous urination
whites: leucorrhoea or thrush
Corall Amber & Ivory: using these powders together seems to be Parkinson's own idea rather than a recipe from the *Pharmacopoeia*

Millefolium

The Vertues

Varieties: As the face and forme of these two *Millefolium* and *Achillea* and all their varieties are very neare in resemblance one unto another, so their vertues even by *Dioscorides* and *Galen* are set downe to bee both alike, and no doubt but either of them that was next at hand, was applied for the same purpose that the other should:

Bleeding: for *Dioscorides* saith that his *Achillea* sodereth or closeth bleeding wounds and preserveth them from inflammations, and stayeth the flux of blood in women being applied in a pessary, as also if they sit over the decoction thereof while it is warme, and is drunke against the bloody flux.

Millfoile or Yarrow hee saith is of excellent use to heale both old and greene wounds, to stay bleedings and to heale Fistulaes: the powder of the dryed herbe taken with Comfrey or Plantaine water doth also stay inward bleedings and put into the nose as I said before will doe the same: the juice thereof put into the eyes taketh away the blood and rednesse therein,

Hair loss: the oyle made thereof stayeth the shedding of the haire:

Decoction: the decoction thereof made in wine and drunke is good for them that cannot reteine their meate in their stomack: it is accounted a good remedy for quartaine Ague to drinke a draught of the decoction warme before the fit, and so for two or three fits together:

Distilled water: the juice of the herbe and flowers taken either in Goates milke or in the distilled water of the herbe, stayeth the running of the reines in men and the whites in women, but it will be the more effectuall if a little powder of Corall Amber and Ivory be put thereto.

Powder: *Matthiolus* doth wonderfully commend the powder of the dryed herbe and flowers against the pissing of blood, so as to an ounce of the herbe a dram of fine Bolarmonacke bee put, and taken three days together fasting in a draught of milke:

Toothache: the roote or the greene leaves chewed in the mouth is said to ease the paines in the teeth.

Matthiolus: Pierandrea Mattioli (1501–77), physician and author
wonderfully commend: proclaim
pissing of blood: haematuria
dram: apothecary's weight, ⅛ oz, 3.89g
Bolarmonacke: [unknown]
three days fasting: without eating
draught: drink

Yarrow *Achillea millefolium* Asteraceae

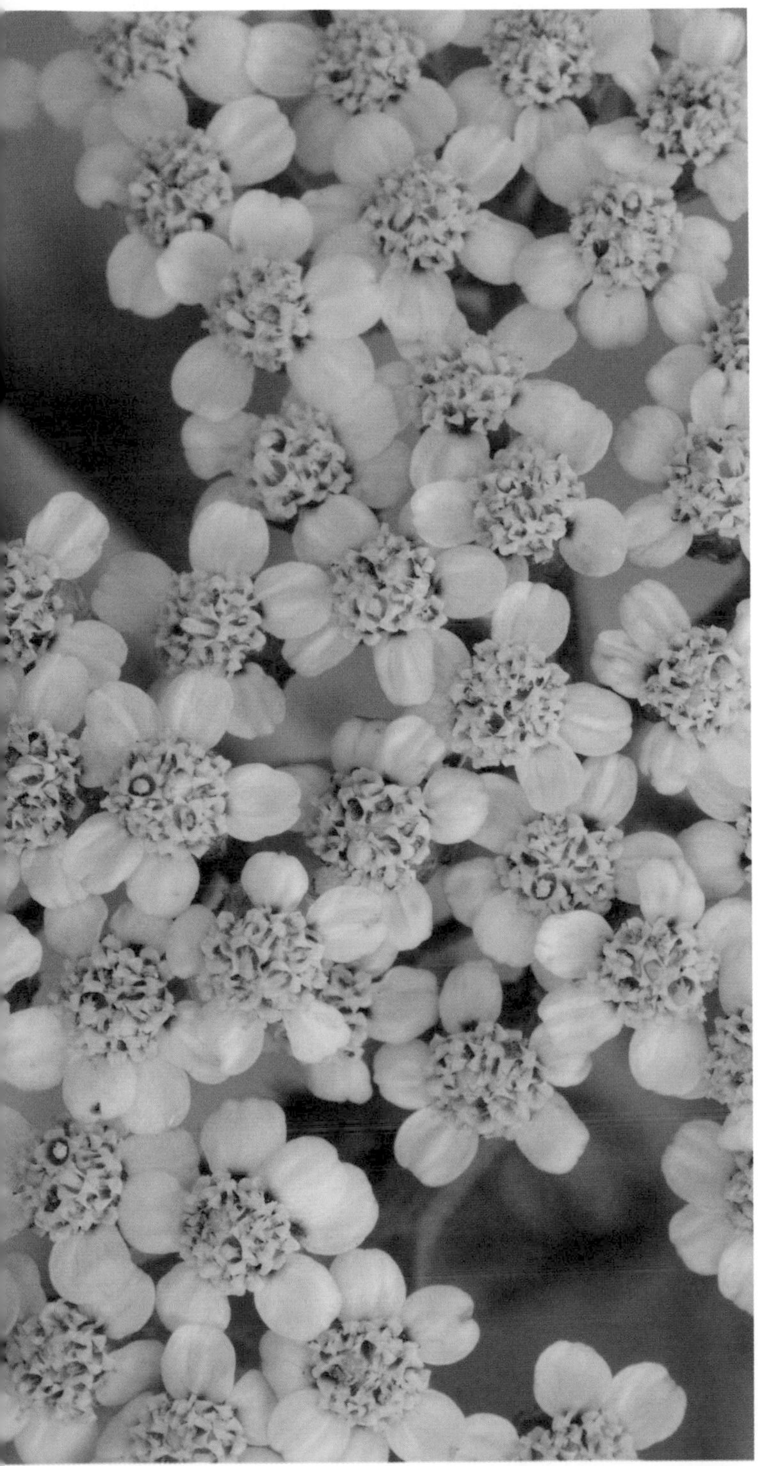

Parkinson talks of the ancient names and uses of yarrow in his 'Names' section. He describes how it was a Trojan war wound herb of Achilles, after whom it was named by Homer. It remains until now a commonly available first-aid herb for bleeding but has multiple other uses, as Parkinson explains.

Varieties: Parkinson describes 10 different kinds of yarrow, and says they can be used interchangeably. He debates with himself whether to differentiate *Millefolium* ('thousand leaves') and *Achillea*, but decides not, as the 'vertues' are the same; even Dioscorides and Galen agree on this. His white Candy yarrow, incidentally, is what we know today as English mace, sneezewort or *Achillea ptarmica*.

Bleeding: Yarrow's remarkable anticoagulant properties are effective on both external and internal wounds, he explains. Note his recommendation of a pessary, or sitting over a warm infusion as a vapour treatment, or a yarrow tea for stopping internal bleeding. The first two are methods worth reviving.

Yarrow is equally useful, he says, for fresh or old wounds; he mentions taking the powder into the nostrils (we have found inserting the fresh leaf handier for nosebleeds). The combination with comfrey (knitbone) and plantain is still used by some herbalists.

Yarrow is often seen as an emotional wound-healer too, a deep re-energizer and releaser of excess heat and toxins. As Irish herbalist Nikki Darrell says, it 'heals our warrior energy'.

Hair loss: We haven't tried a yarrow oil to counter hair loss, but we'd trust him on this.

Decoction: Yarrow is a sweat-inducing herb, in a tea (or in wine, as Parkinson says), and used to raise fevers and as a settling digestive. It also has a role in cleaning the liver – as good as milk thistle, say some herbalists.

Distilled water & powder: We have yet to try his and Matthiolus' intriguing recipes.

Toothache: Chewing the root or leaves is not to everybody's taste but makes a good pain-reliever.

NOTES

These are notes to the Introduction (pp9–21). Place of publication is London, unless otherwise stated. TB and *Theatrum* are abbreviations used for *Theatrum Botanicum*.

1 Sir James Edward Smith wrote in 1819: 'This work [the *Theatrum*] and the herbal of Gerarde were the two main pillars of botany in England till the time of Ray, who indeed gave them fresh importance by his continual reference to their contents.' In A. Rees, *The Cyclopaedia*, vol. 26 (1819) [no pagination]. Reference in Blanche Henrey, *British Botanical and Horticultural Literature before 1800*, 2 vols (1975), I, 79.

2 John Ray ranks 'our Parkinson' with Gaspard Bauhin, Fabius Columna, Prosper Alpinus, Cornutus and other European herbalists: 'Our Parkinson I put into ye number because there be many plants in his work not elsewhere described.' In a letter to John Aubrey, 3 March 1677. Reference in R.W.T. Gunther (ed)., *Further Correspondence of John Ray* (1928), p159.

3 Richard Pulteney, *Historical and Biographical Sketches of the Progress of Botany in England*, 2 vols (1790), I, 148.

4 R.T. Gunther, *Early English Botanists and their Gardens* (Oxford, 1922), pp266–75. The Goodyer Papers in the Magdalen College Archives are now catalogued as MSS 327 and 328.

5 Charles E. Raven, *English Naturalists from Neckam to Ray* (Cambridge, 1947), pp255, 272.

6 Anna Parkinson, *Nature's Alchemist: John Parkinson, Herbalist to Charles I* (2007). See also Anna Parkinson, *Who Do You Think You Are?* (BBC, 2008), pp32–6, with thanks to Wendy Chapman for the reference.

7 Graeme Tobyn, Alison Denham & Margaret Whitelegg, *The Western Herbal Tradition: 2000 years of Medicinal Plant Knowledge* (Edinburgh, 2011). The four herbalists chosen for the 17th century (p2) are Jean Bauhin, Gerard, Parkinson and Culpeper.

8 Benjamin Woolley, *The Herbalist: Nicholas Culpeper and the Fight for Medical Freedom* (2004), p371, n21, points out that Izaak Walton's *The Compleat Angler* has also remained continuously in print, but it was published in 1653, a year after Culpeper's *English Physitian*.

9 Anna Parkinson, *Nature's Alchemist*, pp19–22. *The Oxford Dictionary of National Biography* (*ODNB*) entry on John Parkinson (by Juanita Burnby, 2004) does not offer a place of birth; many earlier accounts stated it was Nottinghamshire. Other historians are now building on Anna Parkinson's research: see e.g. Margaret Willes, *The Making of the English Gardener* (New Haven, 2011), pp175–6.

10 Anna Parkinson has said she would now lay more emphasis on John's mother as an influence on his love of plants (pers. comm., June 2013).

11 Anna Parkinson, *Nature's Alchemist*, p43.

12 In Matthias de l'Obel, *Opera Omnia* (1605); translation in Anna Parkinson, *Nature's Alchemist*, p131.

13 Sir Theodore de Mayerne, English translation from his panegyric in *Paradisi in Sole*.

14 An earlier resident of Cripplegate, the apothecary-surgeon William Bullein, had published his 'Apothecaries' Rules' in 1562. While expected to know Dioscorides and Galen, develop medicines and undertake minor surgery, the apothecary, said Bullein, must never forget he was subject to the College of Physicians, as 'ye Physician's Cook'. Bullein, *Bulwarke of Defence Against All Sickness* (1562). See Penelope Hunting, *A History of the Society of Apothecaries* (1998), p26.

15 Robert Gunther in the 1920s identified a copy of de l'Obel's *Stirpium Observationes* (1576) as belonging to Parkinson, who had annotated it in neat Latin script. The teenage apprentice had chosen to mark his private copy in Latin – a telling response to critics who dismiss Parkinson as lacking academic qualification.

16 Of the 71 apprentices examined that day only a handful were apothecaries and the rest grocers. Anna Parkinson, *Nature's Alchemist*, p85.

17 Richard Bragge in 1594 and Thomas Nicoll in 1597. See Anna Parkinson, *Nature's Alchemist*, pp92, 98.

18 Parkinson had to be watchful to keep his garden intact while all around him the Covent Garden area was being rapidly and expensively developed. Anna Parkinson suggests he may have resisted pressures from the crown to sell or move. See n32 below.

19 The last reference to Richard Parkinson is on 11 June 1646, when Parkinson's old friend John Morris wrote (in Latin) to Johannes de Laet of the loss of 'this young man, very skilled in this Art [of botany], who before the Civil Wars was gardener to the Earl of Newport, on account of his papism'. J.A.F. Bekkers (ed.), *Correspondence of John Morris with Johannes de Laet (1634–1649)* (Nijmegen, 1970), letter 66, p117; English translation, Anna Parkinson, *Nature's Alchemist*, p274. Of Katherine Parkinson, we have no knowledge at all.

20 Morris to De Laet, 11 June 1646; Bekkers, letter 66, p117; translation in Anna Parkinson, *Nature's Alchemist*, p281.

21 St Martins in the Fields, burial register, Westminster Archives, Mf 3, Mf 1546–9. There is no gravestone, but Linnaeus named a semi-arid shrub of the pea family *Parkinsonia*; sadly, *P. aculeata* has become a noxious weed in Australia.

22 The Worshipful Society of Apothecaries of London website, www.apothecaries.org [last accessed 18 March 2014].

23 The royal charter (Letters Patent) of 6 December 1617 lists 122 founder members of the Society. Hunting, *History*, p33. Membership grew slightly once the Society fended off legal challenges by the Grocers, and particularly after the City formally recognized the Society through its grant of full livery status in 1630.

24 Between 1567 and 1609, according to port books, the volume of imported drugs more than doubled. Hunting, *History*, p29. For London's population growth, see figures in Ben Weinreb and Christopher Hibbert, *The London Encyclopaedia* (1983).

25 According to his kinsman, Thomas Delaune, writing in 1681, Gideon de Laune left £90,000 at his death in 1659. Charles G.D. Littleton comments in the *ODNB* (2004) that there was 'a good deal of hyperbole' in the amount. Various historical comparison websites suggest £1 in 1640 is worth from £140 to £278 in 2014, so multiplying by 100 for establishing current sterling values seems conservative, but realistic.

26 See Margaret Pelling and Frances White, Physicians and Irregular Practitioners in London 1550–1640, Database (2004), www.british-history.ac.uk/report.aspx?compid=17693 [last accessed 9 March 2013].

27 In 1624 King James stoutly and successfully defended the Society of Apothecaries, and equally his own championing of it, to Parliament, which had taken up the Grocers' cause: 'I myselfe did devyse this Corporation and doe allow it. The Grocers that compleyned of it, are but marchants.' Hunting, *History*, p35.

28 Bacon especially was playing a dangerous game: he was charged by the House of Lords in 1621 with taking bribes from both sides (£200 from the Grocers' Company and £100 from the Apothecaries, plus a taster of gold and a gift of ambergris). He was imprisoned, fined and banned from Parliament. Hunting, *History*, p266, n12.

29 To explain our own views, we admire the usefulness and even recklessness of Culpeper's 1649 *Pharmacopoeia Londinensis*, but while liking the way his 1652 book *The English Physitian* prioritizes local herbs and is written and priced for everyman, we cannot easily forgive Culpeper for stealing Parkinson's words. See n59 below.

30 In 1635, after many years of silence on Society affairs, Parkinson was called to give evidence in the '*Quo Warranto*' legal dispute with the Grocers. This long-running case was heard in the court of Star Chamber and dragged on unresolved until Star Chamber itself was abolished in 1641. Parkinson condemned the 1618 *Pharmacopeia* as poor, but said it had been rescued by the Apothecaries; the Apothecaries in response had produced their own Schedule and in everyday practice used that instead.

31 In 1640, writing on 'sealed earth' (*Terra lemnia, T. sigillata*) (TB, p1608), Parkinson explains it is not a herb but 'a drugge of much respect and use in physicke', which he wants to describe to 'my Brethren in profession' because it is so often counterfeited. He says: 'for that is the whole scope of my labours in this Worke, viz. to enforme all of the genuine and right things, that they may desire, and know them, and also the best true uses whereunto they serve'.

32 Parkinson's property affairs are as yet untangled, but Anna Parkinson relates how after the *Paradisi* was published Charles I gave Parkinson a lease on a piece of land 'neare the tennis courts in St James Fields' for use as a garden, at 20s a year. Parkinson brought in his fellow Apothecary Stephen Chase, but it appears nothing was built there, and the site lay untouched in 1660. This may well be the 'Physicke garden' land that the Society of Apothecaries came to control in Charles II's reign. See J. Burnby, 'Some Early London Physic Gardens', *Pharmaceutical Historian*, 24(4) (1994), 2–7. Parkinson did have leases on two houses, one in St Martin's Lane and the other in Round Court, Covent Garden. Anna Parkinson, *Nature's Alchemist*, pp214–15.

33 De l'Obel called himself a '*botanographus*', a writer about plants, and he was unusual among the great botanists for organizing publication of his own complete works in his lifetime (his *Opera Omnia* appearing in London in 1605). He passed this insistence on publication to Parkinson. Anna Parkinson, *Nature's Alchemist*, pp129–30.

34 Parkinson often addresses gentlewomen in the *Paradisi* and gives plants the English names they would be familiar with.

35 'Accept, I beseech your Majestie, this speaking Garden': To the Queenes Most Excellent Majestie, *Paradisi*.

36 The Epistle to the Reader, *Paradisi*.

37 Ibid.

38 Long Acre had become one of London's famous gardens, though long since built over. Parkinson quickly had his wall repaired after a storm on 4 November 1636 (we know of this because the bill is preserved by chance in the Goodyer Papers). He was still acquiring plants up to 1640: he writes of the mountain spignel from Germany (i.e. *Meum)* he has received, saying 'when it is better growne up with me … I shall be the better judge' (TB, p889). See John N.D. Riddell, 'John Parkinson's Long Acre Garden 1600–1650', *Journal of Garden History* 6(2) (1986), 112–14. Riddell gives a list of plants in Parkinson's garden, updated by Anna Parkinson (her Appendix, p296). When the parish overseers came to collect the poor rate on 24 December 1640, Parkinson had gone. Anna Parkinson, *Nature's Alchemist*, pp250, 274.

39 Goodyer's visit in 1616, a formative one in Goodyer's life, is recorded in Goodyer MS 327, fo. 107, Magdalen College, Oxford, and in Gunther, *Early English Botanists*, p56.

40 William Broad, translation from Latin in Anna Parkinson, *Nature's Alchemist*, p200.

41 William Atkins, translation from Latin in Anna Parkinson, *Nature's Alchemist*, p201.

42 Parkinson grumbled that 'While I beate the bushe [i.e. paid], another catcheth and eateth the bird' [i.e. Boel had given some of Parkinson's pea plants from Spain to Coys]. Parkinson says he had bought the seedlings, sown them and written up an account for publication, but a 'collateral friend' [probably John Goodyer] had prevented this by giving notes on the peas to Johnson, who now put them in his revision of Gerard (TB, p1064).

43 *Theatrum* as a title was in vogue. Parkinson found Gaspard Bauhin's *Pinax Theatri Botanici* of 1623 formative (see above, p230), and another use of 'Theatrum' might have influenced him to adopt the Latin form. His mentor De Mayerne in 1634 had paid the printing costs of the unpublished insect survey of the late Thomas Moffett (also known as Mouffet and Muffett), *Insectorum … theatrum*. The Moffett papers were sold to de Mayerne by Moffett's colleague, and later Parkinson's, the chemical apothecary Daniel Darnelly. De Mayerne got a bargain as he used several recipes from Moffett's papers to produce commercially successful medicines. Hugh Trevor-Roper, *Europe's Physician: The Various Life of Sir Theodore de Mayerne* (New Haven, 2006), pp215–16, 404n.

44 See Appendix 6, pp246–7, for reproduction of an unaltered sample spread from TB (the edited version is on pp130–1 above).

45 Parkinson's dedication in TB 'To the Kings Most Excellent Maiestie' offers him 'this Manlike Worke of Herbes and Plantes', 'as I formerly did a Feminine of Flowers' to the Queen. These expected customary encomia in TB are harshly judged as demonstrating 'male control of medical practice' and 'genderizing his audience', by Rebecca Laroche, *Medical Authority and Englishwomen's Herbal Texts, 1550–1650* (Farnham, 2009), p28.

47 Parkinson, Epistle to the Reader, TB. One commentator reads it differently: the preface 'practically breeds resentment': Laroche, *Medical Authority*, p40.

48 Parkinson uses an elegant but damning Latin phrase for Johnson's rapid work: 'the rushing dog produces blind puppies' (Epistle to the Reader). In the 'Names' section of 'starre thistle' (*Carduus stellaris*) (TB, p990) he is conciliatory: 'many such faults have passed Mr. *Iohnsons* correction, which I am loth in every place to exhibit'; while the notorious barnacle goose plant, which Johnson kept almost unchanged from Gerard's original, is passed over as 'an admirable tale of untruth' (TB, p1306).

49 The brothers Thomas and Richard Cotes set up as printers in the Barbican, Aldersgate Street, in 1627. Thomas died in 1642 and Richard in 1653, when Richard's widow Ellen took over the

business until at least 1670. Richard was appointed official printer to the City of London in 1642, and in his will of 1652 left his son Andrew the rights in the *Theatrum*; nothing came of this, however. Henry R. Plomer, *A Dictionary of Booksellers and Printers … 1641 to 1667* (1907), pp52–3.

50 Richard Cotes registered the *Theatrum* with the Stationers Company on 3 March 1634: *English Short Title Catalogue*, p215.

51 Rex Jones notes the appearance of another large herbal in 1633, the unrevised reissue of William Langham's *Garden of Health*, coincidentally first published in 1597, the same year as Gerard. Rex Jones, 'Generalogy of a Classic: *The English Physitian* of Nicholas Culpeper', unpublished PhD thesis, University of California, San Francisco, 1984, p110.

52 Parkinson explains he needs a new approach as he is including the 'spices and drougues in our Apothecaries shoppes' (TB, p1564). The new method unfortunately means he relies more on hearsay descriptions for the first time, being unable to examine or grow many of the things he describes. See Appendix 2, p238.

53 Translation in Anna Parkinson, *Nature's Alchemist*, p260.

54 Johnson's Gerard actually cost more in 1633: 42s 6d unbound and 48s bound: Henrey, *British Botanical and Horticultural Literature before 1800*, I, 53. At the other end of the spectrum Culpeper fixed the price of his *English Physitian* (1652) at 3d, so that anyone could afford it.

55 De Mayerne writes in his panegyric to *Theatrum*: 'very recently he [the king] has thought to give you the honourable title First of the King's Botanists for your excellence so that, summoned into the medical family of the Court, you may be obliged to dedicate your work to Your Most Serene Ruler' (translation by Tony Pitman). Normally any medical book needed the imprimatur of the College of Physicians, but the king's approval trumped that.

56 William A. Clarke, *First Records of British Flowering Plants*, 2nd edn (1900) offers an interesting perspective on how many 'firsts' in the British flora these authors named. Turner is counted as 238, Gerard (1597) 182, Johnson (1633) 170, and Parkinson 28. Parkinson's small list includes some surprisingly late first namings, including cock's foot, Scots pine, sea buckthorn, strawberry tree and wintergreen. For full Parkinson list, see Appendix 5, p244.

57 In terms of reputation, copies of Gerard (old and new), Parkinson and Culpeper's herbal were all popular in colonial North America, before locally written and relevant herbals began to be published there in the early 18th century.

58 A good account of Gerard's dishonest and pre-emptive tactics, but which also acknowledges the importance of his *Herball*, is Deborah E. Harkness, *The Jewel House: Elizabethan London and the Scientific Revolution* (New Haven, 2007), pp49–56.

59 A comparison we made of the virtues of two randomly selected herbs in TB and *English Physitian* showed that, for centaury, Culpeper used some 64% of the same words as Parkinson; for lovage, the figure was 82%. If you omit the astrology, always Culpeper's own contribution, the percentages are higher. Further word counts and linguistic analysis will confirm Culpeper's unacknowledged and unreported debt to Parkinson.

[This note was written before seeing a new book chapter by Graeme Tobyn, a Culpeper specialist, who shows with examples how Culpeper was directly copying from Parkinson. Tobyn writes that Culpeper's *English Physitian* 'is substantially indebted to the work of John Parkinson in a way largely unrecognised by researchers'. Graeme Tobyn, 'An Anatomy of *The English Physitian*', in *Critical Approaches to the History of Western Herbal Medicine*, ed. Susan Francina and Anne Stobart (2014), pp87–103, at p99. Thanks to Christine Herbert for the reference.]

60 Raven, *English Naturalists*, p268.

61 Jones, 'Genealogy of a Classic', p114.

62 John Rea's *Flora: Seu, De Florum Cultura. Or, A Complete Florilege* (1676) announces the death of the herbal. In his 'To the Reader', Rea says a Florilege will suit the needs of 'a Florist' better than the 'old method of a Herbal', with its 'old Names, uncertain Places and little or no Virtues'. Rea rejects illustrations, 'especially in Wood, as Mr. Parkinson hath done … such Artless things being good for nothing, unless to raise the price of the Book'.

63 Ray, letter to John Aubrey, May 1678, in Gunther (ed.), *Further Correspondence of John Ray*, p159.

64 Raven, *English Naturalists*, p272.

65 In his study of Galenic medicine as an apprentice and later Parkinson probably made use of Latin translations of Dioscorides and Galen by Thomas Linacre, founder of the College of Physicians (1518). Anna Parkinson, *Nature's Alchemist*, p63. John Goodyer spent his later years trying to finish his own modern version of Dioscorides, but this work was unfinished at his death; it was finally published in an edition by Robert Gunther in 1934.

66 The idea is credited to Robin Fåhraeus, 'The suspension-stability of the blood', *Acta Medica Scandinavica* 55 (1921), 1–228.

67 Plague years in London in Parkinson's lifetime are generally reckoned to include 1585–7, 1593, 1603–4, 1609–10, 1625, 1637 and 1645; the last and most devastating plague, of course, was in 1665. Brian Williams, 'The Cycles of Plague', BA diss., University of Hull, 1996, urbanrim.org.uk [last accessed 3 March 2014]. Sir Theodore offered this advice to physicians faced by the plague: *cito*, *longe*, *tarde*, i.e. get away quickly, go far away and stay away a long time. This periodic desertion by the physicians was much resented by the Apothecaries, who would remain in harm's way, working with masks and wearing pomanders.

68 Parkinson rarely relies on tinctures. Culpeper's *Pharmacopoeia* lists just seven (p70); Culpeper comments that strawberry tincture is 'A gallant fine thing for Gentlemen that have nothing else to do with their money'. It is actually very sweet and tasty!

69 Parkinson had a marked sympathy for female medical issues, as Anna Parkinson notes: *Nature's Alchemist*, pp100–1, while Laroche, *Medical Authority*, p40, sees in the *Theatrum* an attempt to start a new patrilineage of herbalism.

70 Parkinson's mantra is finding out by experience. Superstition, or unexamined knowledge, is his foe: thus, writing on mugwort, he notes 'many … idle superstitions and irreligious relations are set downe, both by the ancient and later Writers, concerning this and other plants, which to relate were both unseemely for me, and unprofitable for you'. He goes on: 'But Oh the weak and fragile nature of man! Which cannot but lament, that it is more prone to beleeve and relye upon such impostures, than upon the ordinances of God in his creatures, and trust in his providence.' This is also as far as he goes in expressing an overtly religious viewpoint (TB, p90).

APPENDIX 1: PARKINSON'S TRIBES

Below is a transcription of the contents page from the *Theatrum*. Parkinson did not add page numbers because the book was printed in sections as he completed the text, and he may have planned to come back to it once the full pagination was known.

He lists 17 Tribes, or classes, and an Appendix. The bracketed numbers are added by us to indicate the number of chapters in each tribe; each chapter might contain a dozen or more species.

His first seven tribes have an apothecary basis in terms of their usefulness; Tribes 8–14 and 16 are botanically descriptive, while 15 and 17 are his 'catch-all' categories. By adopting such a transitional classificatory system, Parkinson has come in for considerable retrospective criticism from post-Linnaean botanical scholars. Richard Pulteney, writing in 1790, argues in Parkinson's defence: 'These are defects common to the age, and Parkinson must not be appreciated by modern improvements but by comparison with his contemporaries.'

As can be seen, the final chapter, of 'Strange and Outlandish Plants' was by far the largest. Plants from overseas kept on arriving in London, and Parkinson would add just one more …

The Classes or Tribes contained in this Worke, are these:

1 Sweete smelling Plants <50>

2 Purging Plants <66>

3 Venemous, Sleepy, and Hurtfull Plants, and their Counterpoysons <35>

4 Saxifrages, or Breakestone Plants <22>

5 Vulnerary or Wound Herbes <113>

6 Cooling and Succory-like Herbes <44>

7 Hot and Sharpe biting Plants <29>

8 Umbelliferous Plants <44>

9 Thistles and Thorny Plants <33>

10 Fearnes and Capillary Herbes <14>

11 Pulses <35>

12 Cornes <26>

13 Grasses, Rushes and Reedes <40>

14 Marsh, Water and Sea Plants, and Mosses, and Mushromes <64>

15 The Unordered Tribe <30>

16 Trees and Shrubbes <107>

17 Strange and Outlandish Plants <149>

An Appendix to The Theater of Plants <about 30; not counted>

APPENDIX 2: APOTHECARY PRICES, 1639

These apothecary prices are taken from Philbert Guibert, *The Charitable Physitian with the Charitable Apothecary*, translated by I.W. (London, 1639), pp45–51. Guibert is named on the title page as Physician Regent in Paris, but the identity of I.W. is not known.

The text does not explain whether I.W. has transposed Paris prices or has adjusted them for London. The difference is unlikely to be radical. The important point here is rather which items an upmarket London apothecary's shop, such as Parkinson's, might stock. It also offers an idea of the comparative costs of typical apothecary items at the time the *Theatrum* was being completed.

I.W. addresses the 'Courteous Reader' by saying he is writing about remedies used by the 'best and faithfullest Physitians', which 'you can easily make your selfe … or cause them to bee made by your servants'. He refers briefly to the medical marketplace: 'You shall buy your Drogues or Medicaments at the Droguists, being chosen by the said Physitian; and your Roots, Hearbes, Seeds, Flowers, &c. at the Herborists or hearbe women in Cheap-side.'

The prices of 152 items are given in pounds, shillings and pence, usually by the pound; in one case, Amber-greece (ambergris) a dramme is specified, and in seven cases, including bezoar, the unit is the ounce. Bezoar, at £2 10s an ounce, is many times the price of the next mostly costly item, saffron. Parkinson says the 'bezar stone' is 'of so high esteeme, even next unto Unicornes horne, and of so much and excellent use in Physicke that I could not leave it out' of the book (TB, p1589). The stone came from the stomach of a goat, he says, and it would resist 'poysons and venomes', and also treat plague. This last use accounts for its extravagant price, but Parkinson questions its efficacy.

This list from Guibert comprises mostly plants, with some foods and many gums and minerals. Most are described systematically in Tribe 17 of the *Theatrum*, and being alphabetically listed there are easily found. Far from Parkinson's final chapter being wacky foreign plants he had barely seen, as some say, we think it is one of his most inclusive and useful for practitioners, which gave the book much of its textbook value.

The basis of this apothecary's list is imported or marketed herbs, with indications of chemical herbalism (quicksilver, fragments of precious stone, litarge), but in a relatively limited presence. What you don't find here are common English herbs. As I.W. points out (p51), 'For the value of roots, hearbes, and other such like you may have them cheape at the Herbarists.' Clearly this book considers expensive imported items to be a cut above simple local herbs and the 'hearbe-women in Cheap-side'.

	£	s	d
Acassia the pound	0	4	2
Acorus the pound	0	10	0
Agaricke the pound	0	18	0
Aloes the pound	0	12	0
Roche Alum the pound	0	3	0
Bitter Almonds the pound	0	1	0
Sweet Almonds the pound	0	0	6
Amber-greece the dramme	0	10	0
Yellow Amber the pound	0	2	6
Angelica the pound	0	6	8
Anniseeds the pound	0	0	10
Quick-silver the pound	0	4	0
Aristolochia round the pound	0	1	0
Aristolochia long the pound	0	1	0
Asarum the pound	0	2	6
Assafætida the pound	0	4	0
Bayberries the pound	0	0	6
Mirtle Berries the pound	0	1	0
Bdellium the pound	0	6	0
Been Album the pound	0	1	8
Been Rubr: the pound	0	1	6
Benjamin the pound	0	6	0
Berberris the pound	0	0	8
Bezoar the ounce	2	10	0
Bithumeis Iudac: the pound	0	4	0
Lign: Aloes the pound	1	4	0
Bol Armoniacke the pound	0	1	4
Borax the pound	0	6	0
Calamus Aromat the pound	0	1	0
Campher the pound	0	6	0
Cantharides the ounce	0	2	6
Cardamom majus the pound	0	4	0
Cardamom minus the pound	0	0	8
Carpobalsamum the ounce	0	0	6
Cassia the pound	0	4	6
Castoreum the pound	0	1	0
Cæruse the pound	0	0	6
White waxe the pound	0	1	4
Yellow waxe the pound	0	1	8
China the pound	0	12	0
Colocynthidos the pound	0	6	0
Colophonia the pound	0	0	4
Red Corall the pound	0	4	6
White Corall the pound	0	3	6
Cortex radic: Cappar: the pound	0	2	6
Cortex radic: Tamarise the pound	0	2	0
Cortex guaiaci the pound	0	0	8
White Costus the pound	0	6	0
Cremor tartar the pound	0	8	0
Christall minerall the pound	0	2	6
Cubebes the pound	0	5	0
Cyperus roots the pound	0	1	4

	£	s	d
Dates the pound	0	1	6
Dictaum: Cret: the pound	0	8	0
White Ellebor the pound	0	0	9
Blacke Ellebor the pound	0	2	0
Olibanum the pound	0	2	6
Common Frankincense the pound	0	0	4
Epithymum the pound	0	2	6
Candied Citron peele the pound	0	3	6
Euphorbium the pound	0	1	6
Fenill seeds the pound	0	1	2
Stæchados the pound	0	1	8
Folium Indum the ounce	0	1	6
Fragments of pretious stones, of Emerauds, Grinads, Saphirs, and Topaz each of them an ounce	0	1	0
Guaicum the pound	0	0	2
Galbanum a pound	0	6	0
Galingall the pound	0	6	0
Gum: Armoniacke the pound	0	2	8
Gum: Arabicke the pound	0	0	10
Gum: Dragant the pound	0	0	10
Grana tinctor: i.Kermes the pound	0	6	0
Hermodacti the pound	0	1	4
Hypocytis the pound	0	4	6
Ialap the pound	0	7	10
Ireos of Florence the pound	0	1	8
Iujubes the pound	0	1	4
Iuncus odoratus the pound	0	6	0
Labdanum the pound	0	3	6
Gum-Lacke the pound	0	6	0
Lapis Calaminaris the pound	0	2	0
Lapis hemacitis the pound	0	10	0
Lapis Luzuli the pound	0	1	8
Lapis spongiæ the pound	0	0	6
Litarge of gold the pound	0	0	6
Litarge of silver the pound	0	0	6
Lupius the pound	0	1	4
Manna Calabrin the pound	0	12	0
Masticke the pound	0	8	0
Mechoachan the pound	0	7	8
Minium the pound	0	0	10
Mirrhe the pound	0	12	0
Muske the dramme	0	15	0
Nux vomica the pound	0	1	6
Cyrpus Nuts the pound	0	0	10
Galls the pound	0	0	8
Opium the pound	0	12	0
Opibalsamum the pound	0	6	8
Opoponax the pound	0	10	0
Orpiment the pound	0	1	4

	£	s	d
Penedes the pound	0	1	6
Navell pitch the pound	0	0	3
Burgundie pitch the pound	0	0	6
Pistaches the pound	0	1	6
Polipodie the pound	0	0	8
Long pepper the pound	0	5	0
Piretrum the pound	0	2	6
Roots of Esula the pound	0	2	6
Licorish the pound	0	1	2
Rubarbe the pound	1	8	0
Saffron the pound	1	12	0
Sagapænum the pound	0	8	0
Dragons blood the pound	0	2	0
White Sanders the pound	0	1	4
Red Sanders the pound	0	1	4
Yellow Sanders the pound	0	6	0
Sarsaparilla the pound	0	6	0
Sassafras the pound	0	1	8
Sacammonie the pound	0	10	0
Sqults the pound	0	1	2
Sebestens the pound	0	1	4
Seeds of Agnus Castus the ounce	0	0	3
Seeds of Ameos the pound	0	6	0
Seeds of Bombas the pound	0	1	8
Seeds of daucus Creticus the pound	0	2	0
Seeds of Levistici the pound	0	0	4
Seeds of Eruca the pound	0	1	0
Seeds of Seseleos the pound	0	0	6
Wormeseeds the pound	0	6	0
Carthamus seeds the pound	0	1	4
Fænugrecke the pound	0	0	4
Linseeds the pound	0	0	6
Seeds of pearle the ounce	0	5	0
Sene the pound	0	4	6
Brimstone the pound	0	0	4
Styrax Calamit the pound	0	6	8
Styrax liquid the pound	0	3	4
White juyce of Licorish the pound	0	2	0
Blacke juyce of Licorish the pound	0	1	8
Sumach the pound	0	0	6
Spica Celtica the pound	0	6	0
Spica Indica the pound	0	8	0
Talc of Venice the pound	0	0	10
Venice Turpentine the pound	0	0	6
Common Turpentine the pound	0	0	8
Tamarinds the pound	0	1	4
Terra Sigillat the pound	0	10	0
Turbith the pound	0	10	0
Verdegrease the pound	0	2	0
Viscus quercin the pound	0	0	8
Xilobalsamum the pound	0	6	0
Zedoaria the pound	1	10	0

APPENDIX 3: PARKINSON REVIVUS, 1880S–1920S

Why did Parkinson's star suddenly shine for forty years between the 1880s and 1920s? Probably because he was enlisted in the cause of English gardening reform. His revival began in 1880 when the garden writer **Mrs Kegan Paul** complained that the massed, carpet planting of the time was boring, and suggested a return to the 'garden of delight' and old-fashioned flowers of Parkinson's *Paradisi*.

The well-known children's author **Mrs Ewing** then took up the theme, publishing a serial story based on the *Paradisi*. Her 'Mary's Meadow' appeared in *Aunt Judy's Magazine for Children* in 1883 and 1884.

Mrs Ewing's story is delightful and still worth reading. In the family library one summer the young heroine Mary finds 'The Book of Paradise'. She says it 'a very old book, and very queer … [though it had] a Latin name on the title-page, it was written in English, and though it seemed to be about Paradise, it was really about a garden and quite common flowers'.

Mary goes on: 'We like queer old things like this, they are so funny. I liked the Dedication, and I wondered if the Queen's Garden was really an Earthly Paradise, and whether she did enjoy reading John Parkinson's book about flowers in the winter time, when her own flowers were no longer '"fresh upon the ground".'

Mary invents roles for other children. They pretend to be Parkinson himself, a Weeding Woman, Queen Henrietta Maria, a Frenchman called Francis le Veau – 'the honestest root-gatherer that ever came over to us' – and the Queen's Dwarf. All these were based on real people of Parkinson's time apart from the Weeding Woman – so, yes, the Queen did have a favourite Dwarf (Jeffery), with his own entourage, and Parkinson did describe his plant-hunter thus.

The characters plan to turn Mary's Meadow into an Earthly Paradise by growing cottage-garden perennials mixed with wild flowers, taking seeds and cuttings and planting them in waste places, hedges and fields. The drama in the story comes with the irascible Old Squire in whose water meadow the children plant some of their paradisiacal flowers. But he repents of his grumpiness in the end and donates the meadow to Mary. All ends happily, after lots of fun gardening by following Parkinson's text.

The series generated an enthusiastic postbag, one correspondent saying her children now went 'Mary-meadowing', planting old flowers everywhere – an early form of guerrilla gardening? Readers suggested a **Parkinson Society**, and this was duly launched in 1884, with Mrs Ewing as first president. Its aims were: 'to search out and cultivate old garden flowers which have become scarce; to exchange seeds and plants; to circulate books on gardening amongst the Members; … and to try and prevent the extermination of rare wild flowers, as well as of garden treasures'.

Reports of the Society, with correspondence on the exchanges of plants and books, were given in *Aunt Judy's Magazine*, but then Mrs Ewing died in 1885. The Society continued for some years under the presidency of Professor Oliver Gilbert of Kew Gardens and the management of Alice Sargant. When Miss Sargant withdrew some years later, the Parkinson Society was absorbed by the Selborne Society.

Another sign of Parkinson's rediscovery was an 1898 **public statue** of him. A civic-minded and successful citizen of Liverpool, Henry Yates Thompson, paid for eight statues to adorn the octagonal Palm House at Sefton Park in the city. He commissioned the eminent French sculptor Léon-Joseph Chavalliaud to make four marble figures to represent gardeners and four in bronze for famous explorers. The gardeners chosen were Parkinson, Linnaeus, Charles Darwin and André Le Notre (the architect of Sefton Park).

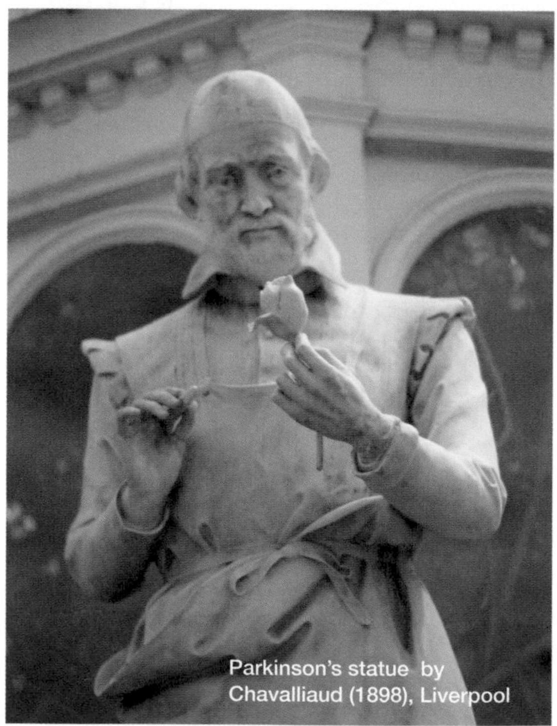

Parkinson's statue by Chavalliaud (1898), Liverpool

At the opening ceremony in 1901 Thompson admitted he hadn't known much about Parkinson, but said a Liverpool gardener, Enoch Harvey, had recommended him as the first of the great gardeners, who could represent the 17th century. An attractive-looking Parkinson, with a working apron, skullcap and leather belt, gazes at a tulip. The statue itself was restored in 2004, a quiet memorial to passing fame.

Parkinson's *Paradisi* was popular enough in the later 19th century for a growing market to develop in scarce 1629 originals. Blanche Henrey's research uncovered the accounts of bookseller Wheldon & Wesley, who had a calf-gilt copy for 12 shillings in 1867 and an inferior copy in 1910 for 13 guineas. The London publisher Methuen surfed the wave of Parkinson popularity with a limited edition for 2 guineas in 1904. Our own copy of the *Paradisi* is the Dover paperback of 1976; there is now an e-book.

This account would be incomplete without mention of **a landmark year in Parkinson studies, namely 1922**. Two unrelated publications emerged that took Parkinson seriously, raised the profile of the *Theatrum* and consolidated the fame of the *Paradisi*.

First was ***The Old English Herbals***, by gardener and writer Eleanour Sinclair Rohde (1881–1950). She entitled her sixth chapter 'John Parkinson, the last of the great English herbalists', and called the *Theatrum* 'the most complete English treatise on plants until the time of [John] Ray'. Rohde makes the interesting point (p151) that Parkinson should have called it a 'book of simples', as he planned; the Latin title, she believes, is 'hard and chilling', and dented the book's popularity.

The other book of that year was ***Early English Botanists and Their Gardens*** by the Librarian of Magdalen College, Oxford, Robert Gunther (1869–1940). Gunther based this on his research and transcripts from the papers of John Goodyer, a gardening friend of Parkinson's and a meticulous hoarder. The Goodyer papers had languished in the college library since being deposited in the 1660s.

Not only did close scrutiny by Gunther reveal that the Goodyer material mentioned Parkinson in many places but there were a number of pages, about 25, that Gunther was able to identify as in a hand he believed to be Parkinson's.

He confirmed this by finding a signature on a scratched-out, undelivered and bad-tempered note to a Mrs Geeres (see below). Under the deletions he discerned Parkinson's faint signature. This was Gunther's 'Rosetta stone', enabling him to verify other papers as by Parkinson.

The excitement at the discovery was laced with disappointment. The pitifully few Parkinson papers contain little of interest that he didn't gather into the vast bulk of the *Theatrum*; some plant 'want' lists (one of which we reproduce in the Introduction); a bill for the rebuilding of his garden wall in November 1636 after a gale, with the labourers' wages precisely recorded; and some notes on Bermudan botany.

On the other hand, after all the elusiveness of other Parkinson records, to have anything at all in his own hand – as you pant up 49 spiralling stone steps to the Magdalen College archives – is inspiring, a supporting arm around the shoulder for Parkinson lovers.

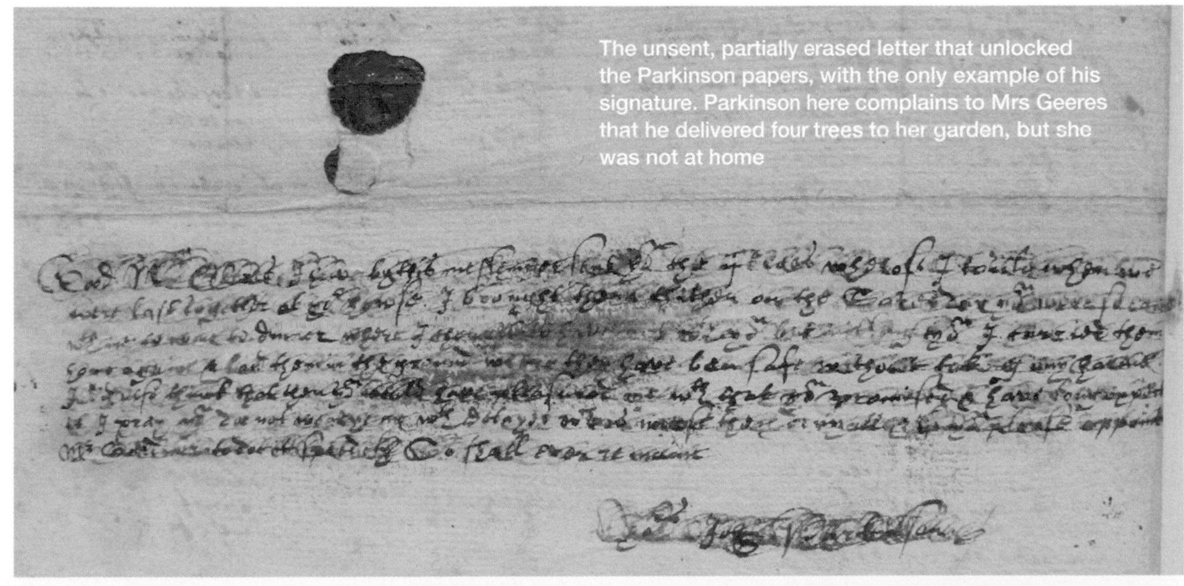

The unsent, partially erased letter that unlocked the Parkinson papers, with the only example of his signature. Parkinson here complains to Mrs Geeres that he delivered four trees to her garden, but she was not at home

APPENDIX 4: A PARKINSON TIMELINE

1564 William Shakespeare born, 23 April 1564

1565

1566

1567 John Parkinson born in Whalley, Lancashire; baptised 26 January 1567

1568 William Turner's *New Herball*, part III, published 1568

1569

1570 Abraham Ortelius publishes the first modern atlas, *Theatrum Orbis Terrarum*, Antwerp, May 1570

1571

1572 Vilcabamba, Peru, the last independent remnant of the Inca Empire, conquered by Spain in 1572

1573

1574 John's first communion, 1574

1575

1576 Martin Frobisher resumes English search for the Northwest Passage, 1576

1577 Francis Drake sets sail around the world in 1577, returning in 1580

1578 Henry Lyte's translation of Rembert Dodoens, *A Niewe herball or historie of plantes,* 1578

1579 Francis Drake lands in what is now California, 17 June 1579 and claims it for Queen Elizabeth I

1580 England signs a commercial treaty with the Ottoman Empire, June 1580

1581

1582 Marriage of William Shakespeare and Anne Hathaway, 29 November 1582

1583

1584 John apprenticed to Francis Slater, 9 November 1584 Sir Walter Raleigh founds the first American colony

1585 Anglo-Spanish War begins

1586

1587 John meets Mary Hutchens, a young widow, 1587 Mary Queen of Scots executed, 8 February 1587

1588 John and Mary issued a licence of engagement on 8 July 1588 Spanish Armada defeated, 8 August 1588

1589

1590 Japan is united by Toyotomi Hideyoshi, 1590

1591

1592 John passes his examination, becomes an apothecary member of the Grocers' Company, 30 January 1592

1593 John takes on his first apprentice, Richard Bragge, 1593

1594

1595 John accused of illicit 'practising', charges dropped Sir Walter Raleigh's first expedition to South America, 1595

1596

1597 John takes on his second apprentice, Thomas Nicholl, 1597 John Gerard's *Herball* published, 1597

1598

1599 The Globe Theatre opens in London, 1599

1600

1601 John's son Richard born, 1601 First performance of Shakespeare's *Hamlet*, 1601

1602

1603 John's daughter Katherine born, 1603 Queen Elizabeth I dies, 24 March 1603, James I and VI becomes king

1604

1605 Gunpowder Plot, 5 November 1605, followed by action against English Catholics

1606 Willem Jantszoon, a Dutch explorer, the first European to sail to Australia, reaches northern coast, 1606

1607

1608

1609 Shakespeare's sonnets published, 1609

1610

1611 Publication of King James Bible, 1611

1612

1613

1614 Sir Walter Raleigh publishes *The history of the world*, 1614

1615

1616 William Shakespeare dies, 23 April 1616 Dirk Hartog lands in western Australia, 25 October 1616

1617 John's wife Mary dies, April 1617 King James I inaugurates Society of Apothecaries, 16 December 1617

1618 John serves on Court of Assistants of the Society, 1617–21 Sir Walter Raleigh executed, 29 October 1618

1619

1620 Pilgrims set sail in *Mayflower*, land at Cape Cod and found the Plymouth Colony, 1620

1621

1622 John resigns his offices in the Society of Apothecaries, 28 January 1622

1623 Jan Carstenszoon discovers western coast of Australia's Cape York Peninsula, 1623

1624 António de Andrade crosses the Himalayas through the Mana Pass, reaches Tibet, 1624

1625 King James I dies, son Charles I becomes king, 27 March 1625

1626

1627

1628 William Harvey's *de Motu Cordis*, describing the circulation of blood, published in Latin, 1628

1629 *Paradisi in Sole* published, 1629 Charles I dissolves parliament, 10 March 1629

1630 Puritans found Boston and ten other settlements in the Massachusetts Bay Colony, 1630

1631

1632 Shah Jahan begins building Taj Mahal in India, 1632

1633

1634

1635 John gives evidence at the 'Quo Warranto' hearings in Star Chamber, 1635

1636 John's garden wall blows down at Long Acre, November 1636 Harvard University founded, 1636

1637

1638

1639

1640 John proclaimed as King's Herbalist; *Theatrum Botanicum* published, early summer 1640

1641

1642 The English Civil War begins as Charles I raises his standard at Nottingham, 22 August 1642

1643 Abel Tasman discovers Tasmania and New Zealand, 1642–43

1644 End of Ming Dynasty in China, 1644

1645 Parliament establishes the New Model Army, 16 February 1645

1646

1647

1648

1649 King Charles I beheaded, 30 January 1649 Culpeper publishes a translation of the London *Dispensatory*

1650 John Parkinson dies, buried 6 August 1650, St Martin in the Fields, London

1651

Appendix 5: Parkinson's 'firsts'

This list of 30 Parkinson's first descriptions of plants in the British flora is adapted from William A. Clarke, *First Records of British Flowering Plants*, 2nd edn (1900). The first two elements are common and scientific names, following Clive Stace, *Field Flora of the British Isles* (Cambridge, 1999); Parkinson's (JP) scientific and common names are from *Theatrum Botanicum* (TB) and *Paradisi in Sole* (Par.); JP's quotes are from these sources

ASARABACCA /*Asarum europaeum* / TB 266 / JP calls it *Asarina Matthioli* or Bastard Asarum of Matthiolus; 'in Somersetshire in our owne Land, found by Dr. Lobel'

AUTUMN SQUILL / *Scilla autumnalis* / Par. 132 / JP calls it *Hyacinthus Autumnalis minor* or lesser Autumne Iacinth; 'I gathered divers rootes for my Garden, from the foote of a high banke by the Thames side, at the hither end of Chelsey, before you come at the Kings Barge-house'

CAREX SYLVATICA / no English name / TB 1171 / JP calls it *Gramen Cyperoides Sylvarum tenuius Spicatum* or Slender eared Wood Cyperus grasse

COCK'S FOOT / *Dactylis glomerata* / TB 1182 / JP calls it *Calamagrostis torosa panicula* or Round tufted Reede grasse; 'not remembered by any Authour before'

CORAL ROOT / Cardamine bulbifera / TB 621 / JP calls it *Dentaria bulbifera* or Bulbe bearing toothed Violet; he identifies two woods in Mayfield, Sussex, in land of 'Mr. Stephen Perkhurst', where it had been found

GREAT SUNDEW / *Drosera anglica* / TB 1053 / JP calls it *Rosa solis sylvestris longifolius* or Long leaved Rosa solis; 'This was sent me by Mr Zanche Silliard an Apothecarie of Dublin in Ireland, which sort wee have growing by Ellestmere in Shropshire by the way sides (the report of Mr. Doctor Coote)'

GREATER POND SEDGE / *Carex riparia* / TB 1265 /JP calls it *Gramen Cyperoides majus latifolium* or The greater sort of Cyperus grasse; 'There are none of these Grasses [he describes 14 sedges in his chapter] used for man or beast that I can learn'

HEATH RUSH / *Juncus squarrosus* / TB 1192 / JP calls it *Oxyschaenos sive acutes Alpinu Cambro britannicus* or Welsh hard or sharpe rushe; 'found by Dr. Lobel in his lifetime, upon a high hill in Wales called Bewrin, in sundry the wet and moorish grounds'

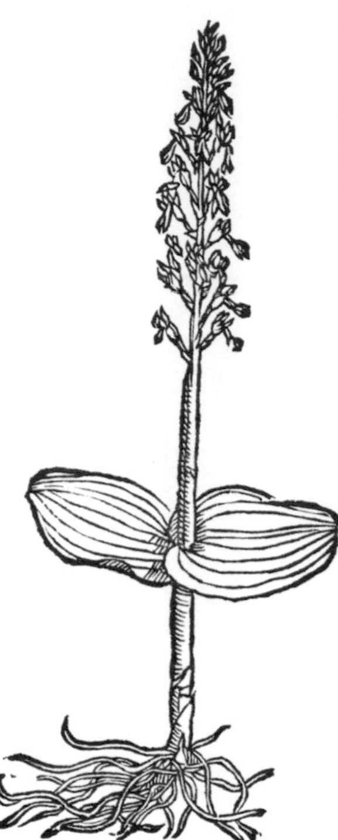
Bifolium sylvestre vulgare seu Ophris.
Ordinary wood Twayblade or Bifoide.

LADY'S SLIPPER / *Cyripedium calceolus* / TB 217 / called by JP *Elleborine major sive Calceolus Mariae* or The great Wilde Hellebor, or Our Ladyes Slipper; grows 'in a wood called the Helkes in Lancashire neere the border of Yorkeshire'

LESSER TWAYBLADE / *Listera cordata* / TB 505 / called *Bifolium palustre* or Marsh Bifoile by JP; found 'not onely in the low wet grounds between Hatfield and St Albans, but in divers places of Romney marsh'

LUNGWORT / *Pulmonaria officinalis* / Par. 248 / JP calls it *Pulmonaria maculosa* or Common spotted Cowslip of Ierusalem; 'found by Iohn Goodier, a great searcher and lover of plants, dwelling at Maple-Durham in Hampshire'

MARSH VIOLET / *Viola palustris* / TB 755 / JP calls it *Viola rural striata Eboracensis* or Yorkshire striped red Violets; he says 'Master Stonehouse a reverend minister of Darfield in Yorkeshiere assured me he found a kind of Wilde Violet neare unto his habitation, whose leaves were rounder and thinner then of others, and the flowers reddish with ladder veins therein'

MOSSY SAXIFRAGE / *Saxifraga hypnoides* / TB 739 / JP calls it *Sedum Alpinum laciniatis Ajugae foliis* or Small Mountaine Houseleeke with jagged leaves; it grows 'upon the mountains of Lancashiere with us as Mr. Hoskes told us'

MOTH MULLEIN / *Verbascum blattaria* / TB 65 / called by JP *Blattaria lutea minor sive vulgaris* or The ordinary yellow Moth Mullein

MOUNTAIN SORREL / *Oxyria digyna* / TB 745 / called by JP *Acetosa Cambro-Britannica Montana* or Mountain Welsh Sorrell; 'no author ever made mention [of it] before now, and scarce is it knowne to any but the Gentleman of Anglesey called Mr. Morris Lloid of Prislierworth that found it on a mountaine in

Wales, and shewed it to Dr. Bonham in his life' [Bonham is named on Parkinson's title page (along with de l'Obel), but this is only reference to him in TB]

OYSTER PLANT / *Mertensia maritima* / TB 767 / JP calls it *Buglossum dulce ex Insulis Lancastriae* or Lancashire buglosse; 'groweth in one of the Iles about Lankashire, there found by Mr. Thomas Hesket'

PALE ST JOHN'S WORT / *Hypericum montanum* / TB 577 / JP calls it *Hypericum majus sive Androsaemum Matthioli*; it grows 'about Bristow and Bath'

REED CANARY GRASS / *Phalaris arundinacea* / TB 1273 / JP calls it *Gramen Arundinaceum acerosa gluma nostras* or Our great Reed grasse with chaffy heads; 'in the low moist grounds by Ratcliffe neere London'

ROMAN NETTLE / *Urtica pilulifera* / TB 440 / JP calls it *Urticaria Romana* or the Romane Nettle; says it is sown in gardens where it is desired, 'but it hath Beene found naturally growing time out of minde, both at the town of Lidde by Romney, and in the streets of the towne of Romney in Kent, where it is recorded that Iulius Caesar landed with his souldiers. … It is reported that the souldiers brought some of the seede with them, and sowed it there for their use, to rubbe and chafe their limbes, when through extreame cold they should be stiffe and benummed.' [It is no longer on the British plant list.]

SCOTS PINE / *Pinus sylvestris* / TB 1539 / JP calls it *Abies*, the Firre tree; 'I have but one sort of Firre to shew you … [grows] in Scotland also, as I have been assured, but not in Ireland or England'

SEA BUCKTHORN / *Hippophae rhamnoides* / TB 1005 / JP calls it *Rhamnus primus Dioscoridis Lobelio sive littoralis* or Sea Buckes thorne with Willow-like leaves

SPIKED WATER MILFOIL / *Myriophyllum spicatum* / TB 1257 / JP calls it *Millefolium aquaticum pennatum spicatum* or Feathered Millfoile; 'onley mentioned by Bauhinus' [i.e. Caspard Bauhinus, *Pinax*, 1623]

STONE BRAMBLE / *Rubus saxatilis* / TB 1015 / JP calls it *Rubus saxatilis Alpinus* or the stony Bramble or Rocke Raspis; it grows 'in stony and rocky places, both in the Ile of Thanet and other places of Kent, as also in Huntingdon and Northamptonshire'

STRAWBERRY TREE / *Arbutus unedo* / TB 1490 / JP calls it *Arbutus* or the Strawberry tree with dented leaves; it 'hath been of late days found in the West part of Ireland … by the name of Cane Apple, with as great judgement and reason as many other vulgar names are'

TREE MALLOW / *Lavatera arborea* / TB 301 / JP calls it *Malva arborea marina nostras* or English Sea tree Mallow; it grows 'in an Island called Dinnie, three miles from Kings Roade, and five miles from Bristow, as also about the cottages neere Hurst Castle, over against the Ile of Wight'

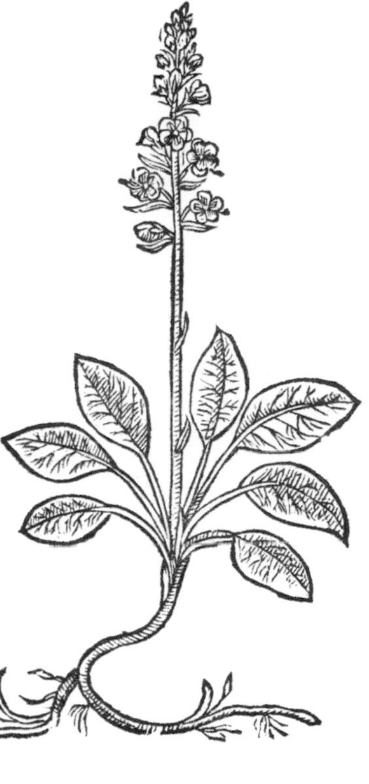
1. *Pyrola nostras vulgaris.* Our ordinary Winter greene.

TUFTED HAIR GRASS / *Deschcampsia cespitosa* / TB 1157 / JP calls it *Gramen Segetum panicula Speciosa* or The great Corne Grasse

WILD TURNIP / *Brassica rapa* ssp. *campestris* / TB 862/ JP calls it *Rapistrum aliud sylvestre non bulbosum* or 'Another Wilde Turnep'; 'found [by JP himself] going from Shoreditch by Bethnall Greene to Hackney … it is not extant in any author before'

WELSH POPPY / *Meconopsis cambrica* / TB 370 / JP's name is *Argemone Cambro-Britannica lutea* or Yellow wild Bastard Poppy of Wales; it grows near the house of 'a worthy Gentleman Sir Iohn Guin'

WINTERGREEN / *Pyrola minor* / TB 508 / JP calls it *Pyrola nostras vulgaris*, 'Our ordinary Winter Greene'; 'groweth in our owne land, yet but in very few places'

WOOD DOCK / *Rumex sanguineus* / TB 1227 / called by JP *Lapathum sanguineum* or Bloodwort; 'a pot-herbe, is planted in Gardens, yet found wild also … more drying' [than other docks]

APPENDIX 6: A SAMPLE FROM THE THEATRUM

Shown at 71% life size. Original page size approx. 235mm x 345mm

port. Of the juice or water of the flowers of Cowſlips, divers Gentlewomen know how to clenſe the skin from ſpots or diſcolourings therein, as alſo to take away the wrinckles thereof, and cauſe the skinne to become ſmooth

may happen thereto, by the ſight of ſuch fearefull *precipices* of ſteepe places, ... lowing their game, and are admitted as good Wound herbes as the former Cowſlips.

CHAP. XXX.

Alchymilla. Ladies Mantile.

VNto the Sanicles ſet downe in the laſt Chapter, I thinke it fitteſt to place this next unto it, becauſe both for forme and quality it is ſo aſſuredly like it, that it is called of divers the greater Sanicle, and will adde thereunto another ſort thereof, which hath not beene formerly well knowne.

1. *Alchymilla major vulgaris.* Common Ladies Mantle.

Our common Ladies Mantle is very like to the former Sanicle, having many leaves riſing from the roote, ſtanding upon long hairy footeſtalkes, being almoſt round, but a little cut in on the edges, into eight or tenne parts, more or leſſe, making it ſeeme like a ſtarre, with ſo many corners and points, and dented round about, of a light greene colour, ſomewhat hard in handling, and as if it were foulded or plaited at the firſt, and then crumpled in divers places, and a little hairy, as the ſtalke is alſo which riſeth up among them, to the height of two or three foote, with a few ſuch leaves thereupon, but ſmaller, and being weake is not able to ſtand upright, but bendeth downe to the ground, divided at the toppe into two or three ſmall branches, with ſmall yellowiſh greene heads, and flowers of a whitiſh greene colour breaking out of them, which being paſt, there commeth ſmall yellowiſh ſeede like unto Poppy ſeede, the roote is ſomewhat long and blacke, with many ſtrings and fibres thereat.

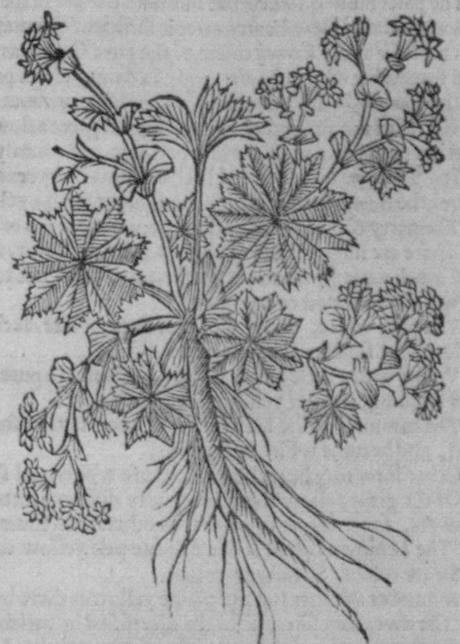

1. *Alchymilla major vulgaris.* Common Ladies Mantle.

2. *Alchymilla minor quinquefolia.* Cinkefoile Ladies Mantle.

This ſmall Ladies Mantle, hath alſo a few ſmaller and ſmoother greene leaves, riſing from the ſmall blacke fibrous roote, ſet upon long footeſtalkes, but divided at the edges into five corners or points, and ſomewhat deepelier dented about the brimmes then the former; from whence two or three ſmall weake bending ſtalkes doe riſe, not halfe a foote high: the flowers that grow at the toppes are ſmaller, but alike according to the bigneſſe of the plant, and of the ſame herby or greene colour.

The Place.

The firſt groweth naturally in many paſtures and wood ſides, both in *Hartford* and *Wiltſhire*, and in *Kent* alſo, as in *Kingwood* neere *Feverſham*, in the paſtures nigh *Tidnam*, and *Chepſtow*, and in other places of this land; the other groweth on St. *Bernards* hill among the *Switzers*.

The Time.

The firſt flowreth in *May* and *Iune*, the other not untill *Auguſt*, but both abide after ſeede time, greene all the Winter after.

The Names.

It was not knowne by name unto the ancient writers, as can be gathered, and although *Brunfelſius* and ſome others thought it to be *Leontopodium* or Lions foote, deceived by the name, becauſe divers nations have ſo called it, from the forme or likeneſſe of the leafe, yet is it not that of *Dioſcorides*, as may plainely appeare by his deſcription thereof. It is uſually called *Alchymilla* by moſt writers, becauſe as ſome thinke the Alchymiſts gave ſuch commendations of it. It is called alſo of *Matthiolus*, *Lugdunenſis*, and others *Stellaria*, from the forme of the leafe, that with the corners reſemble a ſtarre, but there are divers other herbes called *Stellaria* by divers authours, and ſome alſo call this *Pes Leonis*, and *Pata Leonis*: others call it *Sanicula major*, not without good reaſon. *Cordus in hiſtoria de plantis*, calleth it *Droſera*, *Droſium*, and *Pſiadeion* from the *Germane* name *Sinnaw*, becauſe the hollow crumplings and the edges alſo of the leaves, will containe the dew in droppes like pearles, that falleth in the night. *Bauhinus* calleth the other *Alchymilla Alpina Quinquefolia*. The *Italians* call it *Stellaria*, and *Stella herba*. The *French Pied de lyon*. The *Germanes* as I ſaid before *Sinnaw*, and ſome *Lewenfuſſ*, and *Vnſer frawen mantel*. The *Dutch Onſer urawen mantel*. And we in *Engliſh* Our Ladies Mantle, and great Sanicle, and ſome Lions foote, or Lions paw, or *Padelyon* after the *French*.

The

The Vertues.

Ladies Mantle is more cooling then Sanicle, and therefore more proper for those wounds that have inflammations, and more astringent binding and drying, and therefore is more effectuall to stay bleedings, vomitings, fluxes in man or woman of all sorts, and bruises by fals or otherwise, and to helpe ruptures, it helpeth also such maides or women that have overgreat flagging breasts, causing them to grow lesse and hard, being both drunke, and outwardly applyed, and serveth also to stay the whites in them, wherein it is so powerfull that it is used as a surfuling water also, the distilled water drunke continually for twenty daies together, by such women as are barren and cannot conceive, or retaine the birth after conception, through the too much humidity of the matrice, and fluxe of moist humours thereunto, causing the seede not to abide but to passe away without fruite, will reduce their bodies to so good and conformable an estate, that they shall thereby be made more fit and able to retaine the conception, and beare out their children, if they doe also sit sometimes as in a bath, in the decoction made of the herbe. It is accounted as one of the most singular wound herbes that is, and therefore the *Germanes* extoll it with exceeding great praise, and never dresse any wound, either inward or outward, but they give of the decoction hereof to drinke; and either wash the wound with the said decoction, or dippe tents therein, and put them thereinto, which wonderfully dryeth up all the humidity of the sores, or of the humours flowing thereunto, yea although they be fistulous and hollow, and abateth also such inflammations, as often happen unto sores: but for fresh or greene wounds or cuts, it so quickely healeth them up, that it suffereth not any quitture to grow therein, but consolidateth the lippes of the wound, yet not suffering any corruption to remaine behinde: it hath formerly beene much accounted of by Chymists, who have affirmed that the juice hereof will constraine the volubility of Mercury, and make it fixt, from whence as it is thought it tooke the name, but these idle fancies are now quite worne out, as I thinke.

Chap. XXXI.

Solidago Saracenica. Sarasins Consound.

There have beene divers herbes that have beene mistaken and set forth for the right Sarasins Consound, we will therefore shew you here in this place some of them that are not right, with the true one also.

1. *Solidago Saracenica vera Salicis folio.*
The true Sarasins Consound with willow leaves.

The true Sarasins Consound groweth very high sometimes, with brownish stalkes, and other whiles with greene and hollow, to a mans height, having many long and narrow greene leaves snipt about the edges set thereon somewhat like unto those of the Almond, or Peach tree, or Willow leaves, but not of such a white greene colour; the toppes of the stalkes are furnished with many pale yellow starrelike flowers, standing in greene heads, which when they are fallen, and the seed ripe, which is somewhat long, small, and of a yellowish browne colour, wrapped in downe, is therewith carryed away with the wind, the roote is composed of many strings or fibres, set together at a head, which perish not in winter, but abide, although the stalkes dry away, and no leafe appeareth in Winter; the taste hereof is strong and unpleasant, and so is the smell also.

2. *Solidago Saracenica major.*
The greater Sarasins Consound.

This greater *Solidago* differeth not much from the former, rising up with upright hard round hollow stalkes, as high as it, with many darke greene leaves at the first, set at the head of the roote, which afterwards rise up with the stalkes, and are set there without order, somewhat larger then they, and dented about the edges; the flowers are much greater with more and yellower long leaves star-fashion, standing in greene heads many together, wherein after they are past, are contained the seede, which with the downe thereof flieth away with the winde, in the like manner as the former doth, the rootes are composed of a great bush of white strings, or white fibres growing very strongly in the ground, and shooting forth strings on all sides, which produce new plants, encreasing in a small time, and overspreading a great quantity of ground, the head of leaves is somewhat browne at the first shooting out of the ground, and so is the head of the roote before the Spring, and are of a bitter taste, and binding withall.

3. *Solidago Saracenica sive Germanica siliquosa.*
The *Germane* Consound with small cods.

This Consound riseth up with great round wooddy stalkes, to as great an height as the former, or more, but are

3. *Solidago Saracenica sive Germanica siliquosa.*
The *Germane* Consound with small cods.

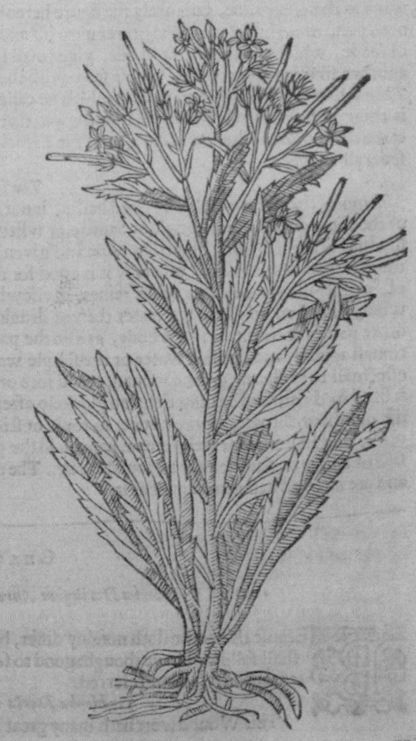

BRIEF BIOGRAPHIES

Andromachus (1st century AD) Name of two Greek physicians, father and son. Andromachus the Elder was born in Crete, and became physician to Emperor Nero. Invented the famous compound medicine and antidote called Theriaca Andromachi, still popular in the 1600s.

Arnoldus de villa nova (1235–c.1315) Catalan botanist, fell foul of Inquisition. Wrote *De Theriaca* (On Treacles). Known to William Turner as Arnold of Newtown.

Avicenna or Ibn Sina (c.980–1037AD) Persian polymath, wrote 450 works, of which 240 have survived. Most are philosophical, with 40 on medicine. His 14-volume *Canon of Medicine* (*Al-Qanoon fi al-Tibb*) was a standard medical text in Europe and the Islamic world until the 18th century.

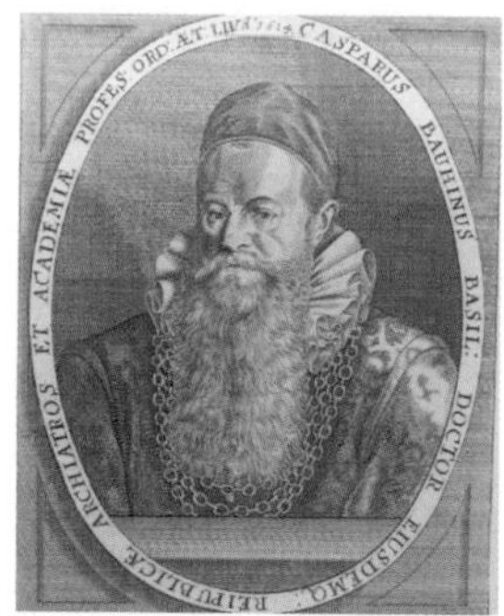

Bauhin, Gaspard (1560–1624) Also known as Caspar Bauhin or Bauhinus. Physician and botanist. His *Pinax Theatri Botanici* (1623) described some 6,000 species, and was heavily used by Parkinson. His brother **Jean** (1541–1613) was also a physician and botanist whose *Historia universalis plantarum*, last of the great European herbals, was published posthumously in 1650.

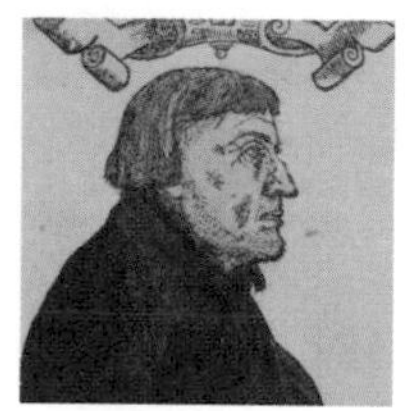

Bock, Hieronymus (1498–1554) Also known as Tragus. Physician, priest, gardener to Count Palatine. Author of *New Kreuterbuch* (1539), in which he proposed his own plant classification system.

Camerarius, Joachim (1534–1598) Camerarius the Younger was a German botanist and physician. Studied medicine in Padua and Bologna. Dean of medical college in Nuremberg from inception in 1592 until his death. Produced an edition of Mattioli's commenatry on Dioscorides (1586).

Coys, William (c.1560–1627) Plant enthusiast with a well-known garden at Stubbers, Essex. His yucca was the first to bloom in England, in 1604; also first ivy-leaved toadflax. John Goodyer made a list of his garden plants (about 450).

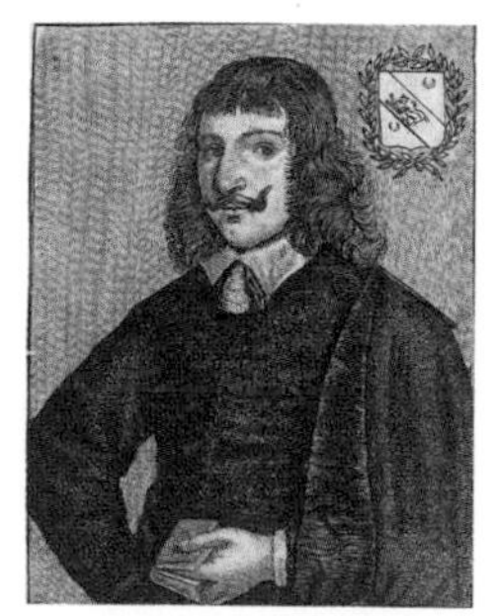

Culpeper, Nicholas (1616–1654) Left Cambridge without graduating, but was an excellent Latin scholar. Apothecary, but did not complete apprenticeship. Politically a radical, opposed to most authority. Offered a free clinic in London. Published first English translation of *Pharmacopoeia Londinensis* (1649); his *English Physitian* (1652) became the renowned *Culpeper's Herbal*; in it he heavily plagiarized Parkinson, but made herbal medicine widely available.

de Laet, Johannes (1581–1649) Resident of Leiden, theologian, scholar in Anglo-Saxon studies and later director of Dutch West India Company. Corresponded with John Morris, 1634–49, though only Morris's letters survive. Invited by Morris to write a poem for Parkinson's *Theatrum*.

de Laune, Gideon (c.1565–1659) Born in Rheims, moved to England with his father, a French Huguenot pastor. Appointed apothecary to Anne of Denmark, queen of James I. Founder member, moving spirit, twice Master and frequent benefactor of Society of Apothecaries, including building of first Apothecaries' Hall.

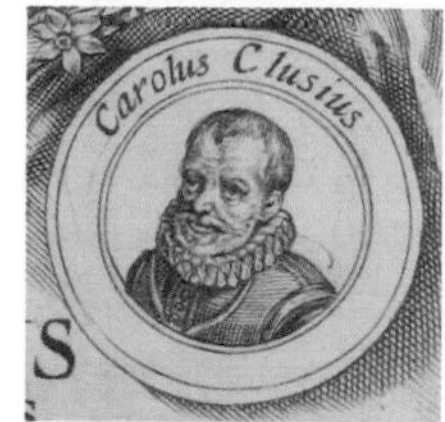

de l'Ecluse, Charles (1526–1609) Also known as Carolus Clusius. Travelled widely in Spain and Portugal, describing the plants in *Rariorum aliquot stirpium per Hispanias observatorum historia* (1576), and *Rariorum stirpium per Pannonias observatorum Historiae* (1583), the first book on Austrian and Hungarian alpine flora. Helped create one of the earliest formal botanical gardens of Europe at Leiden, the Hortus Academicus. Publisher and translator of several contemporary works, and laid foundations of modern Dutch tulip breeding and bulb industry.

de L'Obel, Matthias (1538–1617) Sometimes called Lobel or Lobelius. Flemish plantsman and scholar, studied at Montpellier, settled in England. Gardener to Lord Zouche in Hackney. Dedicated his *Stirpium adversaria nova*, written with Peter Pena (1570), to Elizabeth I. Claimed to be royal herbalist to James I. A mentor of Parkinson, who acquired or used his papers.

de Mayerne, Sir Theodore (1573–1655) Pioneering Swiss Huguenot physician and diplomat. Physician to the French court of Henri IV of France, then the English courts of James I and Charles I, and later to Cromwell. Friend and neighbour of John Parkinson. Made a fortune from selling medicines. Among first doctors to keep patient notes.

Dioscorides, Pedanios (fl. 50–80AD) Greek-speaking Roman physician who studied medicine in Alexandria before joining the Roman army as a doctor. His medical treatise *De Materia Medica* (c.77AD) was the authority on medicinal plants in Europe for the next 1,500 years.

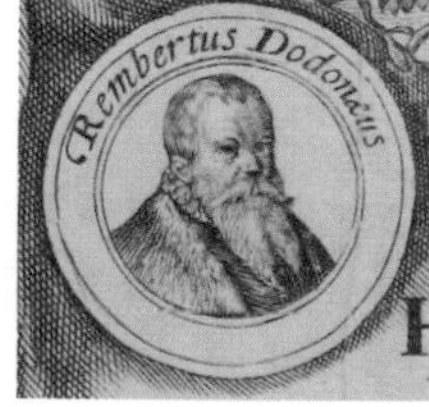

Dodoens, Rembert (1517–1585) French physician and botanist, also known as Rembertus Dodonaeus. Court physician to Emperor Maximillian II in Vienna. His *Cruydeboeck* (1554) was published in Flemish, translated to French by de l'Ecluse and English by Henry Lyte. His *Pemptades Sex* (1583), via the translation of Dr Priest, was the basis for Gerard's *Herball*.

Galen of Pergamon (c.130–200AD) Prominent Greek physician, surgeon and philosopher in Roman empire. Contributed substantially to Hippocratic understanding of pathology. Medical students continued to study Galen's writings until well into the 19th century.

Garrett, James (fl. 1590s–1610) Flemish Huguenot who settled in London. Apothecary and plantsman, who grew first tulips in England. Warned the printer John Norton of the many problems with Gerard's *Herball*. Parkinson often visited his garden.

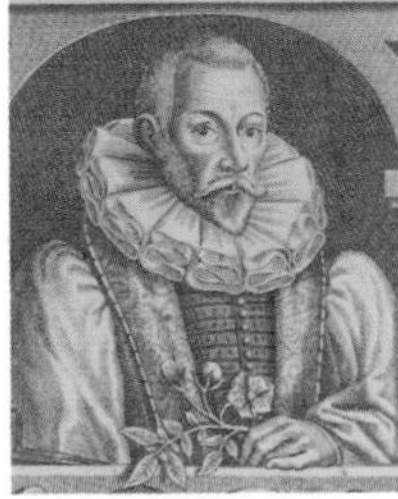

Gerard, John (1545–1612) Chirurgeon, warden of Company of Barber-Surgeons (1597), master (1608). Supervised Lord Burghley's garden in the Strand, was curator of College of Physicians' garden. Owned famous garden in Holborn. Catalogue (1596) the first of any English private garden. Author of famous but flawed *Herball* (1597).

Goodyer, John (1592–1664) Estate manager, Mapledurham, Hants. Grew exotic plants, obsessively recording gardens he visited. Helped Johnson with revision of Gerard's *Herball* (1633). Books and papers gifted to Magdalen College, Oxford. Translated Dioscordes into English for first time; incomplete MS finally published 1934.

Hippocrates of Cos (c.460–c.370BC) Greek physician, founder of Hippocratic School of Medicine; often called father of medicine. The Hippocratic Oath, a seminal document on medical ethics, attributed to him in antiquity, but may have been written after his death.

Johnson, Thomas (c.1600–1644) London apothecary, first to display bananas in his Snow Hill shop (1634). Organized plant-collecting trips, and published pioneering floras in Latin. Edited and expanded Gerard's *Herball* (1633). Died fighting for the king at Basing House, 1644.

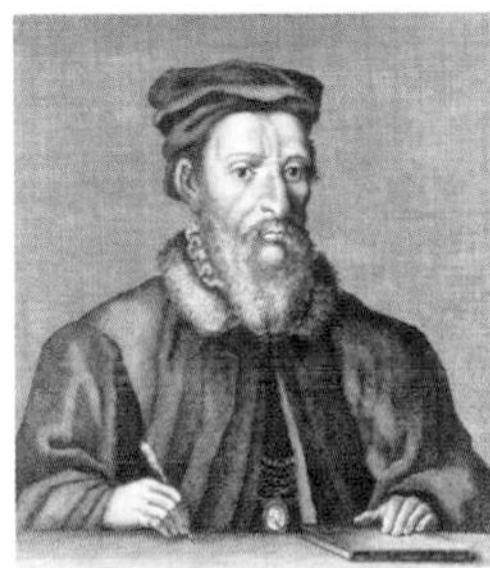

Mattioli, Pietro Andrea/Pierandrea (1501–1577) Also known as Matthiolus. Italian scholar and personal physician to Emperor Ferdinand I. Author of influential commentary on Dioscorides, *Commentarii in VI Libros Pedacii Dioscoridis* (1544), which extended to 61 editions, and said to have sold a phenomenal 32,000 copies.

Mesues or Masawayh (777–857), Syriac physician, personal physician to four caliphs. Composed many Arabic medical monographs, on topics including fevers, leprosy, melancholy, dietetics, eye diseases and medical aphorisms.

Monardes, Nicolás (1493–1588) Spanish physician, wrote first accounts of New World plants, e.g. tobacco, coca, in *Historia medicinal* (1574). English version, *Joyfull newes out of the newe founde worlde* by John Frampton (1577).

Morris, John (1585/90–1658) Son of Peter Morris, Dutch builder of London Waterworks, which supplied family wealth until 1701. A gentleman, with a garden in well-to-do suburb of Isleworth. Wrote three congratulatory poems for *Theatrum*, and helped Parkinson get plants via de Laet from Brazil and West Indies.

Paracelsus (1493–1541) Real name Philippus Aureolus Theophrastus Bombastus Von Hohenheim; influential German–Swiss physician and alchemist, who developed role of chemistry in medicine, introduced opium and arsenic to clinical practice. Opposed to Galen. Published *Der grossen Wundartzney* (Great Surgery Book) in 1536.

Pliny the Elder (c.23–79AD) Roman soldier and cavalry commander. Author of multi-volume *Historia naturalis* (c. 77AD), a collection of information on natural history, much of it hearsay. Died at eruption of Vesuvius at Pompeii.

Robin, Vespasien (1579–1672) Gardener for Henri IV of France, following his father Jean, gardener to Henri III. Planted the Jardin des Plantes at the Louvre Palace. Exchanged plants with Tradescant the Elder and Parkinson.

Slater, Francis (1560–1630) Grocer, with shop in St Mary Colechurch, London. Parkinson his first apprentice. Appointed to Grocer's Court in 1613, did not join Society of Apothecaries, though his son John did in 1620.

Theophrastus (c.372–c.286BC) Studied with Plato and Aristotle. Often called 'father of botany', but published in many other subjects. May have written over 200 works, but only fragments now survive. His *Historia Plantarum* was translated into Latin, 1483.

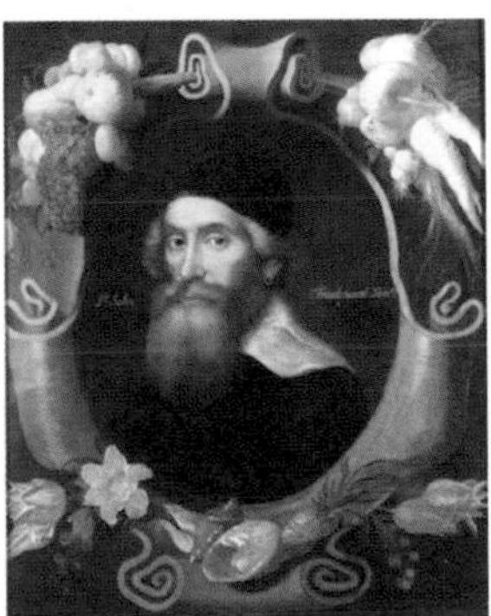

Tradescant, John the Elder (c.1570s–1638) Good friend of John Parkinson. Gardener, collector and traveller. Head gardener to Robert Cecil at Hatfield House; to George Villiers, Duke of Buckingham; and then to King Charles I, as Keeper of his Majesty's Gardens, Vines, and Silkworms at Oatlands Palace, Surrey. Collected seeds and plants on his trips and curiosities of natural history and ethnography. His Ark at Lambeth was the first public museum in England.

Tradescant, John the Younger (c.1608–1662) Travelled to Virginia to collect plants. When father died, succeeded as head gardener to Charles I, to 1642. Published contents of the family's curiosities as *Musaeum Tradescantianum*. Collection is now part of Ashmolean Museum, Oxford.

Turner, William (c.1508–1568) Physician, herbalist, ornithologist. Twice Dean of Wells Cathedral, self-exiled for his protestant views. Known as the father of English botany. Author of three-volume *A new herball*, 1551–68.

A SELECT PARKINSON BIBLIOGRAPHY

A selection of the books that have inspired and maddened us in getting to know John Parkinson (sometimes the same book does both things), with Parkinson-relevant page numbers. Our comments are also offered, in square brackets.

Arber, Agnes, Herbals: *Their Origin and Evolution: A Chapter in the History of Botany, 1470–1670* (Cambridge, 1912; rev. 3rd edn, Cambridge, 1986), pp113–16, 197, 200 [takes a purist line on botanical history, and Parkinson is found wanting]

Bacon, Sir Francis, 'Of gardens', in *The Essayes or Counsells, Civill and Morall*, ed. Michael Kernan (Oxford, 1985) [the famous essay of 1625, which may owe something to Parkinson's example, says Gunther – see below]

Bekkers, J.A.F., *Correspondence of John Morris with Johannes de Laet (1634–1649)* ('s-Gravenhage, Netherlands, 1970) [John Morris's letters are a source for much of what little is known of Parkinson's latter years; in Latin]

Blunt, W. & Raphael, S. *The Illustrated Herbal* (London, 1979), pp166, 169–71 [impressive scholarship, displayed with much affection]

Borodale, Jane, *The Knot* (London, 2012) [a novelist's take on Henry Lyte's efforts to translate Rembert Dodoens' *Cruÿdeboeck*, from the French edn of Charles l'Ecluse; Lyte's *A Nieuwe Herball* appeared in 1578]

Boulgar, G.S. 'A 17thc botanical friendship', *Journal of Botany* 56 (1918), 200–2 [the friendship is the enduring one between John Tradescant the Elder and Parkinson]

Burnby, J., 'Some early London physic gardens', *Pharmaceutical Historian* 24(4) (1994), 2–7 [with accounts of Parkinson's Long Acre garden, among others]

Clark, Sir George, *A History of the Royal College of Physicians of London*, Vol. I (Oxford, 1964), pp216–30 [the official College history]

Clarke, Willam A., *First Records of British Flowering Plants*, 2nd edn (London, 1900) [a source for Appendix 5, p244]

Coleman, Moira, *Fruitful Endeavours: The 16th-Century Household Secrets of Catherine Tollemache at Helmingham Hall* (Andover, 2012) [scrupulous examination of an Elizabethan manor's household accounts, and 42 recipes]

Cook, Harold J., *The Decline of the Old Medical Regime in Stuart London* (Ithaca & London, 1986) [the book that started the 'medical marketplace' hypothesis; Parkinson does not appear in the index]

Culpeper, Nicholas, *Pharmacopoeia Londinensis or the London Dispensatory*, 6th edn (London, 1654; first published 1649; EEBO edn, n.d.) [iconoclastic translation and brave demolition of the Apothecaries' *Pharmacopoeia*, with Culpeper's own additions; available as a printed resource from Early English Books Online]

Desmond, Ray, *Dictionary of British & Irish Botanists and Horticulturalists*, rev. edn (London, 1994), p536 [gives useful sources for further Parkinson studies]

Evelyn, John, *The French Gardiner* (London, 1658) [Evelyn was inspired by Parkinson's *Paradisi*, and added experiences from his French travels to this translation; his first book]

Ewing, Juliana Horatia (Mrs), *Mary's Meadow & Other Tales of Fields & Flowers* (London, 1915 edn [1886]) [the children's story that gave rise to the Parkinson Society]

Francis, Jill, 'John Parkinson: Gardener and Apothecary of London', in *Critical Approaches to the History of Western Herbal Medicine*, ed. Susan Francia and Anne Stobart (London, 2014), pp229–46 [the latest addition to Parkinson studies, focusing on the herbal wisdom of the *Paradisi*]

Gerard, John, *Herball* (London, 1597; rev. Thomas Johnson, 1633, rpt 1636) [the pre-eminent herbal before Parkinson; the charm remains, as do many of the errors, in Thomas Johnson's revision, whose appearance so pained Parkinson]

Guibert, Philbert, *The Charitable Physitian with the Charitable Apothecary*, trans. I.W. (London, 1639) [popular recipes from both physicians and apothecaries; Guibert's list of apothecary prices forms Appendix 2 of this book: see p238]

Gunther, R.T., *Early English Botanists and Their Gardens* (Oxford, 1922), pp265–70 [made sense of the Goodyer papers at Magdalen, gave a voice to early English botanists, and identified Parkinson's papers]

Harkness, Deborah E., *The Jewel House: Elizabethan London and the Scientific Revolution* (New Haven & London, 2007) [buoyant, warm account of a vibrant intellectual community, Lime Street, which Parkinson knew]

Hawks, Ellison & Boulger, G.S., *Pioneers of Plant Study* (London, 1928), pp188–90 [rather condescending and critical of Parkinson, as overly botanic accounts often are]

Henrey, Blanche, *British Botanical and Horticultural Literature before 1800*, Vol. I: *The Sixteenth and Seventeenth Centuries, History and Bibliography* (London, 1975), pp79–82, 161–6 [the authoritative literature survey, with excellent, if critical coverage of Parkinson]

Hill, Thomas, *The Gardener's Labyrinth* (London, 1577; rep. Oxford, ed. R. Mabey, 1987) [charming predecessor to the *Paradisi*, in Mabey's modern edition]

Holmes, Peter, *The Energetics of Western Herbs: An Herbal Reference Integrating Western and Oriental Herbal Medicine Traditions* (Berekely, 1989; rev. 2nd edn, 1993) [ground-breaking integrative herbalism by an admirer of Parkinson]

Hunting, Penelope, *A History of the Society of Apothecaries* (London, 1998) [the fourth, latest and most engaging of the Society's official histories]

Johns, Adrian, *The Nature of the Book: Print and Knowledge in the Making* (Chicago & London, 1998) [amazing and vast survey of the evolution of print and scientific cultures in early modern England]

Jones, Rex Franklin, 'Genealogy of a Classic: *The English Physitian* of Nicholas Culpeper', PhD thesis (University of California, San Francisco, 1984), pp108–15, 129 [a pioneering thesis, with brief account of Parkinson; much of it is now superseded]

Laroche, Rebecca, *Medical Authority and Englishwomen's Herbal Texts, 1550–1650* (Farnham, Surrey, 2009) [a feminist critique of 'masculine' texts, including *Theatrum*]

Morellus, Peter, *The Expert Doctors Dispensatory* (London, 1657) [Morellus was physician to the French king; this English translation was praised by Culpeper]

Parkinson, Anna, *Nature's Alchemist: John Parkinson, Herbalist to Charles I* (London, 2007) [the first biography and at the centre of burgeoning Parkinson studies]

Parkinson, John, *Paradisi in Sole: Paradisus Terrestris* (London, 1629; reprinted as *A Garden of Pleasant Flowers*, New York, 1976) [STC 19300]

Parkinson, John, *Theatrum Botanicum* (London, 1640) [STC 19302]

Pavord, Anna, *The Naming of Names: In Search of Order in the World of Plants* (London, 2005) [A wonderful survey of plant nomenclature from the ancient Greeks to today; Parkinson features but does not fare too well]

Plomer, Henry R., *A Dictionary of the Booksellers and Printers who were at work in England, Scotland and Ireland from 1641 to 1667* (London, 1907) [useful for details of Thomas and Richard Cotes, Parkinson's printers]

Poynter, F.N.L. (ed.), *The Evolution of Pharmacy in Britain* (London, 1965), especially L.G. Matthews, 'Herbals and Formularies', pp187–213; R.S. Roberts, 'The Early History of the Import of Drugs into Britain', pp165–86 [two leading medical historians summarize their findings]

Prest, John, *The Garden of Eden: The Botanic Garden and the Re-Creation of Paradise* (New Haven & London, 1981) [pioneering and ambitious; many unusual illustrations]

Pulteney, R., *Historical and Biographical Sketches of the Progress of Botany in England* (London, 1790, and online) [rescues many botanists from obscurity in his time, including Parkinson; even-handed account of both Parkinson books]

Raven, Charles E., Canon, *English Naturalists from Neckam to Ray: A Study of the Making of the Modern World* (Cambridge, 1947), pp248–73 [still a formidable account, written with impeccable judgement]

Riddell, John N.D., 'John Parkinson's Long Acre Garden 1600–1650', *Journal of Garden History* 6(2) (1986), 112–24 [precedes Burnby (1994), and gives best account of Parkinson's garden]

Rohde, Eleanour Sinclair, *The Old English Herbals* (London, 1992; rpt New York, 1971), pp142–62 [an author who really 'gets' Parkinson's deep delight in gardens and flowers; excellent examples quoted from both books]

Seaver, Paul S., *Wallington's World: A Puritan Artisan in 17th-century London* (London, 1985) [Intellectual biography of a Puritan lathe-turner, compiled from a surviving stash of his personal papers]

Sloan, A.W., *English Medicine in the Seventeenth Century* (Bishop Auckland, 1996), pp96-7 [Short, approachable summary of its subject]

Smith, Sir J.E., 'John Parkinson', *The Cyclopaedia*, ed. A Rees (London, 1819), vol. 26 [no pagination] [confirms that the *Theatrum* was the leading medical textbook until the mid-18th century]

Spurling, Hilary, *Elinor Fettiplace's Receipt Book: Elizabethan Country House Cooking* (Harmondsworth, 1987) [more than well-presented recipes – a cultural history, beautifully edited]

Thomas, Keith, *Religion and the Decline of Magic: Studies in popular beliefs of the sixteenth- and seventeenth centuries* (Harmondsworth, 1971) [Like Trevor-Roper, another historian to envy, for his vast reading, complex but clear arguments and commanding style]

Tobyn, Graeme, Denham, Alison & Whitelegg, Margaret, *The Western Herbal Tradition: 2000 years of medicinal plant knowledge* (Edinburgh, 2011) [The authors take some 30 herbs and see what the leading source books say about them; Parkinson is one of four sources for the 17th century]

Trevor-Roper, H., *Europe's Physician: The Various Life of Sir Theodore de Mayerne*, ed. Blair Worden (New Haven & London, 2006) [posthumous publication of the first full biography of de Mayerne; wonderful prose, a treat to read, even if he has only one sentence on Parkinson: but this is the critical one, confirming Sir Theodore's role in securing Parkinson's elevation as the King's Herbalist]

Willes, Margaret, *The Making of the English Gardener: Plants, Books and Inspiration, 1560–1660* (New Haven & London, 2013), pp175–86 [comprehensive, scholarly but readable modern account]

Woolley, Benjamin, *The Herbalist: Nicholas Culpeper and the fight for medical freedom* (London, 2004) [the subtitle gives the game away, but if it is partisan it is also thorough and entertainingly written]

INDEX

Index, cont.

ACKNOWLEDGEMENTS

Many people have helped us in various ways. We especially thank Ruth Baker, Debs Cook, Jasmine Hastings, Christine Herbert and Dawn Ireland for proofreading, advice and trying out Parkinson's recipes; Anne Chesher and Dr Robin Darwall-Smith of Magdalen College, Oxford Library and Archives, respectively; Nicholas Wood, Honorary Curator, Society of Apothecaries; Dr Sarah Wilmot, outreach curator, John Innes Centre, Norwich; Wendy Chapman for working with us to transcribe from the *Theatrum*, and David Chapman for making a beautiful oak bookstand; Professor William Beinart and Troth Wells for a fabulous garden-grown meal and for help with Oxford's libraries; Sarah and Robin Russell for a home from home near Oxford and for the watercress; Dr Sarah Hawthorn for advice on medical terms; Dr Ron Smith for the seaweed; Dr Janice Swab for sassafras; Mark Naylor for the tomatoes; Oda Seedhouse for being our guide in Peru; Jen Bartlett for all sorts of things; Tony Pitman for Latin translations; Anna Parkinson for encouragement and inspiration.

We thank the British Library, for material on the Parkinson Society, and the Guildhall Library, London, for Society of Apothecaries MSS 8200 (Court Minutes) and 8202 (Accounts).

The opinions expressed here are our own, and we take responsibility for them. We thank the following copyright holders for permission to use illustrations. If we have overlooked any such owner we will gladly amend a future edition of this book.

The Bodleian Libraries, The University of Oxford, for colour frontispiece, *Theatrum Botanicum* [p2]

City of Westminster Archives Centre and St Martin in the Fields, for burials register (Parkinson's burial notice [p11])

The John Innes Foundation Historical Collections, Norwich, for Crispin van de Passe, *Hortus Floridus*, garden [p14]; images of de l'Ecluse and Dodoens [p248]; Bock, *New Kreuterbuch* [p248]; Gerard, 1633 edn of *Herball* [p249]

The President and Fellows of Magdalen College, Oxford, for image of Matthias de l'Obel [p10] and extracts from Goodyer Papers, MS 324 [pp18, 19]

The Wellcome Library, London, for image of Gideon de Laune [p12]; John Evelyn, *The French Gardener* [p16]; Christian Egenolph, *Lustgarten und Pflantzungen* [p19], Matthaeus Merian [p20]; Nicholas Culpeper and Peter Morellus, *The Expert Doctors' Dispensatory* [p21]; image of Gaspard Bauhin [p248]

Wikimedia Commons, for Sir Theodore de Mayerne by Peter Paul Rubens [p10]; John Tradescant the elder by Cornelius de Neve [Public domain], via Wikimedia Commons) [p249]

The Worshipful Society of Apothecaries of London, for Album Amicorum, reformers of 1614 [p13]

All other photographs by Julie Bruton-Seal, apart from Danewort by Willow (Own work) [Multi-license with GFDL and Creative Commons CC-BY-2.5 (http://creativecommons.org/licenses/by/2.5)] [p89]; photo of Parkinson statue by Robin Thomaides [p240]; authors' photo by Tara Ridgewell [p256]

THE AUTHORS

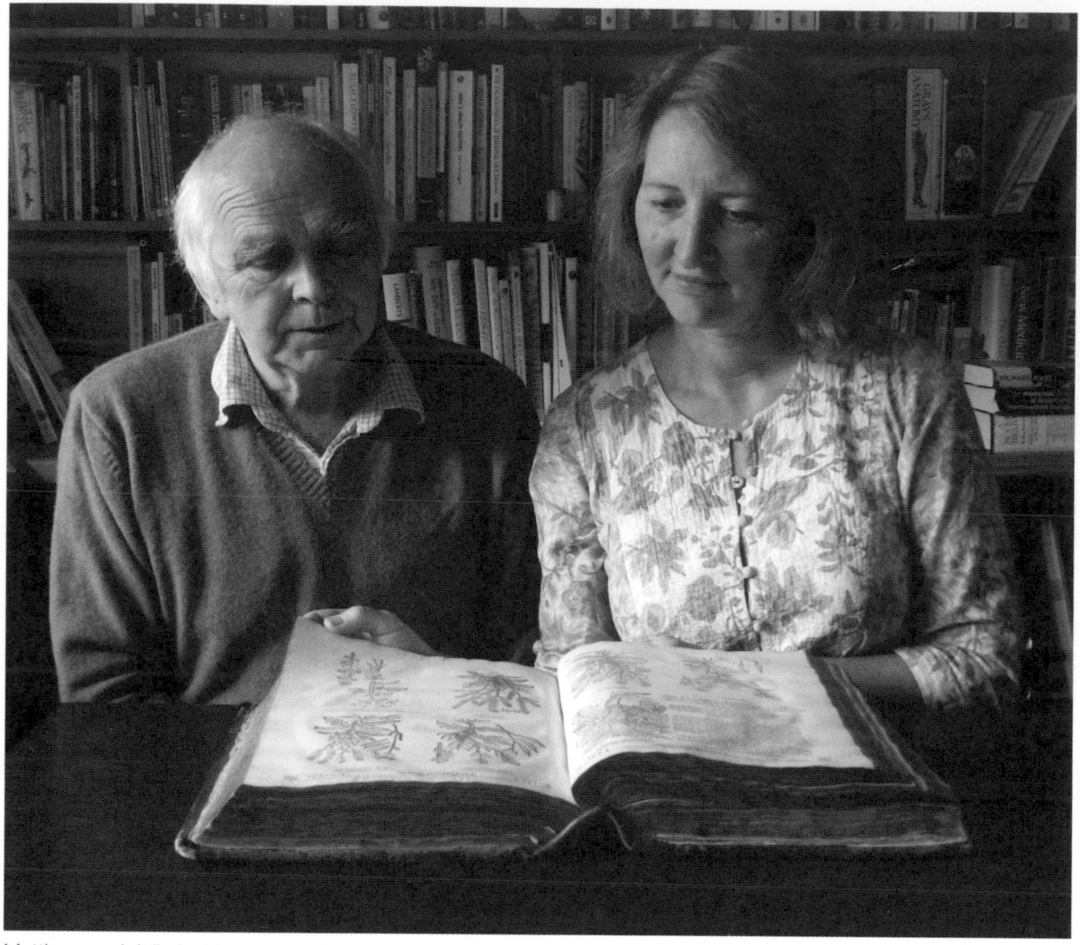

Matthew and Julie looking at the *Theatrum Botanicum*
Photo by Tara Ridgewell. For details of the other books written by Julie and Matthew see their website: www.hedgerowmedicine.com

JULIE BRUTON-SEAL is a practising medical herbalist and natural health practitioner. A council member of the Association of Master Herbalists (AMH), she is also a writer, photographer, artist and graphic designer. Julie co-authored the vegetarian cookbook *Vegetarian Masterpieces* (1988)

MATTHEW SEAL has worked as an editor and writer in books, magazines and newspapers for over forty years, in both the UK and South Africa. He is author of *Survive and Thrive in the New South Africa* (2000), and founded the Professional Editors' Group there in 1993. He has served as publications director of the Society for Editors and Proofreaders (SfEP)

Julie and Matthew teach courses and workshops in herbal medicine: www.hedgerowmedicine.com

For details of the other books written by Julie and Matthew see their website:

www.hedgerowmedicine.com